Food and Animal Borne Diseases SOURCEBOOK

Health Reference Series

Volume Seven

Food and Animal Borne Diseases
SOURCEBOOK

*Basic Information about Diseases that Can
be Spread to Humans through the Ingestion
of Contaminated Food or Water or by Contact
with Infected Animals and Insects, Such as
Botulism, E. Coli, Hepatitis A, Trichinosis,
Lyme Disease, and Rabies, Along with
Information Regarding Prevention and
Treatment Methods and Including a Special
Section for International Travelers Describing
Diseases Such as Cholera, Malaria, Travelers'
Diarrhea, and Yellow Fever and Offering
Recommendations for Avoiding Illness*

Edited by
Karen Bellenir and Peter D. Dresser

Omnigraphics, Inc.

Penobscot Building / Detroit, MI 48226

BIBLIOGRAPHIC NOTE

This volume contains individual publications issued by the Centers for Disease Control and Prevention (CDC), the Food and Drug Administration (FDA), the United States Department of Agriculture (USDA), subagencies of the National Institutes of Health (NIH), and the International Atomic Energy Agency. Selected articles from the USDA's *Food News for Consumers*, and CDC's *Morbidity and Mortality Weekly Report (MMWR)*, are also included. Document numbers where applicable and specific source citations are listed on the first page of each publication.

Edited by
Karen Bellenir and
Peter D. Dresser

Omnigraphics, Inc.

Matthew P. Barbour, *Production Coordinator*
Laurie Lanzen Harris, *Vice President, Editorial*
Peter E. Ruffner, *Vice President, Administration*
James a. Sellgren, *Vice President, Operations and Finance*
Jane J. Steele, *Vice President, Research*

Frederick G. Ruffner, Jr., *Publisher*

Library of Congress Cataloging-in-Publication Data

Food and animal borne diseases sourcebook : basic information about diseases that can be spread to humans through the ingestion of contaminated food or water or by contact with infected animals and insects. . . / edited by Karen Bellenir and Peter D. Dresser.
  p. cm. — (Health reference series ; V. 7)
  Includes bibliographical references and index.
  ISBN 0-7808-0033-8 (Lib. bdg. : alk. paper)
  1. Foodborne diseases.   2. Waterborne infection.   3. Zoonoses
  I. Bellenir, Karen.   II. Dresser, Peter D.   III. Series.
  RC143.F655 1995
  616.9—dc20   95-21240
                                                         CIP

∞

Printed in the United States

Contents

Part III: Disease Information of Special Concern to International Travelers

Indexes

Preface

About this Book

This book contains information about diseases that are transmitted by infectious organisms found in food and water, carried by animals and insects, or are of special concern to international travelers. It consists of numerous individual documents produced by several government agencies including the Centers for Disease Control and Prevention (CDC), the Food and Drug Administration (FDA), the United States Department of Agriculture (USDA), and subagencies of the National Institutes of Health (NIH). In addition, fact sheets produced by the International Atomic Energy Agency describing food irradiation and selected articles from the USDA's *Food News for Consumers* and CDC's *Morbidity and Mortality Weekly (MMWR)* are also included. The documents selected for inclusion were chosen to present basic medical information about food and animal borne diseases and to summarize methods that may be employed to prevent exposure.

How to Use this Book

This book is divided into parts, chapters, and sections. Parts focus on broad areas of interest. Chapters are devoted to single topics within a part. In order to provide complete information about the topics covered in this book, many chapters contain more than one source document. In such instances, individual documents are presented as sections within a chapter. Each chapter containing more than one source document begins with a listing of the chapter contents.

Part I: Food and Water Borne Diseases presents information about commonly occurring bacterial, viral, and parasitic diseases that are transmitted to humans through food and water. Information about the special risks to people with immune system problems is included in Chapter 4. Chapters 5, 6, 7, and 8 focus on various methods that may be employed to prevent food contamination.

Part II: Animal and Insect Borne Diseases offers basic information about the different types of diseases that are transmitted to humans by exposure to infected animals and insects.

Part III: Information about Diseases of Special Concern to International Travelers describes some diseases travelers may encounter. General advice from the U.S. Public Health Service and specific recommendations for disease prevention are also included along with a listing of the geographical distribution of known health hazards.

There are two *Indexes* to help the reader locate needed information. One, a general index, contains listings for diseases, organisms, agencies, and key words for other topics of interest. The second, an index of travel destinations, provides listings for all the countries, states, provinces, cities, and regions mentioned in the text.

Acknowledgements

The editors wish to thank researcher Margaret Mary Missar for her perseverance in locating and obtaining all the documents included in this volume; Bruce the Scanman for his persistence, patience, humor, and hard work; and Mike for his enthusiastic help.

Part One

Food and Water Borne Diseases

Chapter 1

Bacterial Diseases

Chapter Contents

Section 1.1

Botulism

(Source: CDC Document No. 310107, November 19, 1992.)

Botulism is a rare but serious foodborne disease. It is caused by contamination of certain foods by the botulism bacterium commonly found in the soil. There are two different illnesses: adult botulism and infant botulism. An adult may become ill by eating spoiled food containing the botulism toxin. This toxin is produced when the bacteria grow in improperly canned foods and occasionally in contaminated fish. Infant botulism is caused by eating the spores of the botulinum bacterium. For infants one source of these spores is honey.

When contaminated food is eaten by adults, toxin is absorbed from the intestines and attaches to the nerves causing the signs and symptoms of botulism. Early symptoms include blurred vision, dry mouth, difficulty in swallowing or speaking, general weakness, and shortness of breath. The illness may progress to complete paralysis, respiratory failure, and death. When infants eat contaminated food, the spores grow in the intestines and release toxin.

Diagnosis is made by the presence of appropriate neurologic symptoms and by laboratory tests that detect toxin or by culture of *Clostridium botulinum* bacterium from the patient's stool.

Although there are very few cases of botulism poisoning each year, prevention is extremely important. Home canning should follow strict hygienic recommendations to reduce contamination of foods. In addition, because the botulism toxin is destroyed by boiling for 10 minutes, people who eat home-canned foods should consider boiling the food before eating it to ensure safety. A county extension home economist can provide specific instructions on safe home canning techniques. To help prevent infant botulism, infants less than 12 months old should not be fed honey.

Treatment for adults requires care in an intensive care unit; botulism antitoxin can be helpful if given soon after symptoms begin. Treatment for infants requires hospitalization and possibly care in an intensive care unit. Antitoxin is not recommended for infants.

In 1989, 23 adult and 75 infant botulism cases were reported to CDC from 23 states.

Section 1.2

Campylobacter

(Source: CDC Document No. 310104, November 19, 1992.)

Campylobacter is an important cause of foodborne disease in the United States and many other countries. This bacteria causes gastroenteritis, characterized by fever, abdominal cramps and diarrhea which is often bloody. The illness typically lasts 5 to 7 days and usually resolves without antibiotics. Early treatment with the antibiotic erythromycin may shorten the disease. This illness is uncomfortable and even disabling for several days, but deaths are rare. Infections with Campylobacter may provoke a paralyzing neurologic illness called Guillain Barre Syndrome, in a small percentage of cases. There are several different forms of Campylobacter, the most common of which, Campylobacter jejuni, accounts for about 99% of all Campylobacter infections.

These infections are diagnosed when a stool specimen is sent to the laboratory, cultured using special techniques for Campylobacter, and the bacterium is found. It may affect between 2 and 4 million Americans every year.

The most common source of Campylobacter infections is contaminated poultry meat. One third to one half of all raw chicken in the market has Campylobactor organisms on it. People become sick when they eat undercooked chicken or when they inadvertently transfer the organisms from the raw meat or raw meat drippings to their mouth. Simple measures will help prevent people from getting this infection. Poultry should be thoroughly cooked and anything that comes in contact with raw poultry such as hands, knife or cutting boards should be washed with soap and water before they touch any other foods. Campylobacter infections are also acquired from drinking raw unpasteurized milk, travel to foreign countries, drinking untreated water from mountain streams, or contact with infected dogs and cats.

Campylobacter jejuni is common among healthy chickens on chicken farms, where it may spread unnoticed from bird to bird perhaps through their drinking water supplies. When the bird is slaughtered, Campylobacter is transferred in low numbers from the bird's intestines to the meat. Providing safe drinking water to the chickens on the farm has been suggested as one way of reducing the number of Campylobacter infections in humans.

Other forms of Campylobacter are harder to diagnose and appear to be much rarer than Campylobacter jejuni. It is not yet clear what the sources of those infections are.

Section 1.3

Campylobacter Questions and Answers

(Source: USDA Food Safety and Inspection Service, May 1991.)

The Bacteria

What Is Campylobacter?

Campylobacter [pronounced "kamp-e-lo-back-ter"] bacteria are commonly found in the intestinal tracts of cats, dogs, poultry, cattle, swine, rodents, monkeys, wild birds and some humans. The bacteria pass through feces to cycle through the environment and have also been found in untreated water. *Campylobacter jejuni*, the strain associated with most reported human infections, may be present in the body without causing illness.

Is Campylobacter New?

No, *Campylobacter*—under a different name—has been known to cause animal disease for about 80 years. In the 1970's, scientists conclusively proved that *Campylobacter* bacteria could cause human illness as well. However, the bacteria are suspected as the cause of an outbreak of human illness in the early 1940's (*associated with unpasteurized milk*).

Is Campylobacter Tougher Than Other Bacteria?

No. In fact, the bacteria are extremely fragile and are easily destroyed by thorough cooking. They are also destroyed through typical water treatment systems.

Why Are We Hearing about Campylobacter Now?

In 1991, a series on a Washington, D.C., news show and network affiliates increased public awareness of *Campylobacter*. Unfortunately, the series also contained some inaccuracies and misleading statements.

During the 1980's, public health authorities began to learn more about the prevalence of the bacteria in the environment, the illness it can cause, and laboratory techniques for identifying the bacteria. As States increase their reporting of illnesses to the Centers for Disease Control (CDC) and research continues on the organism and the disease, more stories about *Campylobacter* can be expected in the scientific and general media.

The Illness

What Harm Can Campylobacter Bacteria Cause?

The bacteria can exist in the intestinal tracts of people and animals without causing any symptoms at all. However, if people consume bacteria in raw milk, contaminated water, or raw or undercooked meat or poultry, they may acquire a *Campylobacter* infection (*also called campylobacteriosis*). The CDC believes consuming less than 500 *Campylobacter* cells can cause the illness. Infections have also been associated with contaminated water consumed during travel and contact with infected dogs and cats, whose fecal matter on their coats might be transmitted to human hands through petting.

Symptoms of *Campylobacter* infection, which usually occur within 2 to 10 days after the bacteria are ingested, include fever, headache and muscle pain, followed by diarrhea, stomach pain and nausea.

Complications can include meningitis, urinary tract infections and possibly reactive arthritis (*rare and almost always short-term*).

Are More People Becoming Ill from Campylobacteriosis?

No, CDC data do not indicate any rise in the actual number of illnesses. However, reports of illness are going up, as more States recognize that *Campylobacter* infections are a public health concern, and as laboratory techniques for culturing and identifying the bacteria continue to be refined.

Do Many People Actually Die from Campylobacter Infections?

Campylobacter infections are rarely fatal; CDC recorded two deaths from outbreaks (*affecting more than one person at the same time*) over a 9-year period. The estimated death rate per 100,000 cases has actually fallen as more data has been gathered.

Study of epidemiological data from actual illnesses helps the public health community understand and solve public health problems: however, the data are estimates and must be interpreted with great caution.

Who Is Most Susceptible?

Anyone may become ill from a *Campylobacter* infection. However, persons with underdeveloped immune systems (*such as newborns*) or immune systems weakened by chronic illness (*such as AIDS*) or medical treatment (*cancer patients on immunosuppressive therapy*) are believed to be more susceptible to health complications from *Campylobacter* or any other pathogenic bacterial illness. The elderly could also be more susceptible because of weakened immune systems.

Are Campylobacter Bacteria Causing a New Disease?

No. The CDC has tracked outbreaks of the disease caused by the bacteria since 1978, although laboratory-based surveillance did not begin until 1982. Since 1982, States have been asked to report to the CDC each individual finding of the bacteria in human blood or stools. Today, 44 States report such findings to the CDC. FSIS encourages States to report to the CDC so that this problem can be better understood and resolved.

Is Chicken the Cause of This Disease?

No. Foods don't cause illness; bacteria do. Contaminated water, raw milk, and raw or undercooked meat or poultry can all be the "*vehicles*" that carry *Campylobacter* and other bacteria to the human intestinal system. Failure to properly wash hands after contact with infected pets or after bathroom use may also continue the cycle of *Campylobacter* infection. Eating contaminated food or drinking impure water can also be a way to ingest the bacteria.

Campylobacter Control

What Is the Best Way to Prevent Campylobacter Infections?

The best prevention is to follow sensible public health precautions. A recent CDC report ("*Campylobacter* isolates in the United States, 1982-1986" Centers for Disease Control, *"Morbidity and Mortality Weekly Report,"* U.S. Department of Health and Human Services, Vol. 37, No. SS-22.) states, *"Universal pasteurization of milk and proper treatment of all drinking water might prevent 80 percent of the US. outbreaks due to Campylobacter."* The report also noted that improved chicken-handling practices in kitchens would reduce the number of illnesses. To minimize the risk of illness from *Campylobacter* infections or other bacterial illnesses:

- **Don't** drink untreated water from pure-looking mountain streams or lakes.

- **Don't** drink unpasteurized raw milk from farms or other sources.

- **Do** follow the principles of safe food handling, including thorough cooking and rapid, even cooling. Avoid cross-contamination of other foods by thoroughly washing cutting boards (*preferably plastic, not wooden*) and hands after contact with raw meat and poultry.

- *Campylobacter* and other bacteria are destroyed when meat or poultry is cooked to an internal temperature of 160 degrees F, although most people prefer chicken cooked to 180-185 degrees F. Compartments of home freezers generally are not cold enough to destroy bacteria.

Why Can't Campylobacter Be Stopped At the Source?

Campylobacter are and should be stopped at a number of different points in the food chain:

- Good sanitary practices on farms, as recommended by USDA,

minimize the opportunity for the bacteria to spread among animals and birds.

• Pasteurization of milk and treatment of municipal water supplies eliminate another route of transmission for *Campylobacter* and other bacteria.

• USDA enforces a recall policy if ready-to-eat meat and poultry products are contaminated with bacteria that cause illness.

• Raw foods are not sterile, and there are no requirements that they be sterile. Thorough cooking destroys bacteria. Food processing companies are accountable for following good, up-to-date manufacturing practices that minimize the opportunity for spread of *Campylobacter* and other bacteria.

One of the best systems for preventing unsafe foods is called the Hazard Analysis and Critical Control Point (HACCP) approach. USDA is studying how to best apply this preventive system in inspection. (*For information about HACCP, write FSIS Information Office.*)

Bacteria on raw meat and poultry cannot be seen, tasted or smelled. It would not be possible for USDA to inspect for *Campylobacter* or to enforce strict limits for bacteria on raw meat and poultry without (1) a rapid test for *Campylobacter* that could be used in the plant; and (2) the human resources and funding to implement such programs. Scientific experts do not believe these very costly programs would effectively reduce foodborne disease.

USDA is supporting research to learn more about *Campylobacter* in food and how to control it.

Why Have Other Countries, Such As Sweden, Been Able to Solve This Problem?

While Sweden has a rigorous and costly program based on control of *Salmonella*, it also has not been able to eliminate the problem of bacterial foodborne illness. *Campylobacter* infections are only a part of this public health problem.

Sweden has a program under which flocks are destroyed if they carry *Salmonella enteritidis* bacteria. Large numbers of animals have been destroyed under the program. There is more than a 10-fold magnitude of difference in poultry product production between Sweden and the United States. The increased production in the U.S. makes use of control procedures similar to those in Sweden impossible or impractical, at best. Other more effective and practical solutions are being investigated.

What Is USDA Doing to Prevent Campylobacter Infections?

In its commitment to ensure the public has a safe, wholesome food supply, USDA's Food Safety and Inspection Service (FSIS) is constantly working to improve the level of safety and reduce contaminants in the meat and poultry supply. USDA enforces a recall policy on contaminated ready-to-eat products. There is no requirement, however, that raw foods of any kind be sterile.

In addition, FSIS has embraced the Hazard Analysis and Critical Control Point (HACCP) system as the food protection system of the future and plans to work with the entire food industry to establish microbiological controls throughout the complex food-producing chain in order to prevent potential problems.

Finally, FSIS conducts extensive food handling education programs for consumers, institutional food handlers, health care professionals and other groups.

Who Can I Trust on Food Safety?

Every citizen needs to decide for himself or herself whether the Government and the industry are doing their jobs to help protect people from foodborne illness. USDA encourages the public to ask questions and discuss food safety issues with reputable sources, including health care professionals. However, USDA also advises citizens to consider carefully food safety and other health news that appears to frighten more than inform.

The United States has worked hard to achieve one of the best public health systems in the world, including Federal, State and local programs for food safety. We will keep working to improve those systems and to educate the public about safe food handling.

Safe Food Tips to Destroy Campylobacter and Prevent Illness

Most foodborne illness from bacteria on raw meat or poultry can be prevented by proper food handling in home and institutional kitchens.

To keep food safe at home, refrigerate promptly and properly. Freeze raw meat and poultry you can't use within 1 or 2 days. Freezers should register 0 degrees F, and refrigerators, 40 degrees F.

Food should not be thawed at room temperature. Cross-contamination of bacteria to other foods from raw meat and poultry can be prevented by thorough washing of hands, countertops, and utensils.

Campylobacter are very fragile bacteria that are easily destroyed by thorough cooking.

For Safe <u>Microwaved</u> Meat or Poultry...

- First, microwave the food in a covered dish, or under a plastic wrap. Under cover, steam helps kill bacteria and ensures uniform heating.

- Second, rotate the dish or stir the food during microwaving. This is necessary for even cooking.

- Third, check the internal temperature in several places with a temperature probe or meat poultry thermometer. If the internal temperature is at least 160 degrees F for meat and 180 degrees F for poultry, *Campylobacter* and other bacteria will be destroyed.

- Fourth, be sure to observe the *"standing time"* recommended in the microwave recipe. This step is necessary to complete the microwave cooking process before food is served.

For Safe Grilled Chicken or Meat...

- Cook the meat to an internal temperature of 160 degrees F and poultry to an internal temperature of 180 degrees F.

- If you plan to use marinade for dipping or basting on the grill, reserve some in the refrigerator before use on raw meat or poultry. Do not reuse marinades from the raw meat or poultry since they may contain bacteria.

- Transfer cooked meat or poultry to a clean platter— never to the dish that held the raw meat or poultry.

For Safe Precooked Meat and Poultry...

- Precook thoroughly to internal temperatures of 160 degrees F for meat and 180 degrees F for poultry.

- Cool the cooked food rapidly and evenly. Large roasts and whole poultry should be cut into smaller portions, then wrapped separately. Casserole-type dishes should be cooled in shallow, covered pans rather than deep pots.

For Safe Meat and Poultry in Restaurants...

Eat only in restaurants that are clean, follow local public health rules and practice safe food handling. Restaurants that do not follow these rules should be reported to local public health officials. Send back food that is under-cooked.

For More Information....

For more Information about safe food handling, call USDA's toll-free Meat and Poultry Hotline at 1-800-535-4555. You may call from 10 a.m. to 4 p.m., Eastern time, on weekdays.

Helpful Information is also available in an FSIS pamphlet entitled, "*A Quick Consumer Guide to Safe Food Handling.*" Write: Consumer Information Center, Box 574X, Pueblo, CO 81009

Section 1.4

How to Outsmart Dangerous E. Coli Strain

(Source: *FDA Consumer*, January-February 1994.)

Scientists have recently identified a rare but dangerous type of the *Escherichia coli* bacterium. Most *E. coli* are harmless in-habitants of the intestinal tract, but this variant, called *E. coli* 0157:H7, produces toxins in the human gut that are capable of deadly damage.

On Jan. 13, 1993, a physician in Washington state reported a cluster of children with hemolytic uremic syndrome (HUS), the major cause of acute kidney failure in children in this country. There was also an increase in emergency room visits for bloody diarrhea in people of all ages.

Laboratory tests from the stools of infected patients showed *E. coli* 0157:H7. Most infected people had eaten hamburgers from local restaurants of Jack-in-the-Box, a nationwide fast food chain.

Health officials investigated the illness reports and traced the meat in the hamburger patties to one processing plant but were not able to determine the source of the meat. Investigators also discovered that the patties had been undercooked at the restaurant. Thorough cooking would have killed the bacteria, but live, they were free to do their damage.

Reports of illness continued to mount and by the end of February, three children in Washington state and one other in California had died of HUS complications. More than 500 people from Washington, Idaho, California, and Nevada had laboratory-confirmed *E. coli* 0157:H7 infections. Of those, more than 50 people had been infected by person-to-person contact with someone who had eaten the contaminated hamburgers.

As news of the outbreak spread, reports of previous food-borne illnesses involving *E. coli* 0157:H7 were collected and reviewed. One outbreak in 1991, caused by contaminated fresh-pressed, unpreserved apple cider from a southeastern Massachusetts mill, had resulted in the hospitalization of four children with HUS. Another 17 children required medical treatment.

Before the Massachusetts mill incident, it was not common knowledge that this strain of *E. coli* could survive the acid environment of apple cider. Scientists from the national Centers for Disease Control and Prevention and from the University of Georgia continued to study the cider mill outbreak, and published a number of reports in professional journals.

Then, last July and August, several months after the ground beef outbreak in the northwestern states, people who had eaten at two Oregon restaurants of another nationwide chain became ill with confirmed *E. coli* 0157:H7 infections. At press time, public health officials, including Food and Drug Administration scientists, were trying to identify the food source of the contamination.

Bug Not Always Bad

Not all *E. coli* are harmful. *E. coli* is one of several bacterial types that are normal to the human gut and pass through the intestinal tract with feces. It has been known for many years that in healthy people, this group of bacteria and other normal microbial flora reduce the chance of pathogens—harmful bacteria that enter the body through food and water—from colonizing in the intestines and possibly causing illness.

E. coli is also helpful outside the body. In food laboratories, scientists use *E. coli* as an indicator of contamination, explains microbiologist Peter Feng, Ph.D., of FDA's Center for Food Safety and Applied Nutrition (CFSAN). If *E. coli* can be isolated from the suspect food, it implies that the food is contaminated by fecal matter, he says.

Research scientists also put the bug to good use in DNA studies.

"It's because of the knowledge that *E. coli* is a normal intestinal inhabitant that studies of potentially harmful strains were delayed," says CFSAN microbiologist Joseph Madden, Ph.D. "We now know of at least six types of *E. coli*, including 0157:H7, that are particularly virulent and can cause serious illness."

CDC first isolated *E. coli* 0157:H7 in 1975, and in 1982 identified it as the cause of severe bloody diarrhea traced to contaminated ground beef patties during two illness outbreaks in Oregon and Michigan. Since then, CDC has reported about 16 major outbreaks in the United States, with 22 deaths. Most of the fatalities have been young children or elderly people, the two age groups most vulnerable to HUS from *E. coli* 0157:H7.

Reports of outbreaks are increasing, according to CDC, mostly because of public awareness. Physicians have been alerted through professional publications and public announcements to report cases of bloody diarrhea, the most common symptom, to public health officials. Such reporting helps identify clusters of cases.

It is the toxin produced by *E. coli* 0157:H7 in the intestines of humans that damages cells of the intestinal lining. This damage allows blood to pass into the patient's stool. Other symptoms include stomachache, nausea and vomiting.

HUS develops in 2 to 7 percent of *E. coli* 0157:H7 illnesses. In these cases, the toxin enters the patient's bloodstream through the damaged intestinal wall, travels to the smaller arteries that supply the kidneys, and damages the vessels. HUS is fatal in about 3 to 5 percent of the cases.

E. coli 0157:H7 survive refrigerator and freezer temperatures. Once the bacteria get in food, they can multiply very slowly at temperatures as low as 44 degrees Fahrenheit. The actual infectious dose is unknown, but most scientists believe it takes only a small number of this particular strain of *E. coli* to cause serious illness.

E. coli 0157:H7 bacteria can contaminate any food. Undercooked hamburger and roast beef, raw milk, improperly processed cider, contaminated water, and vegetables grown in cow manure have caused illness outbreaks in the United States. Undercooked ground beef has been the food source in most reported cases. Harmful bacteria that are sometimes on the surface of raw meat get mixed through the meat in the grinding process.

Thorough cooking kills *E. coli* 0157:H7. A ground beef dish will be safely cooked when it reaches an internal temperature of at least 160 degrees Fahrenheit. The ground beef should not be pink in the center, and the juices should run clear. All leftovers should be reheated to 165 F.

Besides food-borne transmission, *E. coli* 0157:H7 can be passed from one person to another or through food-to-food cross-contamination. Thorough hand washing with soap and water after using the toilet or changing a baby's diaper can prevent person-to-person transmission. Proper food handling, such as not allowing raw meat juices to mix with cooked food, will help avoid cross-contamination.

Solving the Problem

Food scientists from CFSAN, USDA's Food Safety and Inspection Service, CDC, and state health departments have been working together to track down possible sources of transmission of *E. coli* 1057:H7. Public health officials first needed a laboratory test that would specifically identify 0157:H7. Available laboratory tests identified toxins or toxin genes from *E. coli 0157:H7* that are similar to *Shigella* bacteria, but were not specific for 0157:H7.

This year, FDA's Feng developed a DNA probe that reacts only with *E. coli* 0157:H7 and can specifically identify the organism in about 36 hours. Though this is an improvement, scientists hope for even better tests.

"Faster tests are needed, but we need technology that is more sensitive than what we have today to create a more rapid test," says Feng. "The problem is that sometimes it doesn't take large numbers of

16

the bacteria to make people sick—it can be dangerous in low numbers. In order to find the few cells that might be there, we have to put the suspected contaminated food in a growth medium for hours or days to allow the bacteria to grow. The 0157:H7 bacteria have to multiply to at least 10,000 for current tests to 'see' them. The need for an enrichment process will continue to slow us down until more sensitive technology is available."

USDA recently developed a Pathogen Reduction Program to strengthen efforts to keep harmful pathogens out of the food supply. As part of this food safety initiative, USDA is working with CDC to identify critical control points in meat processing at which contamination might occur. The agencies are preparing recommendations that will help processing plants avoid contamination at these points.

USDA also recently published two new regulations aimed at food safety: One requires labeling on all raw meat and poultry products to give consumers safe handling instructions, and the other specifies the heat-processing, cooling, handling, and storage requirements to be followed by processors of partially and fully cooked uncured meat patties, including veal and pork sausage. (At press time, enforcement of the safe handling labeling for consumers had been delayed.)

In addition, USDA has asked researchers at the University of Georgia to study the possibility of immunizing cattle against *E. coli* 0157:H7. Preliminary research has identified an antigen specific to enterohemorrhagic *E. coli* that may be useful in developing a vaccine.

Although food scientists and public health officials are constantly improving techniques to ensure food safety, Feng reminds consumers that raw foods will never be bacteria-free and even cooked foods can easily be recontaminated. But proper cooking will kill most harmful bacteria. Consumers can help guard against food-borne illness by applying some commonsense food safety rules for storing, cooking and serving foods.

—by Judith E. Foulke

Judith E. Foulke is a staff writer for *FDA Consumer*

Section 1.5

Answering Your Questions on E. coli

(Source: *Food News for Consumers*, Summer Supplement 1993.)

The Meat and Poultry Hotline has received hundreds of calls from consumers about the *E. coli* 0157:H7 organism and how to avoid it at home. Here are some of the most-often-asked questions the Hotline has received since the outbreak made headlines earlier this year.

To What Internal Temperature Should Ground Beef Be Cooked to Destroy E. coli?

Cook the ground beef to at least 160° F. If possible, use a meat thermometer to check that it's cooked all the way through. Otherwise, check visually—red meat is done when it's brown or gray inside. Juices should run clear with no traces of pink.

Is It More Risky to Eat a Rare Hamburger Than a Rare Steak or Roast?

Yes. Undercooked hamburger is more risky because of the kind of handling and preparation hamburger receives. Surface bacteria may be spread throughout the meat during grinding. Also, ground meat is often made with trimmings from several cuts. But this does not mean that we recommend eating other cuts raw or rare either. You should cook ALL meat, poultry and fish to at least 160° F.

What Are the Symptoms of E. coli Food Poisoning?

Symptoms include severe abdominal cramps, followed by watery diarrhea that often becomes bloody. Victims may also suffer vomiting and nausea, accompanied by low-grade fever. In some persons, particularly children and the elderly, the infection can lead to severe complications, including kidney failure.

How Do You Prevent Illness from This Serious Form of E. coli?

Thorough cooking destroys the *E. coli* bacteria. In addition, you should follow these general safe food handling tips:

- After shopping, quickly freeze or refrigerate all perishable foods.

- Never thaw food on the counter or let it sit out of the refrigerator for more than 2 hours. Food should not be off refrigeration over 1 hour in high summer heat (85° F and above).

- Use refrigerated ground meat and patties in 1-2 days; frozen meat and patties in 3-4 months.

- Wash hands, utensils and work areas with hot soapy water after contact with raw meat and meat patties, to avoid cross-contamination. Follow good personal hygiene rules, especially after using the bathroom.

- Cook hamburgers, other meat patties, meat loaf, meat balls (or any dish made with ground meat) until gray or brown inside, or to an internal temperature of 160° F.

- Serve food with clean plates and utensils.

How Can I Tell If The Ground Beef I Buy Is Safe to Eat?

You can't just by looking at it or smelling it. That's why you should always follow the rules mentioned above. If an off-odor is apparent, return it to the store.

Is E. coli a Problem Only with Beef?

No. *E. coli* can appear in raw milk, so only use pasteurized product. Unprocessed apple cider and unchlorinated water can carry the bacteria. And other foods can "pick up" the bacteria from raw meat juices—for example if salad vegetables were chopped on the same cutting board where you had just tenderized steak.

19

What Should I Do When Eating Out in a Restaurant or Fast Food Establishment?

Send back any meat, poultry or fish product that does not appear thoroughly cooked. Ground meat should be gray or brown in the center. Poultry juices should run clear and fish should "flake" with a fork. All cooked food should be served hot.

Does Freezing Kill E. coli?

No! That's why it's important to cook all food thoroughly.

What Is USDA Doing about the E. coli Problem?

USDA has embarked on a number of new initiatives at the farm, meat plant, supermarket and consumer level in order to protect the public. For example, USDA is sponsoring research aimed at keeping food animals from harboring the 0157 bacteria in their systems, which includes efforts to develop a vaccine against the illness. We are working on improved detection methods to keep the bacteria out of meat plants. We are instituting more stringent time and temperature controls in meat processing plants like those that produce hamburger. We are working closely with state and local public health agencies to increase their effectiveness in avoiding and containing outbreaks, and we will soon require that all raw and partially-cooked meat and poultry products have safe handling instructions on the package. These safe handling directions will cover proper cooling and cooking.

—by Herb Gantz

Section 1.6

Listeriosis

(Source: "Preventing Foodborne Listeriosis," USDA Food Safety and Inspection Service, rev. April 1992.)

Listeria are bacteria found frequently in the environment. One *Listeria* species, *Listeria monocytogenes*, can cause the serious foodborne illness listeriosis. Healthy people rarely contract listeriosis, but the illness can be serious for some people, especially the elderly, newborns, pregnant women and those with weakened immune systems.

This backgrounder is written for consumers: To answer questions frequently asked about *L. monocytogenes* and the illness it causes, to describe public health and enforcement activities being conducted by the Federal government to control *L. monocytogenes*, and to outline precautions consumers and other food handlers can take to keep food safe and prevent listeriosis.

The Food and Drug Administration (FDA), the Food Safety and Inspection Service (FSIS) and the Centers for Disease Control (CDC) are working together to provide the public with this information. Pregnant women and immune-compromised consumers may also wish to contact their physicians with questions about listeriosis.

The Organism

Listeria refers to a genus (related group) of bacteria. One species in this genus, *Listeria monocytogenes*, can cause a serious bacterial infection called listeriosis. Usually when public health officials refer to *Listeria*, they are referring specifically to *Listeria monocytogenes*.

Researchers have isolated *L. monocytogenes* from soil, leaf litter, sewage, silage, dust and water. The organism often moves through the animal and human intestinal tract without causing illness, and has been found in many domestic and wild animals, including birds and fish. Because *L. monocytogenes* is widely present in the environment, it would be impossible to prevent animals from coming in contact with the bacteria. However, farmers, animal producers, food processors and food handlers can all take steps to reduce contamination and keep food safe from *L. monocytogenes*.

21

L. monocytogenes is not "new." Since 1911, scientists have known it infects animals, and in 1929 the first case of human infection was detected.

What is new is the recognition that *L. monocytogenes* bacteria may be spread in food. In earlier times, many believed farm animals transmitted *L. monocytogenes* to farm workers. But, when listeriosis appeared in city dwellers, public health authorities realized that animal contact was not always the source of disease transmission.

It has been only in the past decade that researchers have recognized *L. monocytogenes* as an agent of foodborne illness. Fecal contamination is one way the organism is spread to raw agricultural products. For example, farm animals may pick it up from consuming improperly fermented silage, and then vegetables may become contaminated when animal manure carrying the organism is used for fertilizer. Animals in a herd also may pick up *L. monocytogenes* from other animals or manure containing the organism.

L. monocytogenes is a remarkably tough organism. It resists heat, salt, nitrite and acidity much better than many organisms. The bacteria survive on cold surfaces and also can multiply *slowly* at 34 degrees Fahrenheit, defeating one traditional food safety defense—refrigeration. (Refrigeration at 40 degrees Fahrenheit or below stops the multiplication of many other foodborne bacteria. Refrigeration does not kill most bacteria) Commercial freezer temperatures of 0 degrees Fahrenheit, however, *will* stop *L. monocytogenes* from multiplying.

Discrepancies in information available on proper cooking prompted FSIS in 1988 to contract with a private laboratory to conduct research that has become the basis for FSIS regulations on proper cooking of roast beef. Earlier work focused on cooking temperatures and times needed to destroy *Salmonella*. The new study conducted by the laboratory looked at cooking temperatures and times that will destroy *L. monocytogenes*, and confirmed the adequacy of current regulatory cooking standards for eliminating the organism in FSIS regulated products.

In addition, FDA researchers and FDA-funded research have confirmed the adequacy of commercial pasteurization for eliminating the organism in dairy products.

Post-processing contamination, rather than failure of heating or pasteurizing processes, is usually suspected when *L. monocytogenes* is detected on processed products.

Once *L. monocytogenes* were identified as foodborne bacteria that could cause serious illness, scientists began looking at methodology used to detect the bacteria. FSIS scientists developed a more precise method for detection in meat and poultry products. FDA scientists developed a similar method appropriate for dairy products, seafood and vegetables. These methods have steadily improved over the years.

FDA and FSIS developed culture procedures that rely on the presence of antibiotics in the medium, which allow multiplication of *L. monocytogenes* but inhibit multiplication of competing organisms. In 1986, independent laboratories verified the accuracy of the new FSIS method for meat and poultry. The FDA method has also been reviewed and accepted.

As more is learned about the bacteria and their control, new and even better tests are being developed. An example is FDA's gene-probe method.

The Illness

Listeriosis is the disease caused by the bacteria *L. monocytogenes*. Consumers most commonly contract listeriosis by eating food contaminated with the organisms.

Also, the scientific literature contains a few isolated reports of occupational listeriosis; for example, farm workers and veterinarians who work with animals have developed minor skin infections.

Healthy people do not often develop noticeable listeriosis symptoms after eating food containing *L. monocytogenes*. However, some people are very susceptible to the disease.

The highest incidence of listeriosis has been in persons over 60 years old and newborns. One third of infections occur during pregnancy and may lead to spontaneous abortions or serious illness in newborns. Others most at risk include patients with immune systems compromised by cancer, AIDS, or immunosuppressive medications such as steroids; and patients suffering from cirrhosis, diabetes and ulcerative colitis.

The disease symptoms are variable and depend on the individual's susceptibility. Symptoms may be limited to fever, fatigue, nausea, vomiting and diarrhea. However, these symptoms can precede a more serious illness.

The more serious forms of listeriosis can result in meningitis (brain infections) and septicemia (bacteria in the bloodstream). Pregnant women may contract flu-like symptoms of listeriosis; complications can result in miscarriage, stillbirth, or septicemia or meningitis in the newborn. In older children and adults, complications usually involve the central nervous system and blood stream, but may include pneumonia and endocarditis (inflammation of the lining of the heart and valves). Skin contact with *L. monocytogenes* can cause localized abscesses or skin lesions.

It takes from one to six weeks for a serious case of listeriosis to develop, although flu-like symptoms may occur 12 hours after eating *L. monocytogenes* contaminated food. Onset time probably depends on the health of the patient, the strain of *L. monocytogenes* and the dose—or amount of bacteria—ingested.

Four reported outbreaks of listeriosis in North America in the past decade are either known or suspected to have been caused by *L. monocytogenes* in food.

- An outbreak in 1981 in Nova Scotia resulted in 41 cases of listeriosis including 18 deaths; 83 percent of the cases were perinatal (occurring near the time of birth). The outbreak was traced to *L. monocytogenes* on coleslaw that had been made from cabbage grown in a field fertilized with manure from *Listeria*-infected sheep.

- An outbreak in 1983 in Boston resulted in 49 cases of listeriosis including 14 deaths; 14 percent of the cases were perinatal, the remainder in immunocompromised adults; Although pasteurized milk from *Listeria*-infected dairy cows was linked to the outbreak, *L. monocytogenes* was not found in the suspected brand of milk.

- An outbreak in 1985 in Los Angeles resulted in 142 cases of listeriosis including 46 deaths; 85 percent of the cases were perinatal. The outbreak was traced to *L. monocytogenes* on soft, Mexican-style cheese, manufactured with contaminated milk.

- An outbreak in Philadelphia in 1987 resulted in at least 32 cases of listeriosis, including 11 deaths. The cause was never identified.

The Food and Drug Administration funded a Centers for Disease Control (CDC) active surveillance project in 1986. CDC began contacting all acute care hospitals and their respective laboratories in an area that included five states and Los Angeles county.

From the 1986-1987 study results, as well as from findings in studies conducted from 1989-1990, CDC determined that sporadic (non-outbreak) individual cases of listeriosis were associated with soft cheese, undercooked poultry, hot dogs not thoroughly reheated and food purchased from delicatessen counters.

Researchers are not sure how many *L. monocytogenes* organisms it takes to cause illness. The infective "dose" varies, depending on the susceptibility of the individual. However, it is noteworthy that four of the ill persons in the Los Angeles outbreak reported eating the implicated product (highly contaminated soft cheese) only once.

Thorough cooking will destroy *L. monocytogenes* on foods. Nonetheless, FDA and FSIS are committed to reducing contamination of raw foods by *L. monocytogenes* and other potentially harmful bacteria.

From information gathered in its surveillance projects conducted in the 1980s, CDC projects about 1,850 cases of human listeriosis occur annually. Incidence, however, varies from state to state. CDC is now encouraging state health departments to conduct surveillance programs for listeriosis so that outbreaks may be rapidly identified and investigated. As our population ages and more people live longer with malignancies and other immunosuppressive illnesses, many experts believe the number of people at risk for listeriosis is likely to increase.

Surveillance data also indicate that about 425 deaths occur each year in the United States. The probability of death varies greatly depending on the patient's age and status of immune function. About 5 percent of the 9,000 food poisoning deaths each year are due to listeriosis.

Preliminary data suggest that the rate of listeriosis may have declined substantially during 1991 in several areas, perhaps related to intensified efforts to reduce *Listeria* contamination of foods.

Listeriosis can be positively diagnosed, using clinical laboratory techniques, only by culturing the organism from blood or cerebrospinal fluid. Listeriosis can be treated with antibiotic drugs such as penicillin or ampicillin.

What Is the Government Doing?

Neither FSIS nor FDA will accept *any* detectable *L. monocytogenes* on cooked, ready-to-eat food. This is called a "zero tolerance" for the bacteria.

Both agencies have testing programs for *Listeria monocytogenes*. The goal of these programs is to help government and industry identify the causes of contamination in processing plants and to make permanent changes that will reduce *Listeria monocytogenes* contamination, prevent problems and ensure a safe food supply. Both agencies can hold or detain products at the food processing plant, request a voluntary recall of the product or seize products through court order if necessary.

Initially, FSIS regulatory testing programs included selected cooked meat products. Following a CDC report that traced the first case of listerial meningitis to incompletely heated turkey franks consumed by a cancer patient, FSIS expanded the *L. monocytogenes* monitoring program to further prevent the sale of any cooked and ready-to-eat meat or poultry products from which *L. monocytogenes* is isolated, such as cooked sausages (including frankfurters and bologna), cooked roast beef, cooked corned beef, sliced canned ham, sliced canned luncheon meat, jerky, cooked poultry, and poultry and meat salads and spreads.

When a ready-to-eat meat or poultry product is found to contain *L. monocytogenes*, the plant is notified and the product is subject to detention at the plant, voluntary recall or court-ordered seizure. From 1987 through March 1992, 27 FSIS regulated cooked products from 27 firms have been recalled, including frankfurters, bologna and other luncheon meat, chicken salad, ham salad, sausages, chicken, sliced turkey breast and sliced roast beef.

FDA's monitoring programs initially concentrated on cheese and dairy products, both domestic and imported. Later, FDA expanded coverage to include other ready-to-eat foods such as sandwiches, prepared salads and smoked fish. From 1987 to March 1992, 516 products from 105 firms have been recalled.

The agencies' stepped up monitoring and surveillance programs for *L. monocytogenes*, and food industry efforts have helped identify intervention measures aimed at controlling the organism.

Controlling Listeria In the Plant

FSIS and FDA have identified the Hazard Analysis and Critical Control Point (HACCP) system as the most effective strategy for controlling the presence of *L. monocytogenes* and other pathogenic bacteria on food products. In addition to encouraging adoption of this strategy by all who handle food, from farm worker to plant processor to consumer, the agencies are working with industry to design strong HACCP programs. Most of the food industry supports HACCP.

In a HACCP program, points at which food risks are more likely to be introduced are identified, and interventions are introduced where control is possible to reduce the potential for consumption of unsafe products. For instance, insufficient cooking of raw meat, poultry or milk may allow the survival of pathogenic bacteria and present a hazard. Therefore, the agencies require adequate cooking temperatures to destroy the bacteria.

Areas of concern in food processing plants include plant design and layout, equipment design, process control, personnel practices, cleaning and sanitizing procedures, and verification of pathogen control.

Much of the dairy industry has already instituted control measures, based on HACCP principles. Other FDA-regulated industries are following the lead. In 1987, meat companies began to modify production facilities, such as rearranging plant layout and making changes in equipment. An industry working group also developed recommendations for all meat companies based on what is learned, and developed a training video on employee practices and plant hygiene. The poultry industry also instituted improvements.

The food industry, FSIS and FDA have conducted workshops to develop recommendations for controlling risks at critical points. Government and industry, including food processors and grocers, are also working with retail establishments and hotels and other institutions to identify critical control points and interventions to address hazards.

Food Handler Control

Listeria bacteria do not change the taste or smell of a food. As a final check, food handlers—in homes, restaurants and institutional kitchens—must follow basic food safety procedures for destroying any potentially harmful bacteria, thereby avoiding any foodborne illness.

The Centers for Disease Control, FDA, FSIS and the National Advisory Committee on Microbiological Criteria for Foods (which includes food scientists from Federal health agencies, universities and private industry) have developed food handler advice for preventing listeriosis.

Although most people are at very low risk for listeriosis, the risk of listeriosis and other foodborne illnesses can be reduced by following these tips:

- Avoid raw/unpasteurized milk.

- Keep raw and cooked foods separate when shopping, preparing, cooking and storing foods. Otherwise, bacteria in juices from raw meat, poultry or fish might contaminate a cooked food. For instance, transfer cooked meat, poultry or fish to a clean platter—never to the dish that held the raw food of animal origin.

- Wash hands, knives, and cutting boards after handling uncooked foods.

- Wash raw vegetables thoroughly before eating.

- Thoroughly cook all food of animal origin, including eggs. Cook raw meat to an internal temperature of 160 degrees Fahrenheit, raw poultry to 180 degrees Fahrenheit, and raw fish to 160 degrees Fahrenheit or until it is white and flaky. Reheat leftovers thoroughly.

- Read and follow label instructions to "Keep refrigerated" and "use by" a certain date.

- Keep hot foods hot (above 140 degrees Fahrenheit). Do not keep them out for longer than two hours at room temperature—at which *L. monocytogenes* can thrive-before eating.

- Keep cold foods cold (at or below 40 degrees Fahrenheit). Do not keep them out for longer than two hours at room temperature before eating.

- Divide leftovers into small, shallow covered containers before refrigerating, so that they chill rapidly and evenly.

- Keep your refrigerator *clean* and keep the temperature at 34-40 degrees Fahrenheit.

Persons at increased risk for listeriosis such as pregnant women, the elderly, and those with immunosuppressive conditions can decrease the risk by:

- Avoiding soft cheese such as Mexican style, feta, Brie, Camembert and blue cheese. Mexican-style cheeses are soft, white, ethnic (Hispanic-Latin American) cheeses such as Queso Blanco and Queso Fresco. There is no need to avoid hard cheese, processed slices, cottage cheese or yogurt.

- Reheating leftover foods or ready-to-eat foods such as hot dogs *thoroughly* until steaming hot before eating.

- Although the risk of listeriosis associated with foods from delicatessen counters is relatively low, pregnant women and immunosuppressed persons may choose to avoid these foods or to thoroughly reheat cold cuts before eating.

Resources for Consumers

Because listeriosis presents a special risk for pregnant women, newborns, the elderly, and those with weakened immune systems the Federal government has begun a campaign to distribute information about *L. monocytogenes* to government agencies and private groups serving those at risk.

As part of this campaign, FSIS is working with the Administration on Aging to develop fact sheets for the elderly about foodborne illness. FSIS also is working with USDA's Food and Nutrition Service's Special Supplemental Program for Women, Infants, and Children (WIC) to distribute information through WIC clinics. In addition, FSIS distributes several publications that address the problem of listeriosis, especially for those in at-risk groups. These publications include:

- "Is Someone You Know at Risk for Foodborne Illness?"

- "FSIS Facts: Bacteria that Cause Foodborne Illness"
- "A Quick Consumer Guide to Food Handling" (for consumers)
- "Preventing Foodborne Illness: A Guide to Safe Food Handling" (for extension agents and health educators)

You can order these publications from:

> FSIS Publications
> USDA
> Room 1165, South Building
> Washington, D.C. 20250

FDA is participating in educational campaigns and also distributes publications about *L. monocytogenes*. These include:

- *Listeria*, Battling Back Against One Tough Bug"
- "Listeriosis: A Deadly Danger"
- "Guarding Against *Listeria* at Home"
- "Eating Defensively: Food Safety Advice for Persons with AIDS"

You can order copies from:

> Food and Drug Administration
> HFE-88
> 5600 Fishers Lane
> Rockville, MD 20857

In addition, for answers to your food safety questions, call USDA's Meat and Poultry Hotline at 1-800-535-4555. (In the Washington, D.C., area, call 202-720-3333.) Hotline hours are from 10 am. to 4 p.m., Eastern time.

References

1. Carosella, J. (1990) "Occurrence of *Listeria Monocytogenes* in Meat and Poultry." In: Miller, A.J., L. Smith, and G.A. Somkuti (eds.) *Foodborne Listeriosis*. Society for Industrial Microbiology, Washington, D.C.

2. FSIS (1990). "FSIS Directive 10,240.1, Rev.1. "Microbiological Monitoring Program: Sampling, Testing Procedures and Actions for *Listeria Monocytogenes* and *Salmonella*." FSIS, USDA, Washington, D.C. (Available from FSIS Information Office.)

3. National Advisory Committee on Microbiological Criteria for Foods (1991). *"Listeria Monocytogenes."* In: *International Journal of Food Microbiology*, vol. 14. Amsterdam, Netherlands, pp. 185-246. (For further information, contact Executive Secretariat; FSIS, USDA; Room 2801-South Building; Washington, D.C. 20250.)

4. Ryser, E.T. and E.H. Marth (eds.) (1991) *Listeria, Listeriosis and Food Safety*. Marcel Dekker, Inc., New York.

5. Schuchat, A., R. Pinner, K. Deaver, et al. (1991) "Epidemiology of Listeriosis in the United States." In: *Proceedings of the International Conference on Listeria and Food Safety*. ASEPT, Laval, France, pp. 69-73. (Reprinted by the Centers for Disease Control, Atlanta, Georgia.)

6. Lovett, J. and A.D. Hitchins (1989) *"Listeria* Isolation." In: *1987 Supplement to Bacteriological Analytical Manual*, 1984, 6th edition. (Second printing, 1989.) Association of Official Analytical Chemists, Arlington, Va.

7. Schuchat, A., et al. (1992) "The Role of Food in Sporadic Listeriosis: A Case-Control Study of Dietary Risk Factors." In: *Journal of the American Medical Association*, April 14, 1992.

8. Pinner, R W., et al. (1992) "The Role of Foods in Listeriosis: A Microbiologic and Epidemiologic Investigation." In: *Journal of the American Medical Association*, April 14, 1992.

Section 1.7

Paralytic Shellfish Poisoning and Other Shellfish Intoxications

(Source: "Shellfish," CDC Document No. 310108, November 19, 1992.)

Eating shellfish has been related to a number of diseases, including those caused by bacteria, such as vibrios, a variety of viruses including hepatitis A and Norwalk agent, and those caused by toxins. Shellfish foodborne infections caused by bacteria and viruses can be prevented by cooking seafoods thoroughly, storing them properly, and protecting them from contamination after cooking. Traditional methods of cooking seafoods such as steaming clams only until they open, may be insufficient to kill all bacteria and viruses in them. Persons with underlying disease such as liver disease, diabetes, or disorders of their immune system, are at much higher risk than normal persons for acquiring severe or even fatal illnesses from eating raw shellfish. Such person are well advised not to eat raw or undercooked shellfish.

Another source of foodborne infections is shellfish contaminated with toxins. Some of the toxins or poisons that contaminate the shellfish are paralytic shellfish poison, neurologic shellfish poison, diarrheic shellfish poison, and amnesic shellfish poison. Shellfish containing toxin may look and taste normal, and usual cooking methods do not affect the toxin. State shellfish screening programs test shellfish for the presence of these toxins and monitor the safety of shellfish harvest beds.

Paralytic Shellfish Poisoning (PSP) is a foodborne illness caused by eating shellfish that contain concentrated saxitoxin, an alkaloid neurotoxin, or related compounds. These neurotoxins are among the most potent toxins known. They can interfere with sensory, cerebellar, and motor functions. Symptoms usually occur within 30 minutes and high doses can lead to diaphragmatic paralysis, respiratory failure and death. Most victims of paralytic shellfish poisoning in the United States are individuals or small groups who gather shellfish for personal consumption. Paralytic shellfish poisoning has traditionally been considered a danger only in shellfish harvested from cold water but the incidence in tropical areas may be increasing; outbreaks have been reported recently from Central and South America, Asia and the Pacific. Shellfish obtained from waters with toxic algae blooms or "red tide" should not be eaten.

Consumers should be aware of the potential risk to their health, particularly if they eat shellfish from unapproved harvest beds. For normal persons who eat raw shellfish from approved harvest beds the risk is likely to be small, although there is no way to totally eliminate all risk.

Diagnosis of shellfish poisoning is made on the basis of recent food consumption, symptoms and detection of toxin in the uneaten shellfish. There are no laboratory tests to detect toxin within an individual. There are no anti-toxins or antidotes available for treatment of shellfish poisoning, and no other chemotherapy has proven effective. Therefore, treatment is supportive care of infected persons. Ingestion of alcohol increases absorption of the toxin. Evacuation of stomach contents may help by removing remaining toxin-containing shellfish.

The shellfish industry and government regulatory agencies try to control the problem of shellfish contamination at the source by seeing that shellfish are harvested from beds not polluted by sewage. These efforts, however, cannot guarantee that shellfish from unapproved beds do not reach the market. In addition, shellfish-associated infections can be caused by bacteria which are normally present in unpolluted waters.

To prevent outbreaks of paralytic shellfish poisoning and other shellfish intoxications, samples of susceptible mollusks are collected and tested for toxin by state health departments during the appropriate times of the year. Affected growing areas are quarantined and sale of shellfish prohibited. Warning signs posted in shellfish-growing areas, on beaches, and in the news media can warn the public of the hazard.

Due to the monitoring of shellfish beds, shellfish poisoning in the United States is very rare—from 1973 to 1987 only 19 outbreaks were reported with an average of 8 cases per outbreak. Outbreaks on the west coast have been reported between May and October, on the east coast between August and October.

Section 1.8

Salmonella and Food Safety

(Source: USDA Food Safety and Inspection Service, January 1988.)

Chicken, turkey, pork, beef, and other meat and poultry products are important sources of protein and other nutrients. Unfortunately, these foods—like eggs, raw milk, and all raw foods of animal origin—may also carry salmonella and other bacteria. The good news is that these bacteria don't have to cause illness. Routine food safety can destroy salmonella and other bacteria.

The Food Safety and Inspection Service (FSIS) oversees the processing of meat and poultry from the time animals enter the slaughter plant until packaged products leave the plant. FSIS also conducts a comprehensive food safety education program, including a toll-free hotline. FSIS encourages manufacturers to provide "care" information that reminds consumers about thorough cooking and safe handling of meat and poultry products.

Consumers have a right to meat and poultry that is as free as possible of bacteria. However, after more than 20 years of research, it is still economically impossible to produce "salmonella-free" raw meat and poultry. With or without a breakthrough, good sanitation and careful food handling will always be necessary to prevent bacteria on raw products from causing illness—just as toothbrushing is necessary to prevent other bacteria from causing dental cavities.

What Is Salmonella?

This FSIS backgrounder answers common questions about salmonella and offers some tips for safe handling of meat and poultry to prevent foodborne illness.

The salmonella family includes about 2,000 different strains of bacteria, but only 10 strains cause most reported salmonella infections. Strains that may cause no symptoms in animals can make people sick, and vice versa. A salmonella bacterium is a one-celled organism that can't be seen, touched or tasted. The bacteria are common in the intestinal tracts and waste of livestock, poultry, dogs, cats, rats, and other warm-blooded animals.

34

What Is Salmonellosis?

Salmonellosis, or a salmonella infection, is the illness that can occur if live salmonella bacteria enter the body—usually through food. Most reported outbreaks of food-borne illness are caused by bacteria, and salmonellosis is the most common bacterial food-borne illness. Salmonellosis is usually preventable.

How Can Salmonella Bacteria on Raw Meat and Poultry Make People Sick?

First, "food abuse" allows bacteria to survive and often to multiply. For example, if the meat knife is used to cut the salad lettuce without first being washed, the lettuce can be contaminated by any bacteria on the meat. The person who eats the salad then also eats the bacteria.

Next, if the bacteria survive the stomach acid, they reproduce themselves in the small intestine. One cell becomes two, two become four, four become sixteen, and so on. When there are "enough" bacteria, they cause a salmonella infection.

How Many Bacteria Does It Take to Make People Sick?

There is no exact number, but the more bacteria consumed, the more likely a person is to get sick. Healthy adults have eaten food containing millions of bacteria without getting sick. Other people have gotten sick from as few as 10 bacteria in their food.

What Are the Symptoms of Salmonellosis?

According to the Centers for Disease Control, stomach pain occurs within 6 to 48 hours after the food was eaten. Most people get diarrhea, and many people have upset stomachs, chills, fever, or headache. Most people feel better within 3 to 5 days. Many persons with salmonellosis may believe they have the flu and may never see a doctor.

How Many People Get Sick from Salmonellosis?

At least 40,000 salmonella infections are reported every year, but experts believe that between 400,000 and 4 million persons each year actually contract salmonellosis.

How Does the Doctor Know a Person Has Salmonellosis?

The only way to tell for sure is to conduct laboratory tests on the stools of the person who got sick, a process that takes several days.

How Many People Die from Salmonellosis?

Salmonella infections can be life-threatening for the very young, the very old and for persons already weakened by other serious diseases, such as AIDS. Reports show about 2 deaths for every 1,000 known cases of salmonellosis, but experts believe that about 500 persons each year actually die from salmonella infections.

What Foods Are Most Likely to Make People Sick?

Foods don't make people sick—bacteria do. Any raw food of animal origin—meat, poultry, raw milk, fish, and shellfish—may carry salmonellae. The bacteria can survive to cause illness if these specific foods are not thoroughly cooked. The bacteria can also cause illness if they contaminate any other food that comes in contact with the raw food, either directly or by way of dirty hands or dirty equipment. Salmonellosis is a world-wide, food-chain problem that can't be "blamed" on any one food.

Wouldn't Less Bacteria on Animals Mean Less Human Illness?

FSIS and the National Academy of Sciences agree with this logical assumption. However, there will always be some risk of bacterial contamination on raw foods of animal origin. So, food safety will always be necessary to prevent bacteria on raw foods from causing illness.

Are Kosher Chickens Lower in Salmonella Bacteria?

FSIS does not know of any valid scientific information showing that Kosher chickens carry more or fewer salmonella bacteria than other poultry.

Section 1.9

Salmonella Enteritidis:
From the Chicken to the Egg

(Source: *FDA Consumer*, April 1990.)

White, shining, unmarred—a Grade A mystery now lies in the uncracked egg. Is it safe to eat?—9,999 times out of 10,000, yes. But . . .

- In May 1989, six nursing home patients in Pennsylvania died from *Salmonella enteritidis* poisoning after eating stuffing that contained undercooked eggs.

- In July, 21 guests at a baby shower in New York became ill after eating a pasta dish made with a raw egg. One victim was 38 weeks pregnant and delivered her baby while ill. The newborn infant developed *Salmonella enteritidis* blood poisoning and required lengthy hospitalization.

- Last August, a healthy 40-year-old man died, and 14 others were hospitalized, after eating egg-based custard pie contaminated with *Salmonella enteritidis*, which was served at a company party in Pennsylvania. The list goes on.

Public health officials are concerned. More than 49 outbreaks of *Salmonella enteritidis* poisoning took place in nine states and Puerto Rico last year, resulting in at least 13 deaths and more than 1,628 illnesses. According to the Jan. 5, 1990, issue of the Centers for Disease Control's *Morbidity and Mortality Weekly Report*, from January 1985 through October 1989, 189 *Salmonella enteritidis* outbreaks in the United States caused 6,604 illnesses and 43 deaths. Many more illnesses probably went unreported, says Joseph Madden, Ph.D., deputy director of FDA's division of microbiology.

Health investigators suspect that contaminated shell eggs caused nearly half of these outbreaks. The egg connection in these cases was determined by tracing the food eaten by the victims and taking cultures both from patients and foods.

Especially at risk for *Salmonella* poisoning are the elderly, the very young, pregnant women (because of risk to the fetus), and people already debilitated by serious illness, malnutrition, or weakened immune systems. Symptoms of *Salmonella enteritidis* infection usually include diarrhea, vomiting, abdominal pain, chills, fever, and headache. The bacteria can invade organs outside the gastrointestinal tract, causing complications that require lengthy hospitalization, even in healthy people.

Symptoms usually develop 12 to 36 hours after eating the contaminated food. The initial illness also can bring about serious chronic complications.

In 1985, in an incident in Chicago, more than 16,000 people contracted food poisoning from low-fat milk contaminated with *Salmonella* bacteria. Within two weeks, about 2 percent of these patients developed a chronic reactive arthritis condition linked to the infection. Although the *Salmonella* bacteria that made these people ill was not *Salmonella enteritidis*, researchers have found that rats infected with *Salmonella enteritidis* may develop the same arthritic condition. Researchers are concerned that *Salmonella enteritidis* may also cause this complication in humans.

Since 1976, says Robert Tauxe, M.D., a CDC expert on the spread of the disease, the reported rate for *Salmonella enteritidis* infections from food "has increased more than sixfold in the northeastern part of the United States." First noted in the New England states, the infections also appeared in the mid-Atlantic region by 1983, and now have become a problem in the south Atlantic states as well. Recently, outbreaks were reported in Minnesota, Ohio and Nevada.

The problem also has become an international egg to crack. "The U.S. *Salmonella* epidemic," says Tauxe, "is dwarfed by dramatic increases that have been reported from Yugoslavia, Finland, Sweden, Norway, and the United Kingdom." In Britain alone, the number of confirmed *Salmonella enteritidis* cases reported for January through July 1988 (4,424 cases) was more than double the number (2,000) for the same period in 1987.

Source: Intact Eggs

At first, says Tauxe, "we did not have an explanation for this striking increase." The first real clue that intact eggs were a source of the problem came in 1983, when CDC traced a large outbreak caused by *Salmonella enteritidis* to a commercial stuffed pasta product made with raw eggs.

Investigators then reviewed reports of past outbreaks and determined that at least since 1973, *Salmonella enteritidis* outbreaks appeared to be caused by the bacteria in clean, uncracked, Grade A eggs.

"In the 1960s," Tauxe says, "salmonellosis [the disease caused by the *Salmonella* bacteria] associated with chicken eggs was epidemic in the United States. At that time it was determined that eggs were being contaminated by *Salmonella* in chicken feces on the *outside* of the egg shell, which penetrated into the eggs through cracks in the shell." That led to strict rules, established and enforced by the U.S. Department of Agriculture, for washing and sanitizing shells of commercial eggs.

But this new epidemic is associated with *Salmonella enteritidis* in inspected, uncracked and sanitized Grade A eggs. "The infected egg may appear normal," says Tauxe. The contamination comes from the *inside*, not the outside, of the egg.

How Does Contamination Occur?

No one knows how some intact eggs become contaminated with *Salmonella enteritidis*. Poultry researchers, however, suggest that the egg yolk becomes infected before the shell forms.

In fact, Charles Benson, Ph.D., of the University of Pennsylvania, says that in his experiments the bacteria were found not in the white, as when organisms penetrate the egg shell, but only in the yolk. This occurred even though Benson added iron to the white to encourage the bacteria to grow in the albumen, which has antibacterial properties.

Madden believes that in the past 10 years a new strain of *Salmonella enteritidis* that can live in chickens may have evolved. Other researchers are finding that *Salmonella enteritidis* bacteria migrate from the yolk to the white of the egg, where they can survive up to 12 hours. However, it is in the yolk where the bacteria multiply and thrive.

These and other findings, such as ovarian infections in egg-laying chickens, have led to the concept of "transovarian transmission." According to this theory, the infection occurs first in the chicken and is transferred to the egg before the shell is formed.

Researchers also speculate that the infection may be passed from bird to bird in the same flock. For instance, Madden notes that several birds might pick up *Salmonella enteritidis* from the droppings of rodents and sparrows (known carriers of the organism) and spread it among the others. There are also reported cases, Madden adds, of workers picking up the bacteria on their clothing and transmitting *Salmonella* from one chicken house to another.

Only after scientists understand how *Salmonella* is transmitted will they know how to control it. Right now the proposed solution is a long-range plan to prevent spread of the disease by testing flocks and replacing infected ones.

The Voluntary Model State Program

The Northeastern Conference on Avian Diseases in 1987 proposed a voluntary model state program, which FDA and USDA then modified. The program calls for state agriculture, veterinary and health officials to work together to test the poultry flocks in their states for *Salmonella enteritidis*.

There are different levels of flocks in the poultry industry, starting with the grandparents. Only 800,000 birds in the United States, owned by five companies, make up these primary breeders. They produce the multiplier, or parent, flocks, which in turn produce the 230 million commercial, egg-laying hens.

The main targets of this massive, nationwide testing effort are the grandparent and parent birds, based on the theory that the infection is passed from mother to chick. Egg-laying hens that have produced eggs implicated in outbreaks or that are offspring of infected parent birds also should be tested.

Under the plan, blood samples are taken from 300 birds per age group in a flock. (The number of birds in a flock can vary from a few thousand to a hundred thousand.) If blood tests from any of the chickens are positive, state officials must take cultures from birds in that flock. The plan calls for destruction of infected flocks.

Another provision in the plan calls for routine culturing of the hens' cages and litter. Sometimes fertilized eggs don't hatch, and, under the program, every three months 30 embryos from such eggs should also be cultured.

Under the voluntary plan, eggs from infected flocks are to be pasteurized (broken and heat processed) to destroy the bacteria. There is no evidence that *Salmonella enteritidis* survives pasteurization. Pasteurized eggs are used in many commercial food products, such as baked goods.

40

Making Testing Mandatory

The effectiveness of the voluntary program depends upon producers' willingness to test and, if necessary, replace infected flocks. However, according to Madden, the increase and spread of the problem suggest that producers and states are not following the program.

Because of this concern, Madden announced at the annual meeting of the U.S. Animal Health Association on Oct. 31 that FDA is working on a regulation to require mandatory testing. The United States would not be the first to have such a program; the United Kingdom instituted a mandatory plan in March 1989.

The testing program that FDA is reviewing would target both breeder and commercial egg-producing flocks. In addition, the proposed regulation under consideration when this article went to press would tighten requirements of the current program by specifying organ specimen size and culturing media used. "It would leave little room for discretion," says Madden.

Under the voluntary program, producers could choose to send their samples to industry-owned laboratories certified by state agriculture departments under the National Poultry Improvement Program. (NPIP is a cooperative state-federal agriculture program, established in 1935, that already has in place the mechanism for reporting diseases spread by poultry.) Or, producers could choose to send culture samples to private laboratories certified by USDA under the voluntary model program.

USDA responded to the increasing concern over the *Salmonella enteritidis* problem by passing an interim rule on Feb. 16. The regulation, which allows for a 60-day comment period but went into effect immediately, makes testing of primary and multiplier flocks mandatory. Much of the work will be done through NPIP.

Backing of Law

FDA also has the backing of law to attack the *Salmonella enteritidis* problem. The Public Health Service Act authorizes FDA to take steps to "prevent the introduction, transmission, or spread of communicable diseases." Under this provision, the agency can issue regulations requiring flock testing and certification before the eggs can be shipped in interstate commerce.

Another law supports the mandatory program. Under the Food, Drug, and Cosmetic Act, the agency can seize products of a diseased animal. If an egg producer does not want the eggs destroyed, FDA can request a court order requiring that the eggs be pasteurized.

Egg Industry Cooperation

At the same time that FDA and USDA have been working on regulations for mandatory testing, the egg industry has been developing its own quality assurance program. Ken Klippen, vice president of the United Egg Producers (a federation of regional cooperatives representing most of the laying-hen producers in the United States), says that UEP is drafting a new food safety plan. The program will address the *Salmonella enteritidis* problem and will be "a brand new thrust for the industry," says Klippen.

To the producers of the 67 billion eggs marketed in the United States every year, *Salmonella enteritidis* is an economic as well as a public health issue, as FDA acknowledged at the September 1988 public hearing on *Salmonella* and eggs.

Resolving the economic issue will be difficult. Most breeders and egg producers have been seeking USDA indemnification, or reimbursement, for flocks that are destroyed. USDA's responsibility, however, is limited to protecting agriculture, livestock and poultry. For instance, while hens infected with *Salmonella enteritidis* often do not become noticeably sick, in the 1983 avian influenza outbreak sick hens died and there was a significant mortality in the infected flocks. In the avian flu case, says USDA, indemnification was the appropriate response.

67 Billion Eggs

Despite the hard times egg producers are facing, eggs continue to be an inexpensive and important source of protein. According to UEP, the average American eats 250 eggs a year. A survey from the market research group Technical Assessment Systems finds that 90 percent of the population eat eggs in some form each day. (This includes eggs contained in foods like baked items and egg noodles.)

Nearly 5 percent of Americans surveyed said they either ate raw eggs daily or could not specify whether the egg consumed was raw or cooked. Raw and lightly cooked contaminated eggs are causing the illnesses. Thorough cooking kills the bacteria. [See section "Safety Tips: Egg Cooking".]

According to Madden, a person can become ill after eating only a small amount of a contaminated egg. For instance, he says, one New York incident involved a family who cooked three eggs sunny side up. The yolk of one egg broke onto the other eggs during cooking, and all three family members became ill.

Madden explains that the one broken egg was probably responsible for all three illnesses, as it is extremely unlikely that more than one egg per container would be contaminated. In fact, only 1 in 200 eggs from an infected flock may be contaminated. The risk is even lower for all eggs—only 1 in 10,000 eggs on the supermarket shelves are likely to be contaminated with *Salmonella enteritidis*.

Salmonella enteritidis grows quickly, presenting another danger for spread of the disease when a contaminated egg is mixed with clean eggs, such as when eggs are pooled to make scrambled eggs for a group of people. One organism can multiply into millions in an egg stored at 60 degrees for two days. Eggs should always be stored in the refrigerator and only taken out just before use.

Scientists around the country are trying to find out what refrigeration temperatures are most effective for stopping the growth of *Salmonella enteritidis* in eggs. They are also investigating the cooking times and temperatures required to destroy the bacteria.

FDA and USDA officials are conducting a public health campaign to spread information on what they know so far about safe cooking and handling of eggs. Over 50,000 bulletins have been distributed to consumers, food service establishments, and institutions that take care of people particularly vulnerable to *Salmonella enteritidis* infections. For copies of the materials, contact USDA, Agricultural Marketing Service/Information Staff, P.O. Box 96456, Washington, D.C. 20090-6456.

Cold weather seems to slow the growth of *Salmonella enteritidis*. Jack Guzewich, the New York state health department's chief of food protection, notes that in New York 75 percent of outbreaks and 95 percent of illnesses have occurred in the summer. Scientists are working now to solve some of the microbiological mysteries, and officials are trying to resolve the administrative issues before warm weather sets in.

"Are we going to wipe out *Salmonella enteritidis* from the face of the United States?" asks USDA researcher Charles Beard, Ph.D. "I doubt it," he says. "I don't think the rodents and birds would agree to that." Eradicating the bacteria may be impossible, but joint efforts of

FDA, USDA, CDC, and industry are aimed at controlling the spread of this newly recognized danger.

Safety Tips: Egg Cooking

The elderly, patients already weakened by serious illness, and people with weakened immune systems (such as persons with AIDS) are at high risk for death or serious illness from *Salmonella enteritidis*. Nursing home, hospital, and other food institutions serving those in high-risk groups should *strictly* follow these safe egg guidelines, which also apply to all home preparation.

You can't tell a good egg from a bad egg by the way it smells, tastes or looks. But, these precautions can help minimize risks:

- Review recipes, and consider using pasteurized eggs instead of shell eggs whenever possible.

- Avoid serving raw eggs and foods containing raw eggs. Caesar salad, Hollandaise sauce, homemade ice cream, homemade eggnog, and homemade mayonnaise are possible carriers of *Salmonella enteritidis*.

- Lightly cooked foods containing eggs, such as soft custards and French toast, may be risky for those in high-risk groups.

- Cook eggs thoroughly until both the yolk and white are firm, not runny. These cooking times are now recommended by researchers at Cornell University:

  Scrambled—1 minute at 250 degrees Fahrenheit
  Poached—5 minutes in boiling water
  Sunnyside—7 minutes at 250 F or cook covered 4 minutes at 250 F
  Fried, over easy—3 minutes at 250 F on one side, then turn the egg and fry for another minute on the other side
  Boiled—7 minutes in boiling water.

Handling Practices

- Wash hands with hot, soapy water, and wash and sanitize utensils, equipment (such as blenders), and work areas before and after they come in contact with eggs and uncooked egg-rich foods.

- Use only Grade A or better eggs. Avoid eggs that are cracked or leaking.

- Discard the egg if any shell falls into the egg.

- Leave eggs in their original carton, and store them in the main section of the refrigerator—not the egg section in the door, as the temperature in the door is higher.

- Never leave eggs or egg-containing foods at room temperature for more than two hours, including preparation and serving (but not cooking) times.

- When refrigerating a large amount of a hot egg-rich dish or leftover, divide it into several small shallow containers so it will cool quickly.

- Cook scrambled eggs in batches no larger than three quarts. Hold for serving at 140 F or hotter, such as on a steam table. Do not add a batch of just-cooked scrambled eggs to leftover eggs held on a steam table.

—by Dale Blumenthal

Dale Blumenthal is a staff writer for FDA Consumer.

Section 1.10

Outbreak of Salmonella Enteritidis Associated with Homemade Ice Cream—Florida, 1993.

(Source: *MMWR*, September 16, 1994.)

On September 7, 1993, the Epidemiology Program of the Duval County (Florida) Public Health Unit was notified about an outbreak of acute febrile gastroenteritis among persons who attended a cookout at a psychiatric treatment hospital in Jacksonville, Florida. This report summarizes the outbreak investigation.

On September 6, seven children (age range: 7-9 years) and seven adults (age range: 29-51 years) attended the cookout at the hospital. A case of gastroenteritis was defined as onset of diarrhea, nausea or vomiting, abdominal pain, or fever within 72 hours of attending the cookout. Among the 14 attendees, 12 cases (in five of the children and all seven adults) were identified. The median incubation period was 14 hours (range: 7-21 hours); the mean duration of illness was 18 hours (range: 8-40 hours). Predominant symptoms were diarrhea (93%), nausea or vomiting (86%), abdominal pain (86%), and fever (86%). All ill persons were examined by a physician. *Salmonella enteritidis* (SE) (phage type 13a) was isolated from stool of three of the seven patients from whom specimens were obtained.

Eleven of the 12 ill persons had eaten homemade ice cream served at the cookout. No other food item was associated with illness. Testing of a sample of ice cream revealed contamination with SE (phage type 13a).

The ice cream was prepared at the hospital on September 6 using a recipe that included six grade A raw eggs. An electric ice cream churn was used to make the ice cream approximately 3 hours before the noon meal. The ice cream had been properly cooled, and no food-handling errors were identified. The person who prepared the ice cream was not ill before preparation; however, she became ill 13 hours after eating the ice cream. Her stool specimen was one of the three stools positive for SE (phage type 13a).

The U.S. Department of Agriculture's (USDA) Animal and Plant Health Inspection Service attempted to trace the implicated eggs back to the farm of origin. The hospital purchased eggs from a distributor in Florida. However, the traceback was terminated because the implicated eggs from the distributor had been purchased from two suppliers—one of whom bought and mixed eggs from many different sources. Current USDA *Salmonella* regulations limit testing of flocks to one clearly implicated flock.

Reported by: P Buckner, MPH, D Ferguson, HRS Duval County Public Health Unit, F Anzalone, MD, D Anzalone, DrPH, College of Health, Univ of North Florida, Jacksonville; J Taylor, Office of Lab Svcs, WG Hlady, MD, RS Hopkins, MD, State Epidemiologist, State Health Office, Florida Dept of Health and Rehabilitative Svcs. Foodborne and Diarrheal Diseases Br, Div of Bacterial and Mycotic Diseases, National Center for Infectious Diseases, CDC.

Editorial Note: The outbreak described in this report represents the fourth SE outbreak in Florida since 1985; this outbreak is the first in the state to implicate eggs. In the United States, the number of sporadic and outbreak-associated cases of SE infection has increased substantially since 1985; much of the increase can be attributed to consumption of raw or undercooked eggs (*1-3*). During 1983-1992, the proportion of reported *Salmonella* isolates that were SE increased from 8% to 19%. During 1985-1993, a total of 504 SE outbreaks were reported to CDC and resulted in 18,195 cases, 1978 hospitalizations, and 62 deaths (Figure 1.1). Of the 233 outbreaks for which epidemiologic evidence was sufficient to implicate a food vehicle, 193 (83%) were associated with eggs. Of these 193 outbreaks, 14 (7%) were associated with consumption of homemade ice cream. No outbreaks have been associated with pasteurized egg products.

Year	No. outbreaks	No. cases	No. hospitalizations	No. deaths
1985	26	1,166	144	1
1986	48	1,539	131	6
1987	53	2,498	523	15
1988	40	1,010	121	8
1989	77	2,394	175	14
1990	70	2,273	288	4
1991	68	2,346	151	4
1992	59	2,748	229	4
1993	63	2,221	216	6
Total	**504**	**18,195**	**1,978**	**62**

Figure 1.1. Number of reported outbreaks, associated cases, hospitalizations, and deaths caused by Salmonella enteritidis, *by year—United States, 1985-1993.*

After eggs are identified by public health officials as the cause of an SE outbreak, USDA attempts to trace the implicated eggs back to the farm of origin to conduct serologic and microbiologic assessments of the farm. If SE is detected on the source farm, the eggs are diverted to pasteurization, or the flocks are destroyed. Under current regulations, USDA can pursue the traceback only if one farm is identified as the source. During 1990-1993, the success rate of USDA tracebacks to the source farm declined from 86% (19/22 outbreaks) in 1990 to 17% (3/21 outbreaks) in 1993. The rate declined primarily because eggs increasingly have been marketed in shipments containing eggs from multiple sources.

Although 0.01% of all eggs contain SE and, therefore, pose a risk for infection with SE (4), raw or undercooked eggs are consumed frequently. Based on the Food and Drug Administration (FDA) Food Safety Survey conducted in 1993, 53% of a nationally representative sample of 1620 respondents reported ever eating foods containing raw eggs; of these, 50% had eaten cookie batter, and 36% had eaten ice cream containing raw eggs (S. Fein, FDA, personal communication, September 9, 1994). Many persons may eat raw or undercooked eggs because they are unaware that eggs are a potential source of *Salmonella* (3) and that certain foods (e.g., homemade ice cream, cookie batter, Caesar salad, and hollandaise sauce) contain raw eggs.

Consumers should be informed that eating undercooked eggs may result in *Salmonella* infection. In addition, eggs should be refrigerated to prevent proliferation of *Salmonella* if present and should be cooked thoroughly to kill *Salmonella*. Because most serious illnesses and deaths associated with salmonellosis occur among the elderly and immunocompromised persons, these persons in particular should not eat foods containing raw or undercooked eggs. Hospitals, nursing homes, and commercial kitchens should use pasteurized egg products for all recipes requiring pooled eggs or raw or undercooked eggs and should refrigerate all eggs and egg products.

References

1. St. Louis ME, Morse DL, Potter ME, et al. The emergence of grade A eggs as a major source of *Salmonella enteritidis* infections: new implications for the control of salmonellosis. JAMA 1988;259:2103-7.

2. Mishu B, Koehler J, Lee LA, et al. Outbreaks of *Salmonella enteritidis* infections in the United States, 1985-1991. J Infect Dis 1994;169:547-52.

3. Hedberg CW, David MJ, White KE, MacDonald KL, Osterholm MT. Role of egg consumption in sporadic *Salmonella enteritidis* and *Salmonella typhimurium* infections in Minnesota. J Infect Dis 1993;167:107-11.

4. Mason J, Ebel E. APHIS *Salmonella enteritidis* Control Program [Abstract]. In: Snoeyenbos GH, ed. Proceedings of the Symposium on the Diagnosis and Control of *Salmonella*. Richmond, Virginia: US Animal Health Association, 1992:78.

Section 1.11

Shigella

(Source: CDC Document No. 310105, November 19, 1992.)

Shigella is a group of bacteria that has four different species that cause gastrointestinal illness. The illness usually includes fever, abdominal pain, and diarrhea with or without blood in the stools.

Transmission of Shigella is through direct contact with an infected person, or from food or water contaminated by an infected person. The diagnosis is made by culturing the stool.

Handwashing with soap and running water is the single most important preventive measure to interrupt transmission of shigellosis, especially during an outbreak. Because young children are most likely to be infected with Shigella and are also most likely to infect others, a strict policy of supervised handwashing for young children after they have defecated and before they eat is particularly important. Excluding persons with diarrhea from handling food and limiting the use of home-prepared foods at large gatherings will reduce the risk of large outbreaks caused by foodborne transmission.

Treatment with an antibiotic to which Shigella is susceptible decreases the duration of the illness. Antibiotic resistance among Shigella is increasing, and it is important for the clinician to be aware of local resistance patterns. In the outbreak setting, the decision to use antibiotics to treat patients with mild, self-limiting illness should be weighed against the risk of producing resistant strains of Shigella. Prophylactic use of antibiotics is not recommended to prevent illness in persons who are exposed but not ill.

From 1986 to 1988, the reported isolation rate of Shigella in the United States increased from 5.4 to 10.1 isolates per 100,000 persons. As many as 20 times more cases may go unreported. In 1988, state health departments reported 22,796 isolates of Shigella to CDC, the highest number since national surveillance began in 1965. In addition to the recent increase in Shigella isolation rates, many community-wide shigellosis outbreaks have been difficult to control.

Chapter 2

Viral Diseases

Chapter Contents

Section 2.1

Hepatitis A Prevention

(Source: CDC Division of Viral and Rickettsial Diseases, October 1993.)

How is Hepatitis A Spread?

Hepatitis A virus is found in the stool of persons with hepatitis A. The virus is usually spread from person to person by putting something in the mouth that has been contaminated with the stool of an infected person; for this reason, the virus is more easily spread under poor sanitary conditions, and when good personal hygiene is not observed.

Sexual and household contact can spread the virus; casual contact as, for example, in the usual office or factory setting, does not spread the virus.

Can Hepatitis A Be Spread by Food or Water?

People can get hepatitis A by consuming contaminated water or ice; raw shellfish harvested from sewage-contaminated water; and fruits, vegetables, or other foods eaten uncooked that may have become contaminated during handling.

Although infected children younger than 5 years of age usually do not have symptoms of hepatitis A, they easily spread the infection to older children and adults.

Who Is At Risk?

In the United States, hepatitis A virus is present in most communities and can cause isolated cases of disease or widespread epidemics. Especially at risk are

- Persons who share a household or have sexual contact with someone who has hepatitis A.

- Children and employees in child care centers (especially centers that have children in diapers) where a child or an employee has hepatitis A.

52

- Travelers to developing countries where hepatitis A is common and where clean water and proper sewage disposal are not available.

- Residents and staff of institutions for disabled children when a resident or an employee has hepatitis A.

Travelers to developing countries (for example, Mexico) are at risk for hepatitis A. The risk increases with poor or unsanitary living conditions, longer or extended stays, and high incidence of hepatitis A in the area visited.

Travelers to areas with high levels of hepatitis A (contact CDC International Travelers' Health Hotline: 404-332-4555) should avoid drinking water that may not be clean and avoid eating uncooked shellfish or uncooked fruits or vegetables.

What Are the Symptoms of Hepatitis A?

Three of every four persons infected with hepatitis A virus have symptoms. When symptoms are present, they usually develop suddenly and may include fever, tiredness, loss of appetite, nausea, abdominal pain, dark urine, and yellowing of the skin and eyeballs. Adults have symptoms more often than children.

A person is most infectious about one week before symptoms appear and during the first week of symptoms. However, an infected person who has no symptoms can still spread the virus. Unlike some other forms of viral hepatitis, hepatitis A causes no long-term damage and is usually not fatal.

How Can You Prevent Hepatitis A?

Good personal hygiene, e.g., washing hands after using the bathroom, prevents the spread of hepatitis A virus infection.

Can the Virus Be Killed?

The virus is killed by boiling at 85° C (185° F) for 1 minute; cooked foods can still spread the disease if they are contaminated after cooking. Adequate chlorination of water (as recommended in the United States) kills hepatitis A virus.

What Is Immune Globulin and How Can It Prevent Hepatitis A?

No specific treatment exists for hepatitis A. However, immune globulin, a blood byproduct, is used as temporary protection against this disease. When immune globulin is given, a person receives protective antibody from someone who is already immune. Side effects due to immune globulin are rare. Immune globulin produced in the United States has not been associated with any diseases, including AIDS, and can be given to pregnant women and nursing mothers.

Immune globulin is used to prevent hepatitis A both before and within 2 weeks after exposure to hepatitis A virus. If you think that you have been exposed to hepatitis A virus, contact your physician or local health department to determine whether immune globulin is right for you.

Prevent Hepatitis A

- Practice good personal hygiene—wash hands after using the bathroom and before handling food or eating.

- If you think you have been exposed to hepatitis A, ask your physician or local health department if immune globulin is right for you.

- When traveling to areas where hepatitis A is common, avoid drinking water that may not be clean and eating uncooked shellfish or uncooked fruits or vegetables.

- Take immune globulin just before traveling to areas where hepatitis A is common—travelers to even popular tourist areas in Mexico should receive immune globulin before travel.

- If you will be living for a long time in a country where hepatitis A is common, take an increased dose of immune globulin every 5 months to stay protected against hepatitis A.

- A vaccine for long-term protection against hepatitis A is being developed and should become available soon.

For more information on hepatitis A call **CDC Hepatitis Hotline (404) 332-4555** or write

Hepatitis Branch, Mailstop G37
Division of Viral and Rickettsial Diseases
National Center for Infectious Diseases
Centers for Disease Control and Prevention (CDC)
Atlanta, Georgia 30333

Section 2.2

Hepatitis A Cases Up

(Source: *FDA Consumer*, July-August 1990.)

Cases of hepatitis A, a viral disease that attacks the liver, rose 58 percent between 1983 and 1989, according to the federal Centers for Disease Control.

Three of four recent outbreaks of the disease reported in the April 13 issue of CDC's *Morbidity and Mortality Weekly Report* were traced to, or suspected to have been caused by, restaurant food contaminated by employees infected with the disease. The three outbreaks occurred in:

- Seattle—Although CDC never determined the official cause of this May 1989 outbreak, many of the 213 people who got sick reported eating in the same outlet of a Seattle-area restaurant chain. One former employee of the chain and three current employees were among those who came down with the illness; however, none were ill during the period of likely exposure for most of the others who contracted the disease.

- Greensboro, N.C.—An employee of a Greensboro restaurant, who tested positive for hepatitis A, was the probable source of infection for 32 cases of the disease in September 1988, according to CDC.

- Peters Creek, Alaska—An ice-slush beverage sold at a local convenience store was the culprit in 32 cases in the summer of 1988. CDC said the drink was made with water from a bathroom sink, and the utensils used to mix the drink were kept near a toilet.

The fourth outbreak, which affected 61 people from five states, was traced to oysters illegally harvested from polluted waters off the coast of Florida.

To prevent outbreaks of hepatitis A, CDC recommends that food handlers be trained in proper hygiene and food-handling practices— most importantly, good handwashing. It also advises that shellfish be cooked to help prevent infection. (For more information on hepatitis A and other types of hepatitis, see "Hepatitis B: Available Vaccine Safe but Underused" in the May 1990 *FDA Consumer*.)

Section 2.3

Introducing the Norwalk Virus

(Source: *Food News For Consumers*, Winter 1989.)

You say you just learned how to pronounce "salmonella" and don't want to hear any more about food poisoning right now?

That's understandable.

However, the Norwalk virus is rapidly gaining ground as a health threat.

There have been outbreaks from contaminated water, shellfish, cole slaw, salads, baked goods and, recently in Pennsylvania and Delaware, from ice.

Leading food virologist Dr. Dean Cliver at the University of Wisconsin, estimates that Norwalk and other Norwalk-like viruses could account for some 40 percent of all serious, non-bacterial foodborne illness.

What Makes Norwalk Such a Problem?

First, perhaps, the fact that it is a virus. Unlike bacteria, which attack the body like soldiers mounting a pitched battle, viruses are guerrilla fighters.

Viruses don't attack so much as *infiltrate*. They literally invade human cells and turn the cell's genetic material from its normal function to producing the virus itself.

Second, Norwalk is an extremely virulent or infective organism. "With Norwalk" says Dr. Cliver, "we think it normally takes only 100 to 1,000 viral particles to make you sick. And in some cases, it may take just a few."

Another measure of the threat Norwalk poses is its attack rate. "Assuming 100 people are exposed to Norwalk spread by an infected food handler to something served at a large dinner," says Cliver, "you can predict that some 60 to 80 people will become ill. That's an attack rate of 60 to 80 percent. Compared to an attack rate of 20 to 40 percent for most other foodborne illness, you see that Norwalk is quite potent."

A possible explanation of why Norwalk's attack rate is so high is that, while many adults test positive for antibodies to the virus—which means they've already had the illness once—they don't seem to have developed much real immunity. People can get the disease again and again.

What Is the Norwalk Viral Illness Like?

Reports indicate that people normally show symptoms—diarrhea, nausea, vomiting, abdominal pain, headache and fever—within 1 to 2 days after exposure. Symptoms are usually severe enough so that victims call a doctor; some may visit an emergency room. Acute discomfort lasts a day or two.

Serious problems can result from dehydration, and deaths have occurred among the elderly.

Let's Look At Some Actual Case Histories for a Better Idea How the Norwalk Virus Works.

In 1979, the Australians reported Norwalk problems in shellfish. In 1980, there was trouble in Florida oysters and New York clams and oysters.

Then there was the blockbuster buttercream frosting incident. In 1982, one man mixing icing for a Minneapolis-St. Paul area bakery caused some 3,000 illnesses. Investigators said the infected worker mixed the uncooked frosting in a giant vat with his bare arms in the icing up to the elbows.

From 1983 to 1985, there were more shellfish incidents in the U.S., including 888 verified cases in New York State alone. Shellfish are a problem because they feed by filtering nutrients from the water. Unfortunately, they also filter out and store bacteria and viruses.

In a 1986 camping incident, some 135 people on a trip to a South Dakota campground got Norwalk from contaminated water. Apparently sewage was seeping into a well whose chlorination system was not working properly. Even if the chlorination system had been working, though, there still could have been a problem. The Norwalk virus appears to be resistant to chlorine and other sewage-treatment agents.

The virus can even survive freezing! Two related outbreaks in 1987 involved ice produced by a Pennsylvania company that supplied the product to Philadelphia's Franklin Field stadium and to a museum fund-raiser in Wilmington, Del.

The cause of the problem, it turned out, was that the company's wells had been contaminated by flooding from an infected stream.

Well now you've heard the bad news—Norwalk resists chlorine, survives freezing, is highly infective and the body doesn't build immunity to it very well.

The Hopeful Side of Things Is Based On the Virus's Limitations.

"Norwalk," explains Dr. Cliver, "is a very host-specific virus. It multiplies in the cells in the human gut, passes out and can't grow again until it reaches another human gut. It can only *sit* in food. It can't multiply in food as bacteria do."

Norwalk is also killed by thorough cooking. Therefore, other than water contracted infections, says Dr. Shay Fout, a microbiologist for the Food and Drug Administration, there are only three ways Norwalk can spread from food to human hosts:

- Shellfish, vegetables or fruit, infected by human sewage in coastal waters or from seepage and run-off in fields, are eaten raw or undercooked.

- Food that won't be cooked or is only partially cooked becomes contaminated with viral particles from the body of an infected food handler, usually from this persons hands.

- Food is recontaminated after preparation or cooking by contact with viral particles from an infected food handler.

Narrowing the Norwalk Threat

Wash Your Hands Thoroughly

Wash your hands thoroughly in hot, soapy water before preparing food. "This is important advice," says Dr. Fout, because this virus is frequently transmitted from an infected person's hands to the next victim's mouth."

Commercial food preparers should also use a disinfectant on their hands and wear gloves that they change from one operation to the next. "Millions of Norwalk particles can be in a single stool globule on someone s hands," says Dr Cliver.

Don't Drink Untreated Water

Boil water when camping or travelling in suspect areas. This will also protect you from hepatitis and other viruses.

Shellfish

- **Eating raw shellfish.** The elderly, the very young, cancer or AIDS patients, diabetics, and people with liver or chronic digestive diseases are advised not to eat raw shellfish. They are at risk not only for Norwalk but for a number of other serious viral illnesses.

  Healthy persons eat raw shellfish at their own risk. Shellfish are defined as oysters, clams, mollusks, scallops, snails, whelks and cockles.

- **Buy shellfish from reputable, licensed dealers.** This reduces the risk that it was harvested from unsafe waters.

- **Refrigerate shellfish at 32-40°F.** Store live shellfish in a shallow dish covered with damp paper towels. Storing them in water or in an airtight container kills them.

  Use mussels and clams in the shell in 2-3 days; oysters in the shell in 7-10 days. If shells open, tap them. If they don't re-close, discard.

  Freshly-shucked clams. stored in a covered jar, will keep 1-2 days: shucked scallops, 2-3 days: shucked oysters, 5-7 days.

  Commercially frozen shellfish lasts in the freezer up to 6 months: homefrozen shellfish, 3-6 months. Longer freezing cause quality loss.

- **Cooking.** Cover and continue steaming shellfish for 5 minutes after they open.

  Shucked shellfish look plump and opaque when well cooked, which normally takes 4-5 minutes in a boiling mixture. Scallops firm to a milky white. Oysters curl at the edges and may shrink slightly.

- **Leftovers.** Refrigerate cooked shellfish dishes for use in 2-3 days.

—by Mary Ann Parmley

Section 2.4

Viral Gastroenteritis Associated with Consumption of Raw Oysters— Florida, 1993.

(Source: *MMWR*, June 24, 1994.)

During November 20-30,1993, four county public health units (CPHUs) of the Florida Department of Health and Rehabilitative Services (HRS) in northwestern Florida conducted preliminary investigations of seven separate outbreaks of foodborne illness following consumption of raw oysters. On December 1, the HRS State Health Office initiated an investigation to characterize the illness, examine risk factors for oyster-associated gastroenteritis, and quantify the dose-response relation. This report presents the findings of these two investigations.

Preliminary Investigations by the HRS CPHUs

In November 1993, private physicians notified the CPHUs of 20 persons with possible foodborne illness. These 20 ill persons identified seven well meal companions. Raw oysters were the only common food item eaten by all ill persons; no well meal companions had eaten oysters. At the request of the HRS State Health Office, CPHUs initiated active surveillance for cases of raw oyster-associated gastroenteritis among patients of hospital emergency departments, urgent-care centers, and private physicians in northwestern Florida. A case was defined as sudden onset of nausea, vomiting, diarrhea, or abdominal cramps within 72 hours of eating raw oysters. Twenty-five additional cases of gastroenteritis associated with eating raw oysters were detected.

Traceback of implicated oysters by the CPHUs and the Florida Department of Environmental Quality indicated the oysters had been harvested from Apalachicola Bay in northwestern Florida during November 15-23.

Epidemiologic Investigation by the HRS State Health Office

The 45 persons with raw oyster-associated gastroenteritis reported by the CPHUs identified 26 well meal companions who had eaten oysters during the same meal as ill persons, but did not become ill. Of 44 ill persons for whom data were available, 36 (82%) had developed diarrhea; 34 (77%), nausea; 33 (75%), abdominal cramps; 25 (57%), vomiting; 17 (39%), fever; 15 (34%), headache; and 14 (32%), myalgia. The attack rate was 63%. Of the 45 ill persons, 10 were hospitalized for 24 hours or longer. For 30 persons for whom data were available, the median incubation period was 31 hours (range: 2-69 hours). For 26 persons for whom data were available, the median duration of illness was 48 hours (range: 10 hours-7 days); for 13 persons, duration of illness was more than 3 days. No household contacts of ill persons developed gastroenteritis.

No differences were identified between persons who became ill and well meal companions in preexisting medical conditions or medications. Consumption of alcohol or food (e.g., crackers and hot sauce) with the oysters was not associated with risk for illness. Based on the 33 cases for which data were available, a dose-response relation was observed between illness and number of raw oysters eaten (chi square for trend=3.98; p=0.05). The attack rate was highest among raw-oyster eaters who had consumed more than 5 dozen oysters (91%) and lowest among those who had consumed less than 1 dozen oysters (46%).

Paired serum specimens from 10 patients were tested for antibody to Norwalk-like virus by enzyme immunoassay (1); three pairs demonstrated a fourfold or greater rise in titer. Seven stool specimens were examined by electron microscopy (EM) and reverse transcription-polymerase chain reaction (RT-PCR). In four specimens, small round-structured viruses were detected by EM; in one specimen, a Norwalk-like genome was confirmed by RT-PCR (2,3). This Norwalk-like virus strain had a nucleotide sequence distinct from similar viruses in nearly simultaneous outbreaks associated with consumption of oysters harvested along the Louisiana coast (4).

No confirmed evidence of improper handling (e.g., inadequate refrigeration time or temperature) of the implicated oysters was detected. However, three ill persons had purchased oysters from retail establishments that were not licensed seafood dealers.

The National Shellfish Sanitation Program (NSSP) requires fecal coliform testing at least once each month. Fecal coliform testing of water drawn from 39 monitoring sites in Apalachicola Bay on October 3, November 21, and November 24 indicated that water quality in the bay met the criteria of the NSSP (5). No environmental source of pollution was identified. Sanitation procedures at the oyster-processing facilities where seafood dealers purchased oysters met standards set by the Florida Department of Environmental Protection (FDEP). However, based on the epidemiologic evidence of illness associated with oysters harvested from those waters, FDEP temporarily closed the shellfish-harvesting area of Apalachicola Bay during December 1-7. No cases of gastroenteritis related to consumption of oysters harvested after December 7 have been reported.

Reported by: C Davis, A Smith, MD, R Walden, Bay County Public Health Unit, Pananma City; G Bower, K Cummings, B Dean, J Rigsby, Jackson County Public Health Unit, Marianna; P Justice, C Anderson, N Brown, J Minor, Washington County Public Health Unit, Chipley; EF Geiger, MD, V Laxton, District 1 Health Office, Pensacola; L Crockett, MD, W McDougal, District 2 Health Office, Tallahassee; WG Hlady, MD, RS Hopkins, MD, State Epidemiologist, State Health Office, Florida Dept of Health and Rehabilitative Svcs. Food and Drug Administration. Viral Gastroenteritis Section, Respiratory and Enterovirus Br, Div of Viral and Rickettsial Diseases, National Center for Infectious Diseases; Div of Field Epidemiology, Epidemiology Program Office, CDC.

Editorial Note: This report documents outbreaks of viral gastroenteritis in Florida linked to consumption of raw oysters from waters that apparently met the standards for shellfish sanitation. Clinical and epidemiologic features of the outbreaks are similar to recently reported multistate outbreaks of viral gastroenteritis associated with eating oysters harvested in Louisiana (4). RT-PCR with sequencing identified different strains of the virus in the multistate outbreak and the Florida outbreak, suggesting independent sources of oyster contamination.

Although infection with the oysterborne Norwalk-like virus caused no fatalities in this outbreak, raw oyster consumption has been linked in Florida to 30 fatal cases of infection with *Vibrio vulnificus* during 1981-1992 among persons with preexisting liver disease (6). *V.*

vulnificus is a ubiquitous organism found in seawater. In Florida, consumer information statements (required as labels on bags of oysters and in restaurants) emphasize the risk for *Vibrio* infection among persons with underlying liver disease and other preexisting illnesses (6). In addition, these statements suggest that such persons eat oysters fully cooked and consult with their physician if uncertain about whether they are at risk.

States conduct monitoring programs to assure clean oyster beds, legal harvesting, and proper handling of oysters. However, at both the Louisiana and Florida oyster harvest sites, routine fecal coliform water-quality monitoring conducted once each month did not detect oyster-bed contamination. Furthermore, the outbreak reported in Florida was identified in part because of publicity about the larger outbreaks associated with oysters harvested in Louisiana. These findings suggest that monitoring waters for fecal coliforms may be insufficient to indicate the presence of viruses (e.g., Norwalk-like virus). Continued surveillance for outbreaks of gastroenteritis associated with consumption of raw oysters is needed to assess efficacy of the NSSP in preventing human illness. Public health officials should consider raw oyster consumption as a possible source of infection during the evaluation of gastroenteritis outbreaks.

References

1. Monroe SS, Stine SE, Jiang XI, Estes MK, Glass Rl. Detection of antibody to recombinant Norwalk virus antigen in specimens from outbreaks of gastroenteritis. J Clin Microbiol 1993;31:2866-72.

2. Moe CL, Gentsch J, Ando T, et al. Application of PCR to detect Norwalk virus in fecal specimens from outbreaks of gastroenteritis. J Clin Microbiol 1994;32:642-8.

3. Ando T, Mulders MN, Lewis DC, Estes MK, Monroe SS, Glass Rl. Comparison of the polymerase region of small round structured virus strains previously classified in three antigenic types by solid-phase immune electron microscopy. Arch Virol 1994;135:217-26.

4. CDC. Multistate outbreak of viral gastroenteritis related to consumption of oysters—Louisiana, Maryland, Mississippi, and North Carolina, 1993. MMWR 1993;42:945-8.

5. Office of Seafood, Shellfish Sanitation Branch, Food and Drug Administration. Sanitation of shellfish growing areas, part 1. [Section C.3.c]. In: National Shellfish Sanitation Program manual of operations. Washington, DC: US Department of Health and Human Services, Public Health Service, 1992:C8-C9.

6. Hlady WG, Mullen RC, Hopkins RS, *Vibrio vulnificus* from raw oysters: leading cause of reported deaths from foodborne illness in Florida. J Fla Med Assoc 1993;80:536-8.

Chapter 3

Parasitic Diseases

Chapter Contents

Section 3.1

Parasitic Invaders and the Reluctant Human Host

(Source: *FDA Consumer*, July/August 1993.)

Thousands of Milwaukee area residents got an unwanted crash course last April in cryptosporidiosis, a disease most had never heard of until they—or friends or family—contracted it. The culprit was a parasite, *Cryptosporidium*, that had invaded the city's drinking water supply, causing people to become sick with diarrhea and other intestinal symptoms; several died.

Cryptosporidium lives in the intestines of cattle and other animals and is excreted in feces. Health officials suspect the water supply became contaminated from a high level of runoff into Lake Michigan from area dairy farms or slaughterhouses near the water plant's intake pipe. An inadequate filtration system allowed the parasites entry into the water supply.

Cryptosporidiosis is just one of several diseases caused by parasites, which are largely unfamiliar to Americans. But in much of the rest of the world, they are all too well-known. These tiny ravagers—many no larger than a single cell—claim the health and lives of millions of people around the globe.

Parasites live in or on another organism, known as the host, from which they receive nourishment and protection. Some pass successive stages of maturity in hosts of different species, including humans. Parasites are of different types, including protozoa (one-celled animals) and helminths (worms) ranging in size from microscopic eggs to adults up to several feet long. The illnesses they cause range from mild discomfort of short duration to chronic, debilitating disease and death.

People who live in areas where the disease is endemic (constantly present) suffer the devastation most keenly. Hardest hit are developing countries in the tropics, where poor sanitation fosters the parasites and the insects that transfer many of them from one host to another.

A major killer among the parasitic diseases, and perhaps the one best known to Americans, is malaria. It is caused by the protozoa *Plasmodium*, transferred to humans by the bite of the *Anopheles* mosquito. Although malaria is not a significant health problem in the United

States, more than 1 billion people worldwide live in areas where the disease is endemic, and between 125 million and 200 million people are infected at any given time Each year in Africa alone, malaria claims the lives of 1 million children.

Millions more adults and children in Africa, South and Central America, Asia, and parts of Europe suffer from other devastating parasitic diseases as well. For example, African sleeping sickness, caused by the protozoan *Trypanosoma brucei*, is one of the most lethal of all human diseases. It produces fever, enlarged lymph glands, skin lesions, and painful swelling. Neurological symptoms, including tremors, headache, apathy, and convulsions, predominate later in the disease, which can end in coma and death.

Schistosomiasis, a helminthic disease affecting approximately 200 million people between the tropics of Cancer and Capricorn, can produce bladder, intestinal or liver disease that may lead to death. Onchocerciasis (river blindness), found in Mexico, South and Central America, and Africa, results from infection with larvae of the *Onchocerca volvulus* worm, transmitted by flies that breed along fast-moving streams. It causes a skin rash, often with severe and constant itching. Eye lesions lead to blindness in about 5 percent of people infected.

"It is true that parasitic diseases are a much greater problem in other parts of the world," says George Jackson, Ph.D., a microbiologist in FDA's Center for Food Safety and Applied Nutrition, "but they seem to be on the increase in industrialized temperate zone countries, and there are even certain parasitic infections among Native Alaskans."

Life Cycle of Anisakis Simplex

The *Anisakis simplex* parasite matures and reproduces in marine mammals, such as the seal. The parasite eggs pass with the mammal's feces into the water and hatch into larvae. Crustaceans, such as crabs, and other small water creatures swallow the larvae. Larger fish eat the smaller creatures and become infected. Humans eat the fish and become infected, or marine mammals eat the fish and the cycle begins again.

Travelers Play Host

The rising incidence of parasitic diseases in the United States is due in part to increasing international travel. Approximately 8 million

Americans travel to the developing world annually, according to the national Centers for Disease Control and Prevention, and the speed of jet transport permits travelers to return home within the incubation period of every infectious disease. As a result, the agency says, an increasing number of parasitic infections are being diagnosed in business travelers and tourists and are causing considerable disease and occasional death.

One of these diseases is malaria. *Plasmodium* parasites infect red blood cells, causing a spiking fever, possible immune problems, damage to internal organs, and, potentially, death. Certain species of the parasite may lie dormant in the organs for years, until something—perhaps another infection—triggers the disease.

Although once endemic in the U.S. Southeast, malaria was declared eradicated in this country in the 1940s; the last case originating here was reported to CDC in 1957. Yet from 1969 to 1980, the number of cases in civilians reported to that agency rose from 151 to 1,864, and since 1980, the number of cases in travelers has averaged 1,000 annually. Compounding the problem is the fact that malaria has become resistant to the drugs taken to prevent contracting the disease. Once brought in, local transmission is rare, but does occur, since the *Anopheles* mosquito does exist in this country.

Other previously rare and potentially fatal parasitic infections, such as leishmaniasis (which may affect the skin, mucous membranes, or internal organs), schistosomiasis, and onchocerciasis, are also increasing among returning U.S. travelers.

While those particular parasitic diseases are still uncommon in the United States, others are seen here much more often, especially in specific groups of people.

Parasitic Disease and Weakened Immunity

"There are certain parasites we're all exposed to that don't cause us much trouble unless we're particularly vulnerable to them," explains Randolph Wykoff, M.D. "The protozoa that cause pneumocystis pneumonia and toxoplasmosis can be fairly common in the population. Most people have been exposed to them with limited illness, if any."

Wykoff, who is a specialist in tropical medicine and heads FDA's Office of AIDS Coordination, explains that little more than a decade ago these two diseases were seen infrequently—almost exclusively in people with immune systems weakened by cancer chemotherapy, or in malnourished, chronically ill, and pre-term infants.

That changed with the appearance and spread of HIV (human immune deficiency virus) infection. Immune suppression is the hallmark of this infection, which leads to AIDS. HIV-infected patients are vulnerable to many opportunistic infections (infections that would not cause illness in someone with a healthy immune system), including those caused by parasites. Pneumocystis pneumonia, toxoplasmosis, and cryptosporidiosis are responsible for much of the illness and death suffered by people with AIDS.

Parasite Provides First Clue to AIDS

"In fact, it was because of unexplained cases of pneumocystis—an airborne respiratory infection caused by *Pneumocystis carinii*—that AIDS was first recognized in 1981," Wykoff says. "Pentamidine, the drug used to treat the disease, was available only through CDC. When the agency noticed an increase in the number of requests for pentamidine, it began an investigation that eventually led to identification of AIDS as a new disease."

As HIV infections have increased, so has the incidence of pneumocystis pneumonia. According to CDC's *HIV/AIDS Surveillance*, 19,503 new cases of pneumocystis pneumonia were diagnosed in HIV-infected patients in 1992.

Early symptoms are fever, cough, and shallow, rapid breathing. Chest x-ray shows parasitic infiltration of the lungs. As the disease progresses, cyanosis may develop—a bluish discoloration of the skin resulting from insufficient blood oxygen. Pneumocystis is the leading cause of death in people with AIDS, Wykoff says, but adds that control of the disease has improved since the introduction of preventive treatment with aerosolized pentamidine isethionate (NebuPent), approved by FDA in 1989. In 1992, Mepron (atovaquone) was approved to treat the pneumonia, joining Bactrim and Septra (combination products containing trimethoprim and sulfamethoxazole), both approved in 1976. Injectable pentamidine was approved to treat pneumocystis pneumonia in 1984.

"Cryptosporidiosis is another parasitic infection of major concern in HIV-infected and other immune-suppressed patients," says Wykoff, "although it was unknown until relatively recently—the last decade or so—and people are still not sure how common it is."

The parasite infects cells in the intestinal wall and releases a toxin that causes a profuse, watery diarrhea and abdominal cramping.

In healthy people, the disease is self-limiting; symptoms usually last a week or two, and then rapidly abate.

Immune-suppressed patients, however, are unable to clear the infection, and endure unremitting diarrhea. In these individuals, cryptosporidiosis becomes a debilitating wasting disease. According to the American Public Health Association's *Control of Communicable Diseases in Man*, 10 to 20 percent of AIDS patients develop cryptosporidiosis sometime during their illness. No drug is available to effectively combat the parasite, although several are under study. Current treatment is limited to rehydration therapy (replacing and maintaining fluids and electrolytes). Besides drinking plenty of fluids, patients may be given a liquid formula such as Pedialyte (for children) or Rehydralyte (for children and adults), which contains water, dextrose, potassium citrate, sodium chloride, and sodium citrate.

Cryptosporidium is transmitted through the fecal-oral route. Careful hand washing and good sanitation practices are essential in preventing disease spread. Adequate water filtration should prevent waterborne transmission such as occurred in Milwaukee.

Besides immune-suppressed patients, others at increased risk include children, foreign travelers, homosexual men, and close contacts of infected patients, such as family members, health-care workers, and day-care workers.

A third parasitic infection associated with HIV is toxoplasmosis, caused by *Toxoplasma gondii*. As with *Pneumocystis carinii, T. gondii* is common in the U.S. population. An estimated 40 percent of Americans are or have been infected, but most either don't get sick or they develop a relatively harmless illness—slight fever, muscle pain, sore throat, headache, and inflammation of the lymph nodes lasting days or weeks.

But again, infection in immune-suppressed people is much graver. According to CDC, toxoplasmosis is the most common opportunistic infection of the central nervous system in HIV-infected patients, and causes encephalitis (inflammation of the brain) or brain lesions in as many as 30 percent of AIDS patients. Symptoms include paralysis, mental deterioration, severe headache, seizures, and coma, usually ending in death. Toxoplasmosis is acquired by eating raw or undercooked meat contaminated with the parasite, or by exposure to contaminated cat feces. (See [sections], "For Safe Food, Handle with Care" and "Toxo-Tabby.")

Toxoplasmosis and Pregnancy

Toxoplasmosis can also be transmitted to a fetus through the placenta. The fetus is presumed to be at risk only if the mother has a primary, active infection during the pregnancy; a former infection is believed not to be dangerous.

CDC estimates there are between one and three congenital *Toxoplasma* infections per 1,000 live births in the United States each year. Only 10 percent of those infants develop symptoms, but of them, 85 percent develop severe neurologic and developmental problems, and approximately 12 percent die. Of those who have no symptoms at birth, up to 85 percent may develop chronic recurring eye disease and learning disabilities. Toxoplasmosis can also cause miscarriage, stillbirth, and pre-term birth.

Acute toxoplasmosis is usually treated with Daraprim (pyrimethamine) together with sulfadiazine for three to four weeks. Immune-suppressed patients should continue treatment for up to six months or longer, however, and may need reduced dosages throughout their lifetimes to try to prevent recurrence.

More Food-Borne Foes

"There are more than 80 food-borne parasites," says FDA's George Jackson, "but, fortunately, not all are of great significance in this country at this time. However, the food market is becoming international—we're getting not only preserved foods, but fresh foods flown in from all parts of the world."

Jackson says parasites are important not only because of the direct infections they cause, but because of their secretions and excretions. This is particularly true of the helminths. Even if the worms are pulled out of the food, their waste products—biologically active materials—are left behind in the flesh. Studies are getting started to discover what long-term effects they may have on humans.

"Our own habits are also a big factor," Jackson says. "We like to eat raw vegetables in salads and we're eating more raw fish. While most parasites are easily killed by proper cooking, right now we're not doing that well enough."

Probably the best-known-and most serious-food-borne parasitic disease in this country is trichinosis. Larvae of the *Trichinella* roundworm infect pigs and some game animals whose meat ends up on our dinner tables. The incidence of trichinosis has declined, however, with an average of only 44 cases per year from 1984 through 1988 reported to CDC. This is due partly to legislation requiring that garbage fed to pigs be cooked, killing any larvae. The sporadic outbreaks that occur are primarily among new immigrants from Asia.

"There is very little *Trichinella* in pork in Asia," Jackson explains. "Therefore, Asian immigrants do not cook pork as thoroughly as we do."

Trichinosis symptoms vary with individual immunity and the intensity of the infection. The adult worms develop and reproduce in the human digestive tract, where they may cause mild diarrhea. They then die and leave the body in feces. The new generation of larvae may then invade cells of the diaphragm, skeletal muscles or heart, causing serious damage, if present in large numbers.

"If you get a very few worms, you probably will not know it, but if you get a large dose, you will," Jackson says. "The problem is that if it's a subclinical infection, you probably don't need to treat it, and if it's severe, you're in trouble. Once symptoms develop, it's already in the muscles where it causes so much damage."

Treatment is aimed at helping the patient survive the acute infection. Effectiveness of the anthelmintic drug Mintezol (thiabendazole) varies among patients. Those who develop heart or central nervous system problems or who have allergic reactions such as hives and swelling are also given corticosteroids.

New Recipes, New Risks

While trichinosis is on the decline, fish-borne parasitic illnesses are on the rise, corresponding with the growing popularity in this country of raw fish dishes.

Japanese sushi and sashimi, Latin American ceviche, Scandinavian gravlax, lomi-lomi salmon, and other raw fish recipes may tempt our taste buds, but if they're not carefully prepared, our stomachs may revolt.

Seals, dolphins, porpoises, and other large sea mammals are host to a group of parasitic worms called anisakids. The parasites' eggs pass out of the mammal's body in feces. In the water, they hatch into larvae, which are then eaten by fish, such as cod, salmon or herring. When these infected fish reach our mouths raw or undercooked, trouble may ensue.

"Fortunately, the most common symptoms of anisakiasis are more annoying than life-threatening," says Jackson. He explains that the larvae burrow into the mucosa of the stomach or intestine, producing sometimes painful 'attachment ulcers,' and sometimes nausea and vomiting.

"Usually the worms don't last long—we're not their usual hosts—and they die or try to get out of us. They may be coughed or vomited up," he says. "Many people feel a tickling at the back of the throat. They reach back there and pull out this spaghetti-like worm."

In the normal course, the disease usually subsides spontaneously. Sometimes gastroscopy (inserting a tube through the mouth to the stomach) is used to remove the larvae. If chronic illness develops, surgery may be required to remove lesions that have developed.

Jackson says that on rare occasions the larvae penetrate the intestinal wall and go wandering in the body or settling in and affecting other organ systems. After the larvae begin to die, the body responds to their presence with a cellular reaction, which may be misdiagnosed as cancer FDA is working on a new policy to minimize the public's exposure to fish-borne parasites.

"We've decided to try to implement good manufacturing practice levels of allowable parasites on a species group basis," says Jeffrey Bier, Ph.D., research microbiologist in FDA's Office of Seafood. "The policy will be based on species groups because parasites are more visible and more easily detected in the flesh of certain species than in others."

Bier explains that the cods, flounders and sea basses, for example, are similar in the incidence of parasites and in the ease with which the parasites can be detected visually. The process to detect them is candling, in which light is used to look through the flesh of the fish.

Bier says the agency is collecting data on which to base proposed rules for good manufacturing practice levels of parasites for the cod and flounder families.

Day-Care Dilemma

Another parasite gaining ground in this country is *Giardia lamblia*, a protozoan also spread through the fecal-oral route, either directly through person-to-person contact or through contaminated food or water. It infects the small intestine and may cause gas, diarrhea, abdominal cramps, bloating, and, in severe cases, malabsorption and weight loss. Children are infected more frequently than adults, and the parasite is finding a wealth of young hosts in day-care centers.

In random surveys, giardiasis has been identified in 10 to 15 percent of diaper-aged children attending day-care centers, compared with 2 percent of same-age children not attending centers, CDC reports. In addition, approximately 20 to 25 percent of day-care staff and family contacts of infected children also become infected. The agency attributes the spread to poor personal hygiene, closer interpersonal contact, and the children's frequent hand-to-mouth and object-to-mouth behavior.

The simplest and most effective way to prevent the spread of giardiasis is hand washing. Experts advise day-care staff to wash their hands when they start work, before preparing or serving food, after diapering a child, and after going to the bathroom. Similarly, children's hands should be washed when they arrive at the center, before they eat or drink, and after they use the toilet or have their diapers changed. Other common-sense measures—such as cleaning and disinfecting diaper-changing areas after each use, keeping food preparation and diaper-changing areas separate, and keeping children with diarrhea at home—should also be followed.

Giardiasis is not unique to day-care settings. According to CDC, *Giardia* is the most common cause of waterborne outbreaks of intestinal disease in the United States, and the number of such outbreaks has increased significantly in recent years. They occur most often in mountain communities and those that get drinking water from streams or rivers without a water filtration system. Hikers and campers who drink from contaminated lakes, rivers and streams are also frequently affected. Swimming pools have also become contaminated.

Giardiasis seldom causes severe disability, but it is one of the leading causes of diarrheal illness in the United States. FDA has approved Furoxone (furazolidone) and Atabrine hydrochloride (quinacrine hydrochloride) for treatment. Flagyl (metronidazole) is also used.

Though parasitic diseases appear to be increasing in the United States, with proper common-sense sanitation practices and careful food preparation, many of these creatures can be kept at bay.

For Safe Food, Handle with Care

Cook it thoroughly. Cook it thoroughly. Cook it thoroughly! That's the most important thing to know about preventing food-borne illness.

FDA advises consumers to cook pork until it reaches an internal temperature of 71 degrees Celsius (160 degrees Fahrenheit). Fish should be cooked to an internal temperature of 60 C (140 F), flake easily, and be firm and opaque, or dull. If it's translucent, or shiny, it's not done.

"Proper cooking should kill most parasites," says George Jackson, Ph.D., of FDA's Center for Food Safety and Applied Nutrition, "but you've got to be careful that it's not just the outside that's getting all the heat. *Trichinella*, for instance, is on the inside of the meat. Anisakids in fish might be on the outside of the fillet, but they could also be in the fillet."

This is especially important to remember with microwaving, because the food often does not heat evenly. Rotate the dish once or twice during cooking, observe the standing time called for in the recipe or package directions, and check for doneness with a thermometer after removing it from the microwave oven. Insert the thermometer at several different spots.

Raw fish dishes, such as sushi and ceviche, can be safe for most people to eat if they are made with very fresh fish that is commercially frozen and then thawed.

In 1990, FDA issued an advisory to state and local regulatory agencies recommending that fish served raw, marinated, or partially cooked be blast-frozen to minus 35 C (minus 31 F) or below for 15 hours or frozen by regular means to minus 23 C (minus 10 F) or below for seven days.

People with immune disorders should not eat raw fin fish or shellfish because, although freezing kills most parasites, it does not kill bacteria. People with immune disorders need to take extra precautions to thoroughly cook all meat, fish and poultry.

Fruits and vegetables should be scrubbed and washed well to loosen all contaminants on the surface of the produce.

For more information on safe food handling and cooking, call the FDA Seafood Safety Hotline at (1-800) FDA-4010.

For a free copy of the U.S. Department of Agriculture publication "A Quick Consumer Guide to Safe Food Handling," write to Consumer Information Center Item 528Z, Pueblo, CO 81009.

More information on food handling Is available from USDA's toll-free Meat & Poultry Hotline. Call (1-800) 535-4555 from 10 a.m. to 4 p.m. weekdays, Eastern time.

Taxo-Tabby

In addition to cooking meats thoroughly, cat owners need to take additional precautions against toxoplasmosis, because cats are a host for *Toxoplasma gondii*. Cats acquire the parasites from eating rodents, birds, or raw beef.

"Recent studies show that cat ownership is not necessarily a problem," says Randolph Wykoff, M.D., director of FDA's Office of AIDS Coordination, "but people should handle their cat litter boxes appropriately and clean the boxes regularly."

Pregnant women and immune-suppressed individuals should have someone else change litter boxes, if possible. If not, they should wear disposable gloves and wash their hands thoroughly afterward. They should also wear gloves when gardening or doing other activities involving contact with possibly contaminated soil. Cat owners should follow these recommended precautions:

- Feed cats dry, canned or boiled food—never undercooked meat or poultry—and discourage hunting; that is, keep cats as indoor pets only.

- Use disposable plastic liners in cat litter boxes and change the litter daily. (The parasite in the feces is not infectious until two or three days after excretion.) Seal the liner with a twist tie and dispose of it in a plastic garbage bag.

- After emptying, disinfect the litter box with scalding water left in the pan for five minutes. (If a plastic liner is used, disinfecting is not necessary.)

- Wash hands thoroughly after cleaning the litter box.

- Wash hands thoroughly after contact with soil possibly contaminated with cat feces, and especially before eating.

- Cover sandboxes when not in use to prevent stray cats from getting into them.

—by Marian Segal

Marian Segal is a member of FDA's public affairs staff.

Section 3.2

Trichinosis Outbreaks

(Source: *FDA Consumer*, May 1991.)

Two outbreaks in 1990 of trichinosis (infection with *Trichinella spiralis* worm larvae) due to eating undercooked infested pork point up the need for consumers to continue guarding against this preventable, sometimes fatal illness. The U.S. Centers for Disease Control in Atlanta warned in its Feb. 1, 1991, *Morbidity and Mortality Weekly Report* that the risk is particularly high when people routinely eat undercooked pork, as is the practice among Southeast Asian immigrants.

Of the 250 people at a wedding of Southeast Asians last July in Des Moines, Iowa, 90 developed trichinosis—the fourth outbreak since 1975 among the 900,000 immigrants in the United States. The illnesses were linked to pork sausage that was uncooked, which is the customary way to serve that food in Southeast Asian culture. To kill *T. spiralis* larvae, a person must cook pork until it is well done, to 66 degrees Celsius (150 degrees Fahrenheit).

Last November and December, four Virginia counties reported another outbreak of 15 sausage-related cases. One victim denied eating undercooked sausage but was a meat handler in the plant that processed the implicated meat. CDC received reports of 15 additional cases occurring singly in 1990. No deaths were reported.

Trichinosis symptoms are fever, muscle soreness, and upper eyelid swelling. Lab tests show increased eosinophils (white blood cells).

CDC noted that the proportion of cases from commercial pork has declined since 1975, probably because of laws prohibiting feeding raw garbage to pigs, increased use of home freezers, and the practice of thoroughly cooking pork. On the other hand, there has been an increase in the relative importance of another source: wild game—including bear, boar and walrus.

Life Cycle of Trichinella Spiralis

1. Wild or domestic food animal ingests larvae by eating infested farm rats or infested flesh of another animal.

2. Humans eat contaminated meat from the slaughtered infested animal.

3. Larvae grow to adult worms in host's intestine, where they release new larvae able to pass through the intestinal wall.

4. Traveling in the bloodstream, larvae that reach muscle tissue survive by enclosing themselves in protective sacs.

Source: *Morbidity and Mortality Weekly Report*, Feb. 1, 1991.

Section 3.3

Cryptosporidium Infections Associated with Swimming Pools

(Source: *MMWR*, August 12, 1994.)

In March and April 1993, an outbreak of cryptosporidiosis in Milwaukee resulted in diarrheal illness in an estimated 403,000 persons (*1*). Following that outbreak, testing for *Cryptosporidium* in persons with diarrhea increased substantially in some areas of Wisconsin; by August 1, 1993, three of six clinical laboratories in Dane County were testing routinely for *Cryptosporidium* as part of ova and parasite examinations. In late August 1993, the Madison Department of Public Health and the Dane County Public Health Division identified two clusters of persons with laboratory-confirmed *Cryptosporidium* infection in Dane County (approximately 80 miles west of Milwaukee). This report summarizes the outbreak investigations.

On August 23, a parent reported to the Madison Department of Public Health that her daughter was ill with laboratory-confirmed *Cryptosporidium* infection and that other members of her daughter's swim team had had severe diarrhea. On August 26, public health officials inspected the pool where the team practiced (pool A) and interviewed a convenience sample of patrons at the pool. Seventeen (55%)

of 31 pool patrons interviewed reported having had watery diarrhea for 2 or more days with onset during July or August. Eight (47%) of the 17 had had watery diarrhea longer than 5 days. Four persons who reported seeking medical care had stool specimens positive for *Cryptosporidium*.

On August 31, public health nurses at the Dane County Public Health Division identified a second cluster of nine persons with laboratory-confirmed *Cryptosporidium* infection while following up case-reports voluntarily submitted by physicians. Seven of the nine ill persons reported swimming at one large outdoor pool (pool B). Because of the potential for disease transmission in multiple settings, a community-based matched case-control study was initiated on September 3 to identify risk factors for *Cryptosporidium* infection among Dane County residents.

Laboratory-based surveillance was used for case finding. A case was defined as *Cryptosporidium* infection that was laboratory-confirmed during August 1-September 11, 1993, in a Dane County resident who was also the first person in a household to have signs or symptoms (i.e., watery diarrhea of 2 or more days' duration). During the study interval, 85 Dane County residents with stool specimens positive for *Cryptosporidium* were identified. Sixty-five (77%) persons were interviewed; 36 (55%) had illnesses meeting the case definition. Systematic digit-dialing was used to select 45 controls, who were matched with 34 case-patients by age group and telephone exchange. All study participants were interviewed by telephone using a standardized questionnaire to obtain information on demographics, signs and symptoms, recreational water use, child-care attendance, drinking water sources, and presence of diarrheal illness in household members.

The median age of ill persons was 4 years (range: 1-40 years). Reported signs and symptoms included watery diarrhea (94%), stomach cramps (93%), and vomiting (53%). Median duration of diarrhea was 14 days (range: 1-30 days). Swimming in a pool or lake during the 2 weeks preceding onset of illness was reported by 82% of case-patients and 50% of controls (matched odds ratio [MOR]=6.0; 95% confidence interval [CI]=1.4-25.3). Twenty-one percent of case-patients and 2% of controls (MOR=7.3; 95% CI=0.9-59.3) reported swimming in pool A. Fifteen percent of case-patients and 2% of controls (MOR=undefined [6/0]; p=0.02, paired sample sign test) reported swimming in pool B. When persons reporting pool A or B use were excluded from the analysis, the association with recreational water use was not statistically significant (MOR=3.4, 95% Cl=0.8-15.7). Child-care attendance was reported for 74% of case-patients aged <6 years and 44% of controls (MOR=2.9; 95% Cl=0.8-10.7). Two case-patients reported child-care attendance and use of pool A or pool B. No case-patients reported travel to the Milwaukee area during the March-April outbreak, and no associations were found between illness and drinking water sources.

To limit transmission of *Cryptosporidium* in Dane County pools, state and local public health officials implemented the following recommendations: 1) closing the pools that were epidemiologically linked to infection and hyperchlorinating those pools to achieve a disinfection CT value of 9600 (CT=pool chlorine concentration—in parts per million—multiplied by time—in minutes); 2) advising all area pool managers of the increased potential for waterborne transmission of *Cryptosporidium*; 3) posting signs at all area pools stating that persons who have diarrhea or have had diarrhea during the previous 14 days should not enter the pool; 4) notifying area physicians of the increased potential for cryptosporidiosis in the community and requesting that patients with watery diarrhea be tested for *Cryptosporidium*; and 5) maintaining laboratory-based surveillance in the community to determine whether transmission was occurring at other sites (e.g., child-care centers and other pools).

On August 27, pool A was closed and hyperchlorinated for 18 hours; on September 3, pool B closed early for the season. Because many control measures were initiated less than 1 week before many pools closed for the season (after September 5), their impact on transmission could not be evaluated adequately.

Reported by: J Bongard, MS, Dane County Public Health Div, Madison; R Savage, MS, Madison Dept of Public Health; R Dern, MS, St. Mary's Medical Center, Madison; H Bostrum, J Kazmierczak, DVM, S Keifer, H Anderson, MD, State Epidemiologist for Occupation and Environmental Health, JP Davis, MD, State Epidemiologist for Communicable Diseases, Bur of Public Health, Wisconsin Div of Health. Div of Parasitic Diseases, National Center for Infectious Diseases; Div of Field Epidemiology, Epidemiology Program Office, CDC.

Editorial Note: Person-to-person, waterborne, and zoonotic transmission of *Cryptosporidium* has been well documented (2). A marked seasonality has been reported, with peaks occurring in North America during late summer and early fall (*3,4*). Cryptosporidiosis associated with use of swimming pools has been reported previously (*5-7*) but is probably underrecognized. Infection with *Cryptosporidium* resulting from recreational water use may contribute to the observed seasonal distribution.

The March-April 1993 Milwaukee waterborne outbreak stimulated increased testing for *Cryptosporidium* in Dane County, increasing the likelihood of outbreak detection. However, the number of cases described in this report was not sufficient to conduct a stratified matched analysis. Confounding of the associations found for child-care attendance and pool use is possible, although child-care attendance was reported in only one case for each implicated pool.

Cryptosporidium oocysts are small (4-6μ), are resistant to chlorine, and have a high infectivity. The chlorine CT of 9600 needed to kill *Cryptosporidium* oocysts is approximately 640 times greater than required for *Giardia* cysts (*8*). The ability of pool sand-filtration systems to remove oocysts under field conditions has not been well documented, but would not be expected to be effective. Results of an infectivity study suggest that the infective dose among humans for *Cryptosporidium* is low (H. DuPont, University of Texas Medical School at Houston, personal communication, 1994). Because of the large number of oocysts probably shed by symptomatic persons, even limited fecal contamination could result in sufficient oocyst concentrations in localized areas of a pool to cause additional human infections.

This investigation underscores the potential for transmission of *Cryptosporidium* in swimming pools. Health-care providers should consider requesting *Cryptosporidium* testing of stool specimens from persons with watery diarrhea, and public health departments should consider establishing surveillance for *Cryptosporidium* to facilitate prompt recognition of outbreaks. Maintaining the high levels of chlorine necessary to kill *Cryptosporidium* in swimming pools is not feasible; therefore, such recreational water use should be recognized as a potential increased risk for cryptosporidiosis in immunocompromised persons, including those with human immunodeficiency virus infection, in whom this infection may cause lifelong, debilitating illness (*9*).

References

1. Mac Kenzie WR, Hoxie NJ, Proctor ME, et al. A massive outbreak in Milwaukee of Cryptosporidium infection trans-

mitted through the public water supply. N EnglJ Med 1994;331:161-7.

2. Casemore DP. Epidemiologic aspects of human cryptosporidiosis. Epidemiol Infect 1990;104:1-28.

3. Wolfson JS, Richter JM, Waldron WA, Weber DJ, McCarthy DM, Hopkins CC. Cryptosporidiosis in immunocompetent patients. N Engl J Med 1985;312:1278-82.

4. Skeels MR, Sokolow R, Hubbard CV, Andrus JK, Baisch J. *Cryptosporidium* infection in Oregon public health clinic patients, 1985-1988: the value of statewide laboratory surveillance. Am J Public Health 1990;80:305-8.

5. Sorvillo FJ, Fujioka K, Nahlen B, et al. Swimming-associated cryptosporidiosis. Am J Public Health 1992;82:742-4.

6. Bell A, Guasparini R, Meeds D, et al. A swimming pool-associated outbreak of cryptosporidiosis in British Columbia. Can J Public Health 1993;84:334-7.

7. CDC. Surveillance for waterborne disease outbreaks-United States, 1991-1992. MMWR 1993;42(no. SS-5):1-22.

8. Current WL, Garcia LS. Cryptosporidiosis. Clin Microbiol Rev 1991;4:305-8.

9. Navin TR, Juranek DD. Cryptosporidiosis: clinical, epidemiologic, and parasitologic review. Rev Infect Dis 1984;6:313-27.

Chapter 4

Why Immune System Problems Raise the Risk of Foodborne Illness

Picture this: A criminal invades a town, threatening its safety. But before he can do any damage, he's surrounded by police and then hauled off and confined in the local jail.

According to some medical experts, that's a good description of how the human immune system works. It also explains why, when the immune system is weak, people are more vulnerable to invaders like bacteria that can cause foodborne illness.

For those with a weak immune system—pregnant women and very young children, the elderly and people with chronic illnesses— foodborne disease can pose a serious threat to health.

For this reason, USDA's Food Safety and Inspection Service launched an education campaign last year to tell these susceptible people about their risks and how to protect themselves.

However, while many people may realize they face special risks, few really understand why.

How Does the Immune System Work?

What weakens a person's immunity?

The immune system is one of the most important mechanisms for fighting disease and preserving health. Humans have two types of cells that fight invading bacteria and viruses, also known as *antigens*.

Food News for Consumers, Spring 1991.

T cells are white blood cells. They travel through the bloodstream. When they reach some invading antigens, they attack them.

B cells are white blood cells that produce proteins called *antibodies*. These antibodies bind to the invading antigens and help prevent them from doing damage.

One thing that makes the immune system unique is "memory."

Once the body has fought off a particular type of antigen, the body remembers for years, sometimes for life. When that same antigen infects the body again, the immune system often recognizes and attacks it before an infection can even occur. That's why childhood diseases are frequently just that.

Why Very Young Children and Pregnant Women Are More Vulnerable

Children must be vaccinated against an illness or actually contract it before their immune systems develop the memory to counteract that particular invader.

Pregnant women need to know that the unborn child is especially vulnerable too.

While the fetus has some immunities lent by the mother's blood, its immune system is immature and vulnerable. In rare instances, some types of foodborne disease can even cause miscarriage or stillbirth.

After birth, antibodies from the mother are with the child for a few months. As these are lost, the child becomes more vulnerable.

Why Older People Are Vulnerable

Older people may have a weakened immune system for any number of reasons.

Poor nutrition can be a factor.

As people grow older they sometimes lose some sense of smell and taste. As a result, appetites may decrease and vitamin deficiencies increase.

Why is that important? Clinical and animal studies show that dietary components such as protein and vitamins A, D, C and B complex are necessary for healthy immune responses.

Another risk factor for older people is poor blood circulation. That can increase risks because cells from the immune system are carried through the blood. If the blood has trouble reaching the site of an infection, it may go unchecked.

Why the Chronically Ill Are At Risk

Poor blood circulation may also increase infection risks for some people with chronic illness.

Diabetics, many of whom are also elderly, may be vulnerable because they may suffer from poor blood circulation. Diabetics may be vulnerable for another reason too—high levels of sugar in their blood. Blood with a high sugar level may serve as a better growth media for bacteria.

People with *digestive problems* that require them to take antacids are also vulnerable. Acid in the stomach often kills bacteria before they even reach the intestine. Reduce acid and you create a favorable environment for bacteria.

Even people who are taking antibiotics may find they are more vulnerable. The normal intestine has millions of good bacteria. Antibiotics can kill them off, so invading pathogens can more easily gain a foothold.

The bottom line is many different types of people may have a vulnerable immune system and need to take special care to prevent illness that could be caused by mishandling food.

Keys to Preventing Foodborne Illness

Microbiological organisms are everywhere—on our skin, in dirt, on surfaces we touch, and in perishable foods like meat, poultry, fish, eggs and dairy products. But safe food handling can greatly reduce the risk of illness from harmful organisms.

There are three keys to safe food handling:

1. Cook food thoroughly to destroy harmful bacteria.

2. Avoid "cross contamination" by washing anything that touches raw meat or poultry with hot, soapy water (that includes your hands, counters, utensils and cutting boards).

3. And never, never eat anything raw, including raw eggs or seafood.

Health Organizations Can Help Spread the At-Risk Message

Since USDA's Food Safety and Inspection Service (FSIS) launched its educational campaign last spring, more than 40 million Americans have heard that certain people face special risks from foodborne illness.

How can your health organization help? As Joe Carlin, a nutritionist with the Administration on Aging (AOA) says, "FSIS has put all the materials together so all you have to do is copy and go."

The Administration on Aging, part of the U.S. Department of Health and Human Services, provides more than 270 million meals to the elderly each year. In support of the FSIS campaign, AOA distributed the FSIS safe food handling kit to more than 1,600 cooperators.

For a sample copy of the FSIS booklet, "Is Someone You Know At Risk for Foodborne Illness?" write USDA/FSIS-Public Awareness, Rm. 1165 South, 12th & Independence, Washington, D.C. 20250.

—by Dianne Durant

Chapter 5

Preventing Foodborne Illness

Introduction

Today's consumers are purchasing and preparing both traditional and new types of meat and poultry products. People are serving more "keep refrigerated" prepared foods and doing more microwave cooking. To keep pace with new trends, food manufacturers are changing the way they process, package, and distribute their products.

Consumers are concerned, according to recent surveys, about the danger of drug, chemical and pesticide residues in their food. Yet scientific tests have shown that consumers run little risk of health effects from residues in meat or poultry.

The most common foodborne illnesses (a more accurate term than "food poisoning") are caused by a combination of bacteria, naturally present in our environment, and food handling errors made in commercial settings, food service institutions or at home. Ironically, these are also the easiest types of foodborne illnesses to prevent. Proper cooking or processing of raw meat and poultry destroys bacteria that can cause foodborne illness.

As required by law, U.S. Department of Agriculture inspectors check and recheck the safety and quality of meat and poultry from the time animals arrive at the slaughter plant until the final product is ready for distribution. USDA routinely monitors for the presence of

USDA Food Safety and Inspection Service, Home & Garden Bulletin Number 247, September 1990.

microbial contamination in commercially cooked or processed ready-to-eat meat and poultry products to assure that they are safe. Local health departments regulate and monitor conditions in grocery stores, institutions, restaurants, and other establishments that sell food.

However, purchasing, storing, and preparing both traditional and new meat and poultry products present many challenges to consumers—and that's who's responsible for keeping food safe once it leaves the store. By following the guidelines in this book consumers can learn how to properly handle meat and poultry products, as well as other foods, to prevent foodborne illness. Whether dealing with a traditional food or a new product, the basic principles of safe food preparation and storage are the same.

Keeping Food Safe

Most foodborne illness is caused by bacteria that multiply rapidly at temperatures between 60°F and 125°F. To control any bacteria that may be present, it is important to maintain the internal temperature of cooked foods that will be served hot at 140°F or above, and to maintain the internal temperature of foods that will be served cold at 40°F or below.

High food temperatures (160°F to 212°F) reached in boiling, baking, frying and roasting kill most bacteria that can cause foodborne illness. Prompt refrigeration at 40°F or below, in containers that are less than 2 inches deep, inhibits the growth of most, but not all, of these bacteria. Freezing at 0°F or below essentially stops bacterial growth but will not kill bacteria that are already present.

Thorough reheating to an internal temperature of 165°F or above will kill bacteria that may have grown during storage. However, foods that have been improperly stored or otherwise mishandled cannot be made safe by reheating.

To avoid introducing bacteria that can cause foodborne illness, it is important to ensure that everything that touches food during preparation and serving is clean.

The following guidelines highlight the most important food safety rules to keep in mind when shopping for, storing, preparing, and serving food.

Food Temperature and Bacterial Growth

Cooking and canning times and temperatures are usually based on conditions at sea level. At higher altitudes, water boils at lower temperatures. Lower boiling temperatures are less effective for killing bacteria. At altitudes of 1,000 feet or more, cooking or canning times or temperatures must be increased to destroy bacteria.

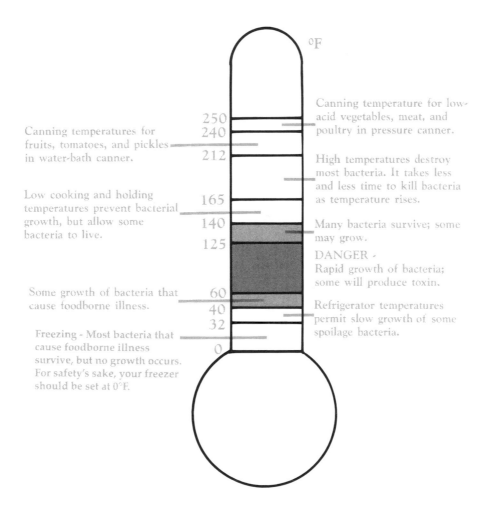

Figure 5.1. Food Temperature and Bacterial Growth

91

Shopping

At the Grocery or Specialty Market

- Buy food from reputable dealers, with a known record of safe handling.

- Buy dated products only if the "sell by" or "use by" date has not expired. While these dates are helpful, they are reliable only if the food has been kept at the proper temperature during storage and handling. Although many products bear "sell by" or "use by" dates, product dating is not a Federal requirement.

- Buy products labeled "keep refrigerated" only if they are stored in a refrigerated case and cold to the touch.

- Buy frozen products only if they are frozen solid.

- Buy packaged precooked foods only if the package is sound— not torn or damaged.

- Avoid cross-contamination. To prevent raw meat and poultry from contaminating foods that will be eaten without further cooking, enclose individual packages of raw meat or poultry in plastic bags. Position packages of raw meat and poultry in your shopping cart so their juices cannot drip on other foods.

- Shop for perishables last. Keep refrigerated and frozen items together so they will remain cold. Place perishables in the coolest part of your car during the trip home. Pack them in an ice chest if time from store to home refrigerator will be more than 1 hour.

Mail Order Foods

- Hard salami and dry-cured country style hams are good choices for ordering by mail because they do *not* require refrigeration.

- However, most other meat and poultry products, as well as many other foods that can be ordered by mail, must arrive as cold as if refrigerated in order to be safe.

- Before ordering such items, ask specific questions about how and when the product will be shipped, and whether a cold source will be included, to ensure that the product will be received cold.

- If you receive a package containing meat, poultry or any other item requiring refrigeration, check the item upon receipt to see if it is as cold as if refrigerated. If it is not, call the mail order company to arrange for a replacement that will arrive cold or request a refund.

Home Storage

Perishable Foods

- Raw meat and poultry should be wrapped securely so they do not leak and contaminate other foods or surfaces. Use plastic bags over commercial packaging or place the product on a plate to contain raw juices.

- Since repeated handling can introduce bacteria to meat and poultry, it's best to leave a product in the store wrap unless it's torn.

- Date any undated products you may have purchased and be sure to use them within the recommended time.

- Refrigerate all products marked "keep refrigerated."

- Eggs should be stored in their carton in the refrigerator.

- Freeze all products with a "keep frozen" label.

- Use a refrigerator thermometer to verify refrigerator temperature at 40°F or below and freezer temperature at 0°F or below.

• Maintain a clean refrigerator and freezer.

• Make sure the arrangement of items in your refrigerator and freezer allows the cold air to circulate freely.

• To minimize dehydration and quality loss, use freezer wrap, freezer-quality plastic bags, or aluminum foil over commercial wrap on meat and poultry that will be stored in the freezer for more than a couple of months.

Cold Storage Chart

These *short* but safe time limits will help keep refrigerated food from spoiling or becoming dangerous to eat. The time limits given for frozen foods are to maintain flavor and texture. It is still safe to eat frozen foods that have been kept longer.

PRODUCT	REFRIGERATOR (40°F)	FREEZER (0°F)
Eggs		
Fresh, in shell	3 weeks	Don't freeze
Raw yolks, whites	2-4 days	1 year
Hardcooked	1 week	Don't freeze well
Liquid pasteurized eggs or egg substitutes		
opened	3 days	Don't freeze
unopened	10 days	1 year
Mayonnaise, commercial		
Refrigerate after opening	2 months	Don't freeze
TV Dinners, Frozen Casseroles		
Keep Frozen until ready to serve		3-4 months

Figure 5.2a. Cold Storage Chart, continued on next page

	Refrigerator (40°F)	Freezer (0°F)
Deli & Vacuum-Packed Products		
Store-prepared (or homemade) egg, chicken, tuna, ham, macaroni salads	3-5 days	Don't freeze well
Pre-stuffed pork & lamb chops, chicken breasts stuffed with dressing	1 day	
Store-cooked convenience meals	1-2 days	If you are going to freeze these foods, do as soon as you get them home, not *after* they've sat in the refrigerator
Commercial brand vacuum-packed dinners with USDA seal	2 weeks, unopened	
Soups & Stews		
Vegetable or meat-added	3-4 days	2-3 months
Hamburger, Ground & Stew Meats		
Hamburger & stew meats	1-2 days	3-4 months
Ground turkey, veal, pork, lamb & mixtures of them	1-2 days	3-4 months
Hotdogs & Lunch Meats		
Hotdogs, opened package	1 week	
unopened package	2 weeks*	In freezer wrap, 1-2 months
Lunch meats, opened	3-5 days	
unopened	2 weeks*	
Bacon & Sausage		
Bacon	7 days	1 month
Sausage, raw, from pork, beef, turkey	1-2 days	1-2 months
Smoked breakfast links, patties	7 days	1-2 months
Hard sausage - pepperoni, jerky sticks	2-3 weeks	1-2 months
Ham, Corned Beef		
Corned Beef	In pouch with pickling juices 5-7 days	Drained, wrapped 1 month
Ham, canned Label says "keep refrigerated"	6-9 months	Don't Freeze
Ham, fully cooked - whole	7 days	1-2 months
Ham, fully cooked - half	3 -5 days	1-2 months
Ham, fully cooked - slices	3-4 days	1-2 months
Fresh Meat		
Beef steaks	3-5 days	6-12 months
Beef roasts	3-5 days	6-12 months
Lamb chops	3-5 days	6-9 months
Lamb roasts	3-5 days	6-9 months
Pork chops	3-5 days	4-6 months
Pork roasts	3-5 days	4-6 months
Veal roasts	3-5 days	4-8 months
Variety meats - Tongue, brain, kidneys liver, heart, chitterlings	1-2 days	3-4 months
Meat Leftovers		
Cooked meat and meat dishes	3-4 days	2-3 months
Gravy and meat broth	1-2 days	2-3 months
Fresh Poultry		
Chicken or turkey, whole	1-2 days	1 year
Chicken or turkey, pieces	1-2 days	9 months
Giblets	1-2 days	3-4 months
Cooked Poultry, Leftover		
Fried chicken	3-4 days	4 months
Cooked poultry dishes	3-4 days	4-6 months
Pieces, plain	3-4 days	4 months
Pieces covered with broth, gravy	1-2 days	6 months
Chicken nuggets, patties	1-2 days	1-3 months

*But not more than one week after the "sell by" date.

Figure 5.2b. Cold Storage Chart

95

Preparation

Keeping It Clean

- Be sure that the food preparation area and all surfaces and utensils that will touch food are clean.

- Always wash hands, with soap and warm water for at least 20 seconds, before beginning food preparation.

- Use rubber or plastic gloves to handle food if there is any kind of skin cut or infection on hands. Gloved hands should be washed just as often as bare hands when working with food.

- Do not sneeze or cough into food.

- Wash fresh fruits and vegetables with plain water to remove surface pesticide residues and other impurities, such as soil particles. Thick-skinned produce may be scrubbed with a brush if desired.

- Do not let juices from raw meat or poultry come in contact with other foods. Wash the cutting board, utensils, counter, sink and hands with hot soapy water immediately after preparing raw meat or poultry. Also use a fingernail brush to clean under nails and cuticles. Keep dish-washing sponges and cloths clean.

- Use cutting boards that are easy to clean—plastic or rubber composition are good choices. Wooden boards may look pretty, but they should only be used for cutting breads because they are porous and difficult to clean thoroughly.

- Don't taste any food of animal origin—meat, poultry, eggs, fish or shellfish—when it's raw or during cooking.

Thawing

- Do not thaw meat or poultry on the counter. Bacteria can multiply rapidly at room temperature.

- The safest way to thaw meat or poultry is to defrost it in the refrigerator. Place the package in the refrigerator immediately after removing it from the freezer.

- Foods that have been thawed in the refrigerator can be safely refrozen.

- For faster thawing, put the package in a water-tight plastic bag submerged in cold water. Change the water every 30 minutes. The cold water temperature slows bacterial growth that may occur on the outer thawed portions while the inner areas are still thawing.

- The microwave oven can be used for quick, safe defrosting. Follow the manufacturer's directions. Foods defrosted in the microwave oven should be cooked immediately after thawing.

Cooking—General Rules

- Cook meat and poultry to the "doneness" temperature given in the chart below.

- To make sure meat or poultry over 2 inches thick is cooked all the way through, use a meat thermometer. Insert the tip into the thickest part of the meat, avoiding fat, bone or gristle. For poultry, insert the tip into the thick part of the thigh next to the body.

- For meat and poultry less than 2 inches thick, look for clear juices and lack of pink in the center as signs of "doneness."

- Cooking temperatures in conventional ovens should be at least 325°F. Do not use recipes that call for cooking without a reliable and continuous heat source.

- Avoid interrupted cooking. Completely cook meat and poultry at one time. Partial or interrupted cooking often produces conditions that encourage bacterial growth.

- When cooking frozen meat or poultry that has not been defrosted, cook it about 1 1/2 times the length of time required for the same cut when thawed.

Cooking Temperature Chart

Cooking food to an internal temperature of 160°F usually protects against foodborne illness. However, some foods are considered more tasty when they are cooked to a higher internal temperature. The higher temperatures in this chart reflect a greater degree of "doneness."

	°Fahrenheit
Eggs & Egg Dishes	
Eggs	Cook until yolk & white are firm
Egg dishes	160
Ground Meat & Meat Mixtures	
Turkey, chicken	170
Veal, beef, lamb, pork	160
Fresh Beef	
Rare (some bacterial risk)	140
Medium	160
Well Done	170
Fresh Veal	
Medium	160
Well Done	170
Fresh Lamb	
Medium	160
Well Done	170
Fresh Pork	
Medium	160
Well Done	170
Poultry	
Chicken	180
Turkey	180
Turkey breasts, roasts	170
Thighs, wings	Cook until juices run clear
Stuffing (cooked alone or in bird)	165
Duck & Goose	180
Ham	
Fresh (raw)	160
Pre-cooked (to reheat)	140
Shoulder	160

Figure 5.3. *Cooking Temperature Chart*

Microwave Cooking

Microwave ovens heat food surfaces rapidly. However, time must be allowed for the heat to penetrate to the center of the food. It is important to be familiar with the information in the owner's manual and take the following steps to ensure that food cooks thoroughly and evenly in the microwave oven:

- Debone large pieces of meat. Bone can shield the area around it from thorough cooking.

- Cover the food to hold in moisture and facilitate even cooking.

- Use the middle-range temperature settings (or 50-percent power) for large cuts of meat or poultry. This allows heat to be conducted throughout the food without over-cooking.

- If the microwave oven doesn't have a turntable, turn the entire dish several times during cooking. Always stir soups, stews, stuffings and gravies several times during cooking.

- Use a temperature probe or meat thermometer to verify that food has reached a safe internal temperature. Check the temperature in several places, avoiding fat and bone.

- When following microwave oven cooking instructions on product labels, remember that ovens vary in power and operating efficiency. Check the cooked product with a meat thermometer to ensure that it has reached a safe internal temperature.

- Allow food cooked in the microwave oven to stand for the recommended time before serving. This is necessary to complete the cooking process.

- Glass cookware, glass ceramic cookware, and waxed paper are safe for microwave cooking. Plastic wrap may be used to cover containers but should not touch the food. Before using other types of containers, wraps or paper products, check to be sure that they are approved for use in the microwave oven. Unapproved materials may melt, burn or contain chemicals that can migrate into food during cooking.

- Do not use the microwave oven for home canning. As the liquid in a sealed glass jar heats and expands, pressure can build up, causing the jar to explode.

Slow Cookers

Slow cookers generally take over 2 hours to heat food to bacteria-killing temperatures. To ensure uniform and thorough cooking:

- Use small pieces of refrigerated (not frozen) meat or poultry.
- Use a recipe that includes a liquid.
- Do not fill the cooker more than 2/3 full.
- Always place the lid on the slow cooker.
- Check the internal temperature to be sure that the food is thoroughly cooked to at least 160°F.

Serving

General Rules

- Always wash hands, with soap and warm water for at least 20 seconds, before serving or eating food.

- Serve cooked products on clean plates, with clean utensils.

- Wash hands, utensils, and other food contact surfaces after contact with raw meat or poultry and before contact with the same food when cooked. For example, if a serving dish is used to hold raw chicken, wash the dish well before using it to serve the same chicken after it's cooked.

- Refrigerate leftovers within 2 hours when the temperature in the food serving area is below 90°F, within 1 hour when the temperature in the food serving area is 90°F or above.

Buffets

- Serve hot food from chafing dishes or warming trays that maintain the internal temperature of the food at 140°F or above.

- For cold foods, nestle the serving dish into a bed of crushed ice.

- Small platters for replenishing the serving table should be prepared ahead and stored in the refrigerator (at 40°F or below) or kept warm in the oven (at a setting of 200-225°F).

- Foods that have been held at room temperature for more than 2 hours during serving should be discarded. Fresh food should not be added to a serving dish or platter containing foods that have already been out for serving.

Traveling, Picnics and Lunches

- When going on a picnic or traveling with food, keep all perishables in a cooler with ice or freeze-pack inserts until serving time.

- Make sure that food is cold or frozen to the touch before placing it in the cooler or cold thermos.

- If soap and water will not be available, take along disposable, wet hand-wipes to clean hands before and after working with food.

- When packing a "bag lunch" that will be eaten within several hours, a small freeze pack insert in an insulated bag is probably all that is necessary to keep the food cold.

- Be sure to put the cooler or lunch bag in the coolest place possible, don't leave it in direct sun or in a warm car.

- A thermos designed for hot foods can be used to keep soup at a safe high temperature for several hours. Just before pouring the soup into the thermos, rinse the thermos with boiling water. Bring the soup to as high a temperature as possible before pouring it in. The soup should be hot to the touch at serving time.

Handling Leftovers

- Wash hands before handling leftovers and use clean utensils and surfaces.

- Refrigerate or freeze leftovers in covered shallow (less than 2 inches deep) containers within 2 hours after cooking. Debone large pieces of meat or poultry and divide them into smaller portions to refrigerate or freeze within 2 hours after cooking. Leave airspace around containers or packages to allow circulation of cold air and help ensure rapid, even cooling.

- When preparing food for later use, refrigerate or freeze it immediately after cooking, in covered shallow containers, so there's no chance of leaving it out for more than 2 hours. Refrigerators and freezers are designed to compensate for the addition of a few temporarily hot foods without allowing other foods to warm up.

- Date leftovers so they can be used within a safe time as shown in the cold storage chart. Avoid tasting old leftovers.

- Remove stuffing from meat or poultry before refrigerating or freezing.

- Before serving, cover and reheat leftovers to 165°F. Soups, sauces, gravies and other "wet" foods should be reheated to a rolling boil.

- When reheating leftovers in the microwave oven, follow the guidelines for microwave cooking.

- If in doubt, throw it out. Discard outdated, obviously spoiled, or possibly unsafe leftovers in garbage disposal or in tightly wrapped packages that cannot be consumed by people or animals.

Special Care for Special Foods:

Some foods require special care either because they are more vulnerable to bacteria that can cause foodborne illness or they have unusual characteristics. This section provides additional information on handling some "special care" foods.

Ground Meat and Ground Poultry

Ground meat (hamburger, pork patties, ground lamb) and ground poultry (chicken patties, ground turkey) receive more handling than roasts, chops, and other cuts or parts. More handling, especially grinding and mixing, increases the likelihood of contamination by bacteria such as *Salmonella, Campylobacter jejuni, Listeria monocytogenes,* and *Escherichia coli 0157:H7.*

To destroy any bacteria that might be present it is important to cook ground meat or poultry thoroughly. Patties should be cooked until they are hot, steaming, and juices run clear, with no evidence of pink color in the center. When preparing a meatloaf or casserole, use a meat thermometer to make sure it cooks to at least 160°F.

If you are using a precooked product it is important to heat it thoroughly before serving, according to the instructions on the container, or as described above.

Ham

Ham is the meat from the leg or shoulder of the pig. It may be "fresh" (uncured), cured, or smoked. Hams are sold plastic-wrapped, vacuum-packaged in plastic, in a can, or country style. When purchasing a ham, read the label carefully. The label will tell you if the ham is cured or smoked, if it is "fully cooked," and if it must be refrigerated.

Hams labeled "fully cooked" can be served cold or reheated to an internal temperature of 140°F. All other hams must be cooked to an internal temperature of at least 160°F before serving.

Both plastic-wrapped and vacuum-packaged plastic-wrapped hams must be refrigerated. A plastic-wrapped ham will keep about 1 week. A vacuum-packaged ham should be consumed by the "use by" date or within 1 week after the "sell by" date.

Both plastic-wrapped and vacuum-packaged plastic-wrapped hams can be frozen. To preserve texture and flavor in the freezer, wrap the ham tightly in an extra layer of freezer paper or plastic and use within 2 months.

Canned hams labeled "keep refrigerated" require refrigeration and, unopened, will keep 6 to 9 months in the refrigerator. Make sure the can isn't showing any bulges, cracks, dents or rust, or leaking any liquid. A canned ham should not be frozen. Shelf-stable canned hams do not require refrigeration and may be stored in a cool, dry place for 2 to 5 years. Country style hams are dry-cured with salt and aged for a distinctive flavor; some are also smoked. Unopened country style hams can be kept up to 1 year without refrigeration. Once the ham is cut, exposing the moist interior, it must be stored in the refrigerator and should be used within 2 to 3 months. After the ham has been soaked, or soaked and cooked, it should be used within 5 days.

Turkey, Chicken and Duck with Stuffing

Bacteria can readily multiply in stuffing. Therefore, it is important to prevent introducing bacteria into stuffing and allowing the bacteria to grow. To safely prepare and serve poultry with stuffing, follow these tips:

- To save time preparing the stuffing, chop and refrigerate perishable ingredients 1 day ahead. Dry ingredients can be premixed the day before and stored separately.

- Combine dry and liquid stuffing ingredients and stuff the bird just before putting the bird into the oven. Stuff the bird loosely, because stuffing expands as it cooks. Extra stuffing may be baked separately.

- *Never stuff a bird that will be cooked in a microwave oven. It may not cook thoroughly.*

- An unstuffed bird takes less time to cook than one that is stuffed. Consider cooking the bird and the stuffing separately. It is usually quicker and the cooking can be more easily controlled.

- To ensure that the bird is fully cooked, insert a meat thermometer into the thickest part of the thigh muscle, without touching the bone, and cook until the thermometer registers at least 180°F.

- After the bird is removed from the oven, check the stuffing for doneness with a meat thermometer. Leave the thermometer in place for about 5 minutes for an accurate reading. To be fully cooked, the stuffing should reach 165°F.

- Remove all the stuffing immediately after cooking and place it in a separate bowl for serving.

- Large amounts of leftover stuffing should be divided into smaller portions for rapid, even cooling.

- Within 2 hours after cooking, debone the bird and divide the meat into smaller portions for storage.

- *Do not thaw commercially frozen prestuffed poultry before cooking.* Carefully follow package directions on the storage and cooking of these products.

Hotdogs and Lunch Meats

Hotdogs and lunch meats are processed to last longer than many other meat and poultry products. However, some bacteria, such as *Listeria monocytogenes*, can grow slowly under refrigeration. Therefore, it is important to use, freeze, or discard these products within the recommended length of time.

Hotdogs and lunch meats will keep in the original vacuum-sealed pouch for 2 weeks. They should never be kept longer than 1 week after the sell-by date, unless frozen. When freezing these products, do so as soon as possible after purchase. Freezing may lead to loss of flavor and texture after 1 to 2 months.

Watch the liquid that often forms around hotdogs. If it's cloudy, it can be a sign that spoilage bacteria have started growing. Discard hotdogs with cloudy liquid.

Once a package of hotdogs or lunch meat is opened, rewrap it well and plan to use hot dogs in 1 week, lunch meats in 3 to 5 days.

It is advisable to thoroughly reheat hotdogs and lunch meats that will be consumed by pregnant women, the very young, the elderly, and others with incomplete or impaired immune systems.

Prepared, Refrigerated Foods

New food packaging techniques are making it possible for processors to offer prepared foods that can be refrigerated for longer periods than consumers are used to. Increased refrigerated storage times are facilitated by vacuum packaging or modified atmosphere packaging where oxygen in the package is replaced with gases such as carbon dioxide or nitrogen. These techniques slow spoilage, discoloration, and the growth of harmful bacteria.

This new packaging is being used for products as diverse as fully cooked roast chicken, tuna spread, and ravioli. It offers many advantages to consumers but emphasis must be placed on proper handling to avoid potential food safety problems:

- Foods may be processed 4 to 6 weeks before the "sell by" or "use by" date. However, these dates assume that the product is refrigerated properly throughout its shelf life.

- Bacteria such as *Listeria* and *Yersinia* can grow slowly under refrigeration.

- Many of these foods do not require additional cooking or thorough heating before consumption. Therefore, if the product was mishandled, any bacteria that could have multiplied would not be destroyed.

To use refrigerated, prepared foods safely:

- When purchasing, make sure that the food is cold.
- Also check the "sell by," or "use by" date on the package.
- Read the label and follow storage and cooking or heating instructions carefully.
- Use these foods within the recommended length of time.
- When freezing these products, do so as soon as possible after purchase.

Eggs and Egg-Rich Foods

Due to the possibility of contamination with *Salmonella enteritidis* or other bacteria, it is important to handle all eggs and egg-rich foods properly.

- Buy grade AA or A eggs with clean, uncracked shells.

- Do not buy unrefrigerated eggs.

- Refrigerate eggs in the original carton.

- Cook eggs thoroughly—until the yolk is not runny and the white is firm. Cook scrambled eggs until firm.

- Avoid foods that contain raw eggs, such as Caesar salad or homemade mayonnaise, ice cream or eggnog. Commercial mayonnaise, ice cream and eggnog are safe, since they use pasteurized eggs and the pasteurization kills bacteria.

- Avoid foods that contain lightly cooked eggs such as chilled chocolate mousse or soft meringues that are only slightly cooked.

- Eggs and egg-rich foods should never be kept out of the refrigerator for more than 2 hours, including serving time.

- To ensure safe Easter eggs, do not leave hard-cooked dyed eggs at room temperature for more than 2 hours. Hard-cooking an egg destroys much of its natural protection and makes it more susceptible to bacterial growth.

Marinades

When using marinades to flavor and tenderize meat, poultry, or fish, follow these guidelines:

- If the recipe calls for basting cooked food with marinade, reserve a portion of marinade for this purpose before combining the marinade with raw meat, poultry, or fish.

- Marinate in a glass or plastic container. Marinades often contain acidic liquids such as wine, lemon juice, or vinegar which react with metal.

- Marinate in the refrigerator.

- Avoid cross-contaminating other foods by thoroughly cleaning any utensils, bowls, or surfaces that the marinade comes in contact with after it is combined with raw food.

- Do not save marinades that have been combined with raw food, unless they will be immediately cooked in a sauce. Bring the marinade to a rolling boil before adding any other ingredients. Then cook the sauce to at least 160°F.

Mayonnaise

A couple of important facts about mayonnaise:

Adding commercial mayonnaise to food does not increase the chances that it will cause foodborne illness. Commercial mayonnaise is made with pasteurized eggs. Most commercially prepared mayonnaisses contain ingredients, such as vinegar, lemon juice and salt, that slow bacterial growth.

Mayonnaise separates when frozen and becomes an oily mess upon defrosting, so don't try to freeze mayonnaise or any salad made with it.

Shelf-Stable Products

Shelf-stable products packaged in plastic containers, foil packages, waxed paper cartons, metal cans, and glass jars have extended, but not infinite, shelf lives. Commercial packaging is done under carefully controlled conditions, but there are still limits to how long it will preserve food. Here are some tips on using these products wisely:

- Check the labels on unfamiliar products that look shelf stable to be sure that they do not require refrigeration. Also check the package for a "sell by" or "use by" date.

- Store shelf-stable products in a cool (below 85°F), clean, dry place.

- When storing products in the pantry, place newly purchased packages behind older ones, so each package can be used within its recommended shelf life.

- Carefully check package condition before use. Most foods in plastic, foil or paper that has been punctured or torn should be discarded. An exception would be rice or noodles with no visible contaminants, such as pests or mold.

- In general, high-acid canned foods (e.g. tomatoes, grapefruit, pineapple) can be stored in the cabinet for 12-18 months; low-acid canned foods (e.g. stew, carrots, spinach) will keep 2 to 5 years, without losing quality.

- As a safety precaution, boil all low-acid home-canned foods for at least 10 minutes before serving. Add 1 minute of boiling time for every 1,000 feet above sea level.

- Leaking, bulging, badly dented, or rusted cans; cracked jars or jars with loose or bulging lids; food with a foul odor, or any container that spurts liquid when you open it may indicate the presence of *Clostridium botulinum*. If possible, avoid opening such foods. NEVER TASTE THEM.

- Report any suspect commercially canned foods according to the instructions [at the end of this chapter].

- To dispose of suspect home-canned products, it is best to enclose the food, in its original container, in a heavy garbage bag marked "POISON" and place the bag in a trash container that is not accessible to homeless people, children or animals.

- If a suspect canned food is opened in your kitchen, thoroughly scrub the can opener or other utensils, containers, counters, etc., that might have contacted the food or its container. Discard any sponges or cloths used in the cleanup. Wash your hands thoroughly. Promptly launder any clothing that might have been splattered upon.

Power Outages/Appliance Failure

Following these steps will help keep food safe during power outages or when the freezer or refrigerator is not working:

- If the appliance will be working again within a couple of hours, just minimize opening of the freezer and refrigerator doors.

- A fully stocked freezer will usually keep food frozen for 2 days after losing power. A half-full freezer will usually keep food frozen for about 1 day. If the freezer is not full, quickly group packages together so they will retain the cold more effectively.

- Separate raw meat and poultry items from other foods. If the raw meat and poultry begin to thaw, this will prevent their juices from getting onto other foods.

- If the power will be out for a longer period than the freezer will maintain the cold, dry ice may be placed in the freezer.

  CAUTION: Never touch dry ice with bare hands or breathe its vapors in an enclosed area. Dry ice is frozen carbon dioxide, a gas that settles in low areas and is lethal to breathe in high concentration.

- In the refrigerator, food will usually keep 4 to 6 hours, depending upon the temperature of the room. If the power will be out for a longer time, block ice may be placed in the refrigerator.

When the freezer is operating again, use the following guidelines to decide what to do with foods that were stored in the freezer:

- If ice crystals are still visible and/or the food feels as cold as if refrigerated, it is safe to refreeze. Raw meats and poultry, cheese, juices, breads and pastries can be refrozen without substantially compromising quality. Prepared foods, fish, vegetables and fruits can be refrozen safely, but quality may suffer.

- If the food thawed or was held above 40°F for more than 2 hours it should generally be discarded because bacteria may multiply to unsafe levels under these conditions. The only foods that should be refrozen are well-wrapped hard cheeses, butter and margarine, breads and pastries without custard fillings, fruits and fruit juices that look and smell acceptable, and vegetables held above 40°F for less than 6 hours.

When the refrigerator is operating again, use the following guidelines to decide what to do with foods that were stored in the refrigerator:

- Fresh meats, poultry, lunch meats, hotdogs, eggs, milk, soft cheeses, and prepared or cooked foods should be discarded if they have been held above 40°F for more than 2 hours because bacteria can multiply to unsafe levels under these conditions.

- Fresh fruits and vegetables are safe as long as they are still firm and there is no evidence of mold, a yeasty smell or sliminess. Juices, opened containers of vinegar and oil salad dressings, ketchup, pickles, jams and jellies, and well-wrapped hard cheeses are safe as long as there is no evidence of mold growth, and they look and smell acceptable. Well-wrapped butter and margarine can usually be kept as long as they do not melt, but should be discarded if rancid odors develop.

To remove spills and freshen the freezer and refrigerator, wash them with a solution of 2 tablespoons of baking soda dissolved in 1 quart of warm water. To absorb any lingering odors, place an open box or dish of baking soda in the appliance.

Spoilage and Mold

Spoilage

When foods have not been stored properly, or have simply been kept too long, signs of deterioration by microorganisms that cause food spoilage become evident. In general, it is best to discard any food that exhibits an uncharacteristic color, odor, texture or flavor.

Mold

If there is only a small area of mold on a piece of hard block cheese, hard salami, or a dry cured country ham, the food can be salvaged by cutting out an inch of the product surrounding and below the moldy area. Keep the knife out of the mold itself and re-cover the food in fresh wrap.

Any other visibly moldy foods—soft cheeses, sour cream, hotdogs, lunch meats, baked chicken, soft fruits and vegetables, bread, cake, flour, rice, peanut butter, etc.—should be discarded. To avoid spreading mold spores, gently wrap the food or place it in a bag before discarding. Be sure to examine other items that the moldy one may have contacted. Clean the refrigerator or container that held the item as necessary.

Parasites

Parasites are organisms that depend on nutrients from a living host to complete their life cycle. There are several parasites that can infect humans through the food chain.

Trichinosis

Humans may contract trichinosis, caused by *Trichinella spiralis*, by eating undercooked pork or game that is infested with trichina larvae. Much progress has been made in reducing trichinosis in grain-fed hogs, and human cases are on the decline.

Thorough home cooking will destroy any live trichina larvae that may be present in pork or other meat. Other proven trichina destruction methods—used by industry under carefully controlled conditions—include curing, pickling, freezing, and, of course, cooking and canning.

Toxoplasmosis

Toxoplasmosis, caused by *Toxoplasmosa gondii*, is a common parasitic infection in cats that can be transferred directly to humans through cat feces, or indirectly through improperly cooked meat or poultry. It is a particular risk for the pregnant woman. The consequences of infection are most severe for the infant who acquires the parasite from an infected mother before birth.

To prevent infection, cook meat, particularly lamb and pork, thoroughly. Pregnant women should limit their exposure to cats that may be infected, wash hands after handling cats, and have someone else change the cat litter box.

Bacteria That Can Cause Foodborne Illness

A few types of bacteria are responsible for most cases of foodborne illness. Unlike microorganisms that cause food to spoil, they do not usually advertise their presence—they cannot be seen, smelled, or tasted.

Some people are more vulnerable to foodborne bacterial illness than others. The very young and very old are generally most at risk. Others at risk include those with underlying health problems and the malnourished. Genetic differences may make some persons more susceptible than others. For certain types of infections, pregnancy or antibiotic use may be a factor.

Salmonella

Sources: *Salmonella* bacteria continually cycle through the environment in the intestinal tracts of humans and animals. Salmonellae are often found in raw or undercooked foods, such as poultry, eggs and meat. They may spread to other foods through cross contamination. *Salmonella enteritidis* has been linked to Grade A shell eggs. Unpasteurized milk can also contain *Salmonella* bacteria.

Disease: About 40,000 cases of salmonellosis are reported each year. Symptoms include stomach pain, diarrhea, nausea, chills, fever, and headache that normally appear 6 to 48 hours after eating and may last 3 to 5 days. Infants and young children, the ill, and the elderly may be seriously affected.

Prevention: Thoroughly cook all meat, poultry, fish, and eggs. Avoid contaminating cooked foods with juices from raw foods. Don't drink unpasteurized milk.

Staphylococcus aureus (Staph)

Sources: Staph bacteria are found on our skin, in infected cuts and pimples, and in our noses and throats. They are spread by improper food handling. Staph can multiply rapidly at warm temperatures to produce a toxin that causes illness. Staph bacteria prefer cooked food high in protein. They also grow well in foods high in sugar or salt, which inhibit the growth of more sensitive microorganisms.

Disease: Symptoms of staph intoxication include nausea, vomiting, and diarrhea that usually appear 30 minutes to 8 hours after eating and may last a day or two. The illness is usually not serious in healthy people.

Prevention: Wash hands and utensils before preparing and serving food. Refrigerate, in shallow, covered containers, cooked foods that will not be served immediately. Don't let prepared foods—particularly cooked and cured meats and cheese and meat salads—sit at room temperature more than 2 hours. Thorough cooking destroys staph bacteria, but staph toxin is resistant to heat, refrigeration, and freezing.

Clostridium perfringens

Sources: *Clostridium perfringens* bacteria are present throughout the environment—in the soil, the intestines of humans and animals, and sewage. *Clostridium perfringens* is anaerobic (grows only where there is little or no oxygen) and may be present as either a vegetative cell or a spore. The vegetative cells produce the toxin that causes illness. While thorough cooking will kill the vegetative cells, some of the spores may survive. At temperatures between 70°F and 120°F the spores can become vegetative and produce toxin. *Clostridium perfringens* is called the "cafeteria germ" because it often strikes food served in quantity and left for long periods on a steam table or at room temperature.

Disease: Symptoms of *Clostridium perfringens* enteritis include diarrhea and gas pains that appear within 9 to 15 hours and usually last about 1 day. Elderly people and ulcer patients can be affected more seriously.

Prevention: Divide large portions of cooked foods such as beef, turkey, gravy, dressing, stews, and casseroles into smaller portions for serving and cooling. Keep cooked foods hot (at an internal temperature of 140°F or above) or cold (at 40°F or below). Reheat leftovers thoroughly (to an internal temperature of at least 165°F) before serving.

Campylobacter jejuni

Sources: *Campylobacter jejuni* may be present in raw or undercooked meat, poultry, or shellfish. Other sources include unpasteurized milk, untreated drinking water and infected pets.

Disease: Symptoms of campylobacteriosis include fever, headache and muscle pain followed by diarrhea (sometimes bloody), abdominal pain and nausea that appear 2 to 10 days after eating and may last 1 to 10 days.

Prevention: Thoroughly cook all meat, poultry and fish. Thoroughly clean hands, utensils and surfaces that touch raw meats. Don't drink unpasteurized milk or untreated water.

Clostridium botulinum

Sources: *Clostridium botulinum* bacteria are present throughout the environment—in soil and water. Like *Clostridium perfringens*, *Clostridium botulinum* is anaerobic (grows only where there is little or no oxygen) and may be present as either a vegetative cell or a spore. The vegetative cells produce the toxin that causes illness. While thorough cooking will kill the vegetative cells, some of the spores may survive. At temperatures above 38°F the spores can become vegetative and produce toxin. The risk of botulism has long been associated with canned foods that are not processed to a high enough temperature to kill all the spores. More recently, it has been associated with cooked foods held at room or warm temperatures for an extended time under conditions where oxygen is limited—mounded cooked onions in butter, potatoes wrapped tightly in foil, meat pies and vacuum packaged foods.

Disease: Botulism toxin affects the nervous system and can be fatal if not treated. Symptoms appear 12 to 48 hours after eating and include double vision, droopy eyelids, trouble speaking and swallowing, and difficult breathing. Without treatment, a patient can die of suffocation because the nerves no longer stimulate breathing. There are antitoxins, which have reduced the number of deaths from botulism, but patients may suffer nerve damage, and recovery is often slow.

Prevention: Divide large portions of cooked foods into smaller portions for serving and cooling. Keep cooked foods hot (at an internal temperature of 140°F or above) or cold (at 40°F or below). Reheat leftovers thoroughly (to an internal temperature of at least 165°F) before serving. Outbreaks of botulism are rarely associated with commercially canned products. Home canners should follow established guides for canning.

Do not taste food from leaking, bulging, or damaged cans; from cracked jars or jars with loose or bulging lids; from containers that spurt liquid when opened; or any canned food that has an abnormal odor or appearance. Discard suspect home-canned foods according to the instructions [previously given]. Report any suspect commercially canned foods according to the instructions [at the end of this chapter].

Listeria monocytogenes

Sources: *Listeria monocytogenes* bacteria are found frequently in the environment. They are common in the intestines of humans and animals, and in milk, soil, leafy vegetables, and food processing environments. Listeria bacteria can grow slowly at refrigeration temperatures.

Disease: Listeriosis is a rare but potentially fatal disease. Symptoms in adults include the sudden onset of flulike symptoms such as fever, chills, headache, backache, and sometimes abdominal pain and diarrhea. Symptoms in newborns include respiratory distress, refusal to drink, and vomiting. Possible complications of listeriosis include meningitis or meningo-encephalitis, which affects tissues around the brain or spine, and septicemia, which is blood poisoning. Listeriosis can cause spontaneous abortions and stillbirths.

Prevention: Avoid raw milk and cheese made from unpasteurized milk. Pregnant women and other high-risk groups are advised to follow "keep refrigerated" labels and carefully observe "sell by" and "use by" dates on processed products, and to thoroughly reheat frozen or refrigerated processed meat and poultry products before consumption.

Escherichia coli 0157:H7

Sources: Several strains of *Escherichia coli* bacteria, frequently associated with fecally contaminated water, have long been known to cause diarrhea in infants and travelers. The specific serotype 0157:H7 produces a toxin that can cause hemorrhagic colitis. Raw or rare ground beef and unpasteurized milk have been involved in some illnesses.

Disease: Symptoms of hemorrhagic colitis include severe abdominal cramps, followed by diarrhea (often bloody), nausea, vomiting, and occasionally a low-grade fever. A possible complication is hemolytic uremic syndrome (HUS), a urinary tract infection that is a leading cause of acute kidney failure in children. Symptoms generally begin 3 to 4 days after the food is eaten, last up to 10 days, and often require hospitalization.

Prevention: Thorough cooking and reheating, good sanitation, and refrigeration at 40°F or below are all important.

Yersinia enterocolitica

Sources: *Yersinia enterocolitica* bacteria are common in swine and swine waste. They have been isolated from many wild and domesticated animals, seafood, milk, fruit, and vegetables. *Yersinia* bacteria can grow slowly at refrigeration temperatures.

Disease: Symptoms of yersiniosis include abdominal pain that mimics appendicitis, fever, diarrhea (often bloody), and sometimes vomiting. Symptoms occur within 1 to 7 days after ingestion and last 1 to 2 days. Children are most at risk for contracting the disease. The aged and those with weakened immune systems are most at risk for complications such as arthritic or anemic conditions, heart problems, and occasionally meningitis.

Prevention: Thorough cooking and reheating are essential control measures, along with sanitation and personal hygiene.

In Case of Foodborne Illness

The following are general guidelines to follow if foodborne illness is suspected:

Preserve the Evidence

- If a portion of the suspect food is available, wrap it securely in a heavy plastic bag and place it on ice in a secure container marked "DANGER". Write down the name of the food, when it was consumed, and the date of the illness. Store the container away from children, pets, and other foods, in a location where it will not be mistaken for edible food.

- The sample may be useful to medical personnel treating the illness and/or health authorities tracking the problem.

- If available, also save the container, wrapping and any metal clips used on the original package. This is where the Establishment number, which indicates the plant that a meat or poultry product is from, is shown.

Seek Treatment

- As with any illness, judgement should be used to determine if and when to seek professional medical advice or care.

- Keep in mind that it is important to drink liquids such as water, tea, apple juice, bouillon, or ginger ale to replace fluids lost through any episodes of diarrhea or vomiting.

- *If symptoms are severe, or the victim is quite young, pregnant, elderly, or has a chronic illness, professional medical advice or care should be sought immediately.*

Call the Local Health Department If:

- The suspect food was served at a large gathering.

- The suspect food is from a restaurant, delicatessen, sidewalk vendor, or other commercial or institutional kitchen.

- The suspect food is prepared and packaged in a retail grocery store.

- The suspect food is a commercial product.

Try to Have the Following Information Available When Calling:

- Your name, address, and daytime phone number.

- The name and address of the event, party, or establishment where the suspect food was consumed or purchased.

- The date that the food was consumed and/or the date of purchase.

- If the suspect food is a commercial product, have the container or wrapping in hand for reference while on the phone. Most meat and poultry products have a USDA or State inspection stamp and a number that identifies the plant where the product was manufactured. Many products also have a code indicating when the item was produced. This information can be vital in tracing a problem to its source.

Other Authorities to Call

- Foodborne illness involving a USDA-inspected meat or poultry product may also be reported to the toll-free Meat and Poultry Hotline at 1-800-535-4555. (See below for more information.)

- Foodborne illness involving other products that cross State lines may be reported to the nearest Food and Drug Administration office, listed in the local phone book.

- Foodborne illness involving products that are sold only within the State may be reported to the State health department or the State department of agriculture.

USDA's Meat and Poultry Hotline 1-800-535-4555

The U.S. Department of Agriculture operates a toll-free Meat and Poultry Hotline to address specific consumer food safety concerns on an individual basis. The Hotline is staffed by home economists who can answer questions on topics such as proper food handling, how to tell if a particular food is safe to eat, and how to better understand labels.

The nationwide toll-free number is 1-800-535-4555. The Hotline can be reached from 10 a.m. to 4 p.m. Eastern time, Monday through Friday. Callers in the Washington, DC, metropolitan area should call (202) 447-3333. Both phone numbers provide access to a telecommunications device for the deaf.

When calling to report a faulty product or foodborne illness, please refer to [the instructions above]. Be sure to preserve the product, if possible, and notify the local health department *before* contacting the Hotline.

The local Extension Service office, listed in the phone book under county government, is also an excellent source of food safety information.

—by Susan Rehe

Chapter 6

Food Handling Information

Chapter Contents

Section 6.1

Answers to Your Food Handling Questions

(Source: *Food News for Consumers*, Summer 1991.)

What Consumers Want to Know About Chicken & Turkey

Do bacteria from poultry contaminate the counter and every-thing they contact? Can bacteria pass from object to object or into cuts on my hands?

Poultry, like all raw foods of animal origin, carries salmonella and other bacteria. It should be handled carefully to prevent cross con-tamination. Never let raw poultry or its juices contact cooked foods or foods that will be eaten raw like salad ingredients.

Salmonella bacteria must be *eaten* to cause illness. They cannot enter the body through a cut on your hand. Refrigeration slows the growth of salmonella and thorough cooking destroys it.

After I left the grocery, I did more shopping. The turkey roast was in my van for 3 hours on a 90-degree day. Is it safe?

Absolutely not. Don't leave poultry in a hot car for more than 30 minutes. The supermarket should be your last stop before heading home, and perishable foods, like turkey, should be the last you choose before checkout. Unload perishables from your car first and refriger-ate them immediately.

Sometimes when I buy chicken, it looks frozen. But by the time I get it home, it is defrosted. Is it safe to freeze?

Yes. What you have observed is only frozen surface tissues. The entire chicken is not frozen. Processors quickly chill and store fresh chicken at 28 to 32°F to prevent the rapid growth of bacteria and in-crease its shelf-life.

122

I've had a thawed turkey breast in the refrigerator 8 days. Is it safe to cook? I'm 90 and I don't want to get sick.

Senior citizens, pregnant women, very young children and people who suffer from chronic illnesses are especially vulnerable to foodborne bacteria.

But for persons of any age, 8 days is too long to refrigerate raw or cooked poultry. The safe time limit for refrigerating raw poultry is 1-2 days; 3-4 days if it's cooked.

Your turkey may have begun to spoil. Even without spoilage indicators like an off-odor or sticky surface, harmful bacteria may be present. Discard it.

I'm concerned about the dark color of meat around the bones of chicken. How do you prevent it?

First, it's perfectly safe to eat chicken meat that turns dark during cooking. The darkening around bones occurs primarily in young broiler-fryers 7 to 9 weeks old. Since their bones have not calcified completely, pigment from the bone marrow can seep through the porous bones. When the chicken is cooked, the pigment turns dark.

Try buying a more mature 5 to 7 pound baking hen or debone chicken before cooking.

Handling and Storing Poultry Safely

- Store raw poultry in the refrigerator (40°F) 1 or 2 days only before cooking or freezing. Store whole birds in the freezer (0°F) up to 1 year; parts up to 9 months; giblets 3 to 4 months.

- Before cooking poultry, throw away packaging and rinse product under cool running water. Cut on a nonporous cutting board.

- Wash board, utensils and counter with detergent and hot water immediately.

- Set oven temperature no lower than 325°F. For doneness, cook breasts to an internal temperature of 170°F and dark meat or whole birds to 180°F, or until juices run clear and flesh is tender.

123

• Refrigerate leftovers within 2 hours after cooking.

—*by CiCi Williamson,* Certified Home Economist

What Consumers Want to Know About Red Meat

Why is prepackaged ground beef often red on the outside, but a greyish brown on the inside?

This color difference is a natural phenomenon. Red meat contains a pigment called oxymyoglobin. When meat is exposed to air this natural pigment combines with oxygen to produce the red color referred to as "bloom." The inside portion of the meat, while perfectly safe, may be darker due to lack of oxygen.

I always thought that pork should be cooked to a final internal temperature of 170°F. A friend told me that USDA changed its recommendation to 160°F several years ago. Is this true?

Yes. To prevent confusion, USDA now recommends that fresh pork (as well as other meats, poultry, fish and egg products) be cooked to a minimum internal temperature of 160°F.

While cooking meat to a temperature of 160°F normally assures safety, many people prefer the taste of pork cooked to 170°F. That was the reason for the earlier recommendation—taste not safety.

How long is it safe to keep a smoked ham in the refrigerator? Will a vacuum-packaged ham keep longer?

Both plastic-wrapped and vacuum-packaged hams must be refrigerated. A plastic-wrapped ham will keep about 1 week. The smoking process adds flavor but does not preserve the ham. A vacuum-packaged ham should be consumed by the "Use-by" date or within 1 week after the "Sell by" date listed on the package.

How long is it safe to keep fresh meat in the refrigerator? I was always told to use it within several days, yet supermarkets seem to keep meat for a week or so. Why the difference?

Ground beef and poultry should be used within 1-2 days. Red meats can be stored in the home refrigerator for 3-5 days. Commercial refrigerators can safely store meat for longer periods because they are significantly colder than home refrigerators. Meats are held in commercial refrigerators/lockers in the back of the store until rotated out to display cases for consumer purchase.

What is sodium erythorbate? I've seen this word listed on packages of many luncheon meats.

Sodium erythorbate is an accepted curing agent. It is also used to prevent undesirable color changes from occurring in processed meats. The additive is required in some meat products to prevent the formation of nitrosamines linked to cancer development. Sodium erythorbate is made from sugar and is chemically related to Vitamin C.

Handling and Storing Red Meats

- Keep raw meat under constant refrigeration. Wrap it securely so that packages do not leak and contaminate other foods or surfaces.

- Don't thaw food on the kitchen counter. Bacteria multiply rapidly at room temperature.

- Wash hands and utensils after contact with raw meat. Wash cutting boards or other work surfaces. Bacteria, often present on raw foods, can spread to other foods if you aren't careful.

- Cook red meat to 160°F. Use a meat thermometer to check that it's cooked all the way through. Red meat is done when it's brown or grey inside.

- Freeze or refrigerate leftovers promptly. Divide leftovers into shallow containers for rapid, even cooling.

—by Pat Moriarty, Registered Dietitian

What Consumers Want to Know about Deli Foods

I don't know how long I've had some deli cold cuts in my refrigerator. If they smell good, are they safe to eat?

You can't see, smell or taste the bacteria that cause foodborne illness. If the cold cuts have been opened and refrigerated more than a week, discard them.

CAUTION: If meat is slimy or sticky, has an off-odor or is discolored, food spoilage and, possibly, foodborne bacteria could be present. Do not use it.

Generally you can freeze cold cuts that won't be used soon after purchase.

The store clerk was handling some raw meat and didn't wash his hands before picking up my deli meat to slice it. Is it safe?

Whether you're a clerk or a home cook, you should always wash your hands before and after touching raw meat. Bacteria from raw juices can cross-contaminate cooked foods.

Since cold cuts are usually eaten without further cooking, any bacteria would not be destroyed. Eating a sandwich made at this deli could be risky.

The potato salad I just purchased at the deli tastes spoiled. Where should I complain?

Potato salad is not a product under USDA jurisdiction. Foods purchased at food service establishments and supermarkets are regulated by your state and local health departments.

Contact these officials listed in your phone book.

Processed deli meats like cold cuts or a sealed carton of chicken salad are inspected by the USDA. If you have a concern about this type of product, call the Hotline at 1-800-535-4555.

The sliced ham and roast beef I bought from the deli shimmers with green iridescent colors. Does this mean it is spoiled?

Not necessarily. Meat contains fat, iron and many other compounds. When light hits a slice of meat, it splits into colors like a rainbow. There are also various pigments in meat compounds which can give it an iridescent or greenish cast when exposed to heat and processing.

Spoiled meat would probably also be slimy or sticky and have an off-odor.

Is it safe to buy uncooked pre-stuffed meats from the deli?

The USDA recommends against purchasing previously stuffed whole poultry products because these items are highly dense and perishable. Cold storage may not stop bacteria from growing in the stuffing inside the bird's cavity. But smaller products like stuffed pork chops or chicken breasts are safe to buy.

Handling and Storing Deli Foods Safely

- Buy only deli foods that are stored at safe temperatures and handled in a sanitary manner. Don't buy deli foods displayed at room temperature.

- Deli-sliced bologna and salami remain safe 3 to 5 days in your refrigerator; sliced turkey, chicken and roast beef, 2 to 4 days. Freeze if not used by then.

- Store vacuum-packaged cold cuts and hotdogs 2 weeks unopened, 1 week opened. For foods with a "Sell-by" date, simply use them within five days of purchase. If the product has a "Use-by" date, observe that.

- Salads and cooked fresh deli foods are more perishable. Use them within 1 or 2 days. Any foods with stuffing should be used on the day of purchase!

—*by CiCi Williamson,* Certified Home Economist

What Consumers Want to Know about Shelf-Stable, Canned and Packaged Foods

How long is it safe to keep canned goods?

Low-acid canned goods such as canned meat and poultry, stews, corn, carrots and peas can be stored in the cabinet 2-5 years. High-acid foods like tomato-based products, fruits, juices, vinegar-based salad dressings and sauerkraut should be used within 9-18 months. Store canned goods in a cool (below 85° F), clean, dry place.

I have several cans of food that accidentally froze. Are they still safe to use?

Frozen canned goods, whether left in a car, basement or cabin, can present health problems. Seams on cans may be compromised when cans freeze and the contents swell. The cans should be moved immediately to a refrigerator and allowed to thaw. After thawing, cook and use the food or cook and refreeze. If the cans were not thawed in the refrigerator, or if you suspect that the foods may have frozen and thawed more than once, discard them.

My neighbor stores leftover food right in the can. I thought this was dangerous because lead can leach into food.

It is always best to transfer leftover food to a storage container intended for refrigerator use. Food left in the can may develop an off-taste as the food reacts with metals used in the can. However, this is a quality issue, not a safety issue. Fortunately, lead has nearly been eliminated as a metal used in the U.S. canning industry. According to the National Food Processors Association, the percentage of food packed in lead-soldered containers dropped from 90.3% in 1979 to 3.07% in the first quarter of 1990.

I've started buying the new shelf-stable entrees to take to work and heat in the microwave. How long can I expect to safely keep these products on my kitchen shelf?

Many new types of packaging use plastic or paper containers instead of metal cans or glass jars. Think of these new plastic and paper type containers as "flexible cans." Like cans, the contents have been heat treated (sterilized) to make them shelf-stable. Assuming there are no breaks or tears in the package, these products should maintain top quality for over a year if stored in a cool, dry place.

Meat and poultry products come in so many different kinds of packages these days. How can I tell if a package requires refrigeration?

Read the label carefully. If refrigeration is necessary for safety, the label must say "KEEP REFRIGERATED." If the package was purchased off the shelf, chances are the product will not require refrigeration until opened.

Shelf-stable Handling Tips

- Store shelf-stable products in a cool, dry place.

- Do not store canned goods in any location such as a garage or cabin where; the temperature may drop below 32°F or go above 85°F.

- Place newly purchased packages behind older ones, so each package can be used within its recommended shelf-life.

- Check labels carefully to make sure that the product does not require refrigeration. Check to see if a "Sell-by" or "Use-by" date is on the container.

- Use high-acid canned goods within 18 months. Use low-acid canned goods within 2-5 years. Home canned goods should be used within 1 year.

- Do not use cans or glass jars with dents, cracks, or bulging lids.

—*by Pat Moriarty,* Registered Dietitian

USDA's Meat and Poultry Hotline handles calls on the handling of perishable foods. Hours are 10-4 weekdays, Eastern Time. Dial 1-800-535-4555. Washington, D.C. area residents call 1-202-447-3333.

Section 6.2

The Egg Handling Handbook

(Source: *Food News for Consumers*, Summer 1992.)

It's a whole new situation with eggs today. Eggs have been implicated in an increasing number of cases of foodborne illness. The real culprits? Mishandling as well as bacteria lurking inside some shells.

The bacteria is *Salmonella enteritidis*. The problem surfaced in the Northeastern United States a few years ago and is now moving across the country.

Salmonella is found more frequently in the yolk which can support bacterial growth. Egg whites are less likely to harbor bacteria but may still be a problem. The U.S. Department of Agriculture does not recommend eating raw or undercooked egg yolks, whites or products containing them.

"Most egg-borne illness is a result of leaving eggs out at room temperature, pooling eggs and incomplete cooking," said Betsy Crosby, a home economist in the Poultry Division of USDA's Agricultural Marketing Service.

Pooling occurs most often in food service establishments where many eggs are cracked into one bowl for later use, and the bowl may be left out at room temperature for a long period of time. Salmonella from one egg can contaminate the whole bowl, and the bacteria can multiply quickly at room temperature.

The good news is that the proper storing, handling and cooking of eggs can prevent foodborne illness. There are also ways to satisfy people who are reluctant to give up "runny" eggs and recipes traditionally made with raw eggs.

You can continue to enjoy eggs and egg-rich foods if you follow these safe handling guidelines.

Safe Handling of Eggs

At the Store

Choose Grade A or AA eggs with clean, uncracked shells. Shop at a reputable grocery. *Buy only eggs that have been kept refrigerated,* never those sitting out at room temperature. Any bacteria present in eggs can grow rapidly outside refrigeration.

If the egg carton has a date printed on it, make sure it hasn't passed.

Get eggs into a 40°F home refrigerator as soon as possible. Leave eggs in their original carton in a colder section of the refrigerator, not in the door. Do not wash eggs prior to storage because that will remove the protective coating applied at the packaging plant.

Refrigerator Storage

Fresh shell eggs can be kept safely in the refrigerator 3 to 5 weeks from the *date of purchase*, not from the date on the carton.

If eggs get cracked on the way home, break them into a clean container, cover tightly, refrigerate them and use within 2 days.

Sometimes recipes require separated eggs and you may have either the whites or the yolks left over. Refrigerate egg whites in a tightly closed container and cover yolks with cold water before storing for up to 4 days.

Freezer Storage

For longer storage, you can freeze eggs after beating yolks and whites together. Or freeze separated whites by themselves. To freeze yolks separately, mix 4 yolks with a pinch of salt and 1 1/2 teaspoons of sugar or corn syrup. Store frozen eggs up to 6 months.

If eggs freeze accidentally in their shells, keep them frozen until needed; then defrost in the refrigerator. Discard eggs whose shells cracked during freezing.

Handling Eggs

Wash hands, utensils, equipment and work areas with hot, soapy water before and after they come in contact with eggs and raw egg-rich foods. Avoid keeping eggs out of the refrigerator for more than 2 hours, including time for preparing and serving (but not cooking).

Serve cooked egg dishes immediately after cooking, or refrigerate at once for serving later. When refrigerating a large amount of a hot food, divide it into several shallow containers so it will cool quickly. Use within 3 to 4 days, or freeze for longer storage.

Fancy Egg Recipes

The egg is found in every cuisine of the world. In fact, one of the first known recipes featured eggs. To prepare "Ova Mellita," or sweet eggs, ancient Romans were directed to beat eggs with honey and cook the mixture in an earthenware dish. From its title, we get the modern word "omelette."

This recipe is still safe to make. However, some other recipes in their current forms are not.

Caesar salad was created in 1924 by Italian chef Caesar Cardini who owned a restaurant in Tijuana, Mexico. Made with a raw egg dressing, it's not safe today.

Neither is **Hollandaise sauce**, created by a French chef to honor the dairy products for which Holland is famous. The hot butter and lemon juice in the recipe don't destroy bacteria potentially present in the egg yolks.

To update these recipes as well as **homemade mayonnaise, salad dressings and uncooked egg-rich sauces**, use pasteurized eggs or egg substitutes.

In some markets, you may find refrigerated, frozen and dried pasteurized egg products or egg substitutes. These products are eggs which have been removed from the shells and commercially heated to destroy bacteria but are not cooked. This process cannot be done at home.

These products are safe to use in recipes that call for raw or lightly cooked eggs. Try them to see if they work to your satisfaction.

Everyday Eggs

Many "old favorite" recipes were written before salmonella made eggs a problem. Other recipes may have been written by cooks uninformed about the danger of eating raw eggs.

"Unless an egg recipe is cooked thoroughly, there's no 100% guarantee of its safety," says USDA's Betsy Crosby.

"You can find articles in scientific journals where laboratories have tested the role acidity has in destroying bacteria, for example—by adding lemon juice to eggs. This can be effective but it's difficult to duplicate in the home. Be prepared to evaluate the safety of recipes based on USDA recommendations."

For optimal safety, eggs should be thoroughly cooked so both yolks and whites are firm. This advice is particularly important for those people most at risk for foodborne illness—the elderly, the very young, pregnant women and those with weakened immune systems.

People unwilling to give up their favorite "**runny**" eggs can *minimize* their risk by cooking or microwaving an egg until the white is completely firm and the yolk begins to thicken but is not hard.

Fried eggs should be cooked 2 to 3 minutes on each side or in a covered pan 4 minutes. **Scrambled eggs** should be cooked until firm throughout. **Poach eggs** in boiling water 5 minutes or boil them in the shell 7 minutes.

Lightly cooked foods such as French toast should be avoided for those in the high-risk groups.

Egg mixtures are safe if they reach 160°F. So recipes such as eggnog can be made safe if the raw eggs are heated with liquid or another ingredient contained in the recipe. *Use a thermometer to check the temperature of egg mixtures.*

An additional safety check for egg dishes such as **quiche** and casseroles is that a knife inserted in the center comes out clean.

Egg-rich desserts: Some recipes such as **chiffon pies** and **fruit whips** are made with raw beaten egg whites. These cannot be guaranteed safe. Either substitute whipped cream or use pasteurized dried egg whites available in cake decorating departments.

To make **key lime pie** safely, heat the lime juice with the raw egg yolks in a pan on the stove, stirring constantly, until the mixture reaches 160°F. Then combine it with the sweetened condensed milk and pour filling into baked pie crust. Top with meringue. Bake all **meringue-topped pies** at 350°F for at least 15 minutes.

Simmer small **poached meringues** in liquid 5 minutes or until firm. **Dry meringue shells** are safe as are **divinity candy** and **7-minute frosting**, made by combining hot sugar syrup with beaten egg whites.

For other recipes like ice cream and soft custard, you can use fresh eggs if you start with a cooked base. Heat gently until the mixture coats a metal spoon.

For further information about handling and cooking eggs safely, call USDA's Meat and Poultry Hotline at 1-800-535-4555 weekdays from 10 a.m. to 4 p.m. Eastern time. Washington, D.C. area residents call 202-720-3333.

—by CiCi Williamson, Certified Home Economist

Section 6.3

A Microwave Handbook

(Source: *Food News for Consumers*, Winter 1993.)

The popularity of microwave cooking continues to grow—almost every American household possesses at least one oven. Yet, concerns about the safety of cooking meat and poultry products in the microwave persist. Even the cookware and plastic wraps used in the ovens have come under question.

Plus, there are traits, unique to microwave cooking, that affect how completely food is cooked. "Cold spots" can occur because of the irregular way the microwaves enter the oven and are absorbed by the food.

Since we have traditionally relied on thorough cooking to kill bacteria that may be present in food, consumers should take simple, yet effective steps to ensure even cooking when using a microwave.

How to Microwave Safely

Defrosting

- *When using the microwave to defrost foods, plan to finish the cooking immediately.* Some areas of larger food items may begin to cook during the defrost cycle, raising the temperature to a point where bacteria can flourish.

- *Remove food from store wrap prior to thawing.* Foam insulated trays and plastic wraps are not heat stable at high temperatures. They can melt or warp from the food's heat, possibly causing chemicals to migrate into the food.

- *Don't defrost or hold food at room temperature for over 2 hours.* It is easy to forget all about a food item thawing in the microwave oven. Set a timer to sound an alert when the thawing time is up.

Cooking

- *Debone large pieces of meat.* Bone can shield the meat around it from thorough cooking.

- *Arrange food items uniformly in a covered dish* and add a little liquid. Under the cover, steam helps kill bacteria and ensure uniform heating. Either plastic wrap or a glass cover works well. Many recipes suggest venting a small area, allowing some steam to escape. Plastic wrap shouldn't touch the food.

- *Cook large pieces of meat at 50% power for longer periods of time.* This allows the heat to reach deeper portions without overcooking outer areas. Commercial oven cooking bags can also help even out cooking and provide a tender product.

- *Move the food inside the dish several times during cooking.* Stir soups or stews. If you don't have a turntable, turn the entire dish during cooking. This is especially important for foods like casseroles that can't be stirred.

- *Do not cook whole, stuffed poultry in the microwave.* The bones and density of the bird do not allow even cooking. Microwaves may not thoroughly cook the moist stuffing deep inside the bird either.

- *Never partially cook food.* If planning to combine microwave cooking with conventional roasting, broiling or grilling, transfer the microwaved foods to conventional heat immediately.

- *Use a temperature probe or meat thermometer to verify the food has reached a safe temperature.* Check the temperature in several places, avoiding fat and bone. It should reach 160°F for red meat; 180°F for poultry.

- *Make allowances for oven wattage variations.* Because ovens vary in power and operating efficiency, make sure food is done. Use a meat thermometer and visual signs to check doneness. Juices should run clear, and meat should not be pink.

- *Observe the standing time in the recipe.* It is necessary to complete the cooking process.

Warming Precooked Foods

- *Cover precooked foods with microwave-safe plastic, waxed paper or a glass lid.* This will keep moisture in and provide even cooking.

- *Heat leftovers and precooked food to at least 165°F.* Food should be very hot to the touch and steaming before it is served.

- *Use caution when warming baby food.* Stir toddler foods thoroughly and taste-test them yourself for child-safe temperatures. Shake milk or formula in a bottle before tasting as it can become extremely hot.

What Utensils, Wraps and Cookware Should Be Used in the Microwave?

Glass and glass ceramic cookware are safe for microwave cooking. But what about other materials?

- *Use only those containers and products that have been approved for microwave use.* These items are designed to withstand the high temperatures possible when cooking foods that have a high fat or sugar content.

- *Avoid the use of cold storage containers.* Margarine tubs, whipped topping bowls and cottage cheese cartons, for example, have not been approved for microwaving. High heat could cause chemicals to transfer into the food.

- *Waxed paper is safe.* Other paper goods such as towels, plates and napkins have not been tested for use in cooking. If using these items, for optimal safety, use only plain white paper goods.

- *Never use brown grocery bags and newspapers.* These contain recycled materials and metals which could start a fire.

- *Avoid letting plastic wrap touch foods during microwaving.* It's fine to cover utensils with plastic wrap, but unless the wrap is a heavy-duty type, it could melt in contact with hot foods.

- *Oven cooking bags are safe for use in the microwave.* They are made from tough nylon material. Oven bags also promote even cooking, which helps meat reach safe temperatures throughout.

- *Follow package directions when heating microwavable foods with special browning or crisping devices in the package.* Never try to reuse these special browning devices. Don't eat from a package that becomes "charred" in cooking. Handle carefully, they become very hot to the touch.

- *Do not re-use trays and containers provided with microwave convenience products.* They have been designed for one-time use with that specific food only.

—by Susan Coney,
CiCi Williamson, and
Marilyn Johnston.

Section 6.4

Microwave-Safe For Baby

(Source: *Food News for Consumers*, Winter 1992.)

It's 2 a.m. You grope toward the glow of the night light and scoop up the wailing baby. Finding a nurser half-filled with formula from the 10 o'clock feeding, you zap it in the microwave and sigh with relief as the toothless gums close on the nipple.

But this silence could come at a high price. You may have put your baby at risk from burn injuries or food poisoning.

Heating Bottles in the Microwave

Studies show that microwaves heat baby's milk and food unevenly. Resulting "hot spots" can scald a baby's mouth and throat.

Dr. Madeline Sigman, R.D., a food scientist at Pennsylvania State University, is completing a study on microwaving infant formula. She said, "When formula is microwaved, heat accumulates in the top of the bottle. So shake well and test the temperature by shaking some of the liquid on top of your hand. The wrist is one of the areas least sensitive to heat. Don't test there."

Playtex, Evenflo and Gerber unanimously recommend against microwaving formula in nursers with disposable plastic inserts. Hot spots in milk heated in these bottles may weaken the seams, causing the plastic to burst and spill hot milk on the baby.

To heat a bottle with a disposable insert, place it under hot tap water until the desired temperature is reached. This should only take a minute or two. Or heat water in a pan, remove it from heat and set the bottle in it.

Hard plastic and glass baby bottles can be warmed in this same manner or in the microwave if you remove the cap and nipple first. For 8 ounces of milk or formula at refrigerator temperature, microwave on high 30 seconds. Let stand for a minute.

As with other warming procedures, shake the liquid to even the temperature and test before using.

Heating Solid Foods

Microwaving solid baby foods in the jars is not recommended. Robert F. Schiffmann, a leading expert in microwave product development, presented a paper at the International Microwave Power Institute annual symposium in 1990 documenting uneven heating.

He measured the temperature of various baby foods in jars at three depths and nine spots. The center of the foods reached 170 to 200°F. The coolest place, 48°F, was next to the glass sides. So pulling the jar out of the microwave could lead you to believe the food is not too hot.

However, if the foods are transferred to a dish, Schiffmann found they could be microwaved if stirred and taste-tested for temperature before feeding.

"Babies should not be fed foods heated higher than 90 to 120°F," according to the Gerber Products Company. In the microwave, this temperature is reached when 4 ounces of solid food in a dish are heated for about 15 seconds on high power. Always stir, let stand 30 seconds and taste-test before using. Food that's "baby-ready" should feel lukewarm to you.

Since fats heat faster in a microwave than other substances, do not microwave baby food meats, meat sticks or eggs. These foods have a high fat content which can cause splattering and overheating.

Handling Baby Foods Safely

Back to that early morning bottle: your baby might get food poisoning if you give him or her leftovers from a previous feeding. Harmful bacteria from the baby's mouth can be introduced into the formula where it can grow and multiply even after refrigeration and reheating.

The same thing can happen if a baby is fed straight from a jar of baby food. Saliva on the spoon contaminates the remaining food.

Milk, formula or food left out of the refrigerator more than 2 hours may be unsafe. Also, you should not leave a bottle in the crib with an older baby where it might be imbibed over many hours.

Even a small "dose" of harmful bacteria can make a tiny baby sick.

Follow the manufacturer's recommended procedure for preparing bottles before filling with formula or milk. Observe the "Use-by" dates on formula cans.

See our baby food storage chart for holding times. Don't feed a baby anything kept longer.

If making homemade baby food, use a brush to clean areas around blender blades or food processor parts. Old food particles can harbor harmful bacteria that may contaminate other foods.

Use detergent and hot water to wash and rinse all utensils (including the can opener) which come in contact with the baby's foods.

If using commercial baby foods, check to see that the safety button on the lid is down. If the jar lid doesn't "pop" when opened, do not use. Discard jars with chipped glass or rusty lids.

To freeze homemade baby food, put the mixture in an ice cube tray. Cover with heavy-duty plastic wrap until the food is frozen. Then pop food cubes into a freezer bag or airtight container and date it. Store up to 3 months. One cube equals a serving.

Small jars can also be used for freezing. Leave about 1/2 inch of space at the top because food expands when frozen.

When traveling with baby, transport bottles and food in an insulated cooler. Place the ice chest in the passenger compartment of the car. It's cooler than the trunk. On airplanes, placing frozen gel packs in an insulated bag should keep the food safe.

If leaving the baby in the care of a sitter or family member, give explicit instructions for warming and handling bottles and food. Don't assume the person knows about baby foods and your appliances.

Nutrition Issues

There's no nutritional reason that food and formula should not be microwaved. However, overheating liquids or foods by any method can cause some nutrient destruction.

Parents interested in health foods may consider using honey as a sweetener to entice babies to drink water from a bottle. Honey is not safe for children less than a year old. It can contain the botulinum organism that could cause illness or death.

Consult your doctor about your baby's nutrition requirements. When it's a question about baby food safety, call the USDA Meat and Poultry Hotline at 1-800-535-4555, 10 to 4 weekdays. Washington, D.C., area residents, call 202-720-3333.

—by CiCi Williamson, C.H.E.*
and Grace Cataldo, C.H.E.*

*Certified Home Economist

SAFE STORAGE OF BABY FOOD

NOTE: Don't leave baby food solids or liquids out at room temperature for more than 2 hours.

	REFRIGERATOR	FREEZER
LIQUIDS		
Expressed breast milk	5 days	3 to 4 months
Formula	2 days	not recommended
Whole milk	5 days	3 months
Reconstituted evaporated milk	3 to 5 days	not recommended

SPECIAL HANDLING:
1. For shelf storage of unopened cans of formula, observe "Use by" dates printed on containers. Store evaporated milk up to 12 months.
2. Heat liquid in disposable bottles in hot tap water, not in the microwave.
3. If heating glass or hard plastic bottles in the microwave, remove the cap and nipple first.
4. Shake bottle before testing the temperature on top of your hand.
5. Discard any unused milk left in a bottle.

	REFRIGERATOR	FREEZER
SOLIDS - opened or freshly made		
Strained fruits and vegetables	2 to 3 days	6 to 8 months
Strained meats and eggs	1 day	1 to 2 months
Meat/vegetable combinations	1 to 2 days	1 to 2 months
Homemade baby foods	1 to 2 days	3 to 4 months

SPECIAL HANDLING:
1. Observe "Use by" date for shelf storage of unopened jars.
2. Check to see that the safety button in lid is down. If the jar lid does not "pop" when opened or is not sealed safely, do not use.
3. Do not heat meats, meat sticks, eggs or jars of food in the microwave.
4. Transfer food from jars to bowls or heating dish. For 4 ounces of food, microwave on high 15 seconds; stir and let stand 30 seconds.
5. Stir and test the temperature of the foods before feeding baby.
6. Don't feed a baby from the jar.

Section 6.5

Daycare and Food Safety—Emerging Issues

(Source: *Food News for Consumers*, Winter 1992.)

The numbers alone will stop you. By 1999, the experts say, 8 out of 10 American children will be in daycare.

Could this pose a health risk? "Yes," said Dr. Larry Pickering, a recognized authority on pediatric infectious diseases at the University of Texas in Houston.

"Pre-school youngsters are particularly prone to foodborne and other infectious diseases," Pickering explained. "Young children have immune systems too immature to give much protection. You've got kids at close quarters sharing toys and blankets. There are diapering and food activities, and children this age constantly put everything in their mouths. It's an ideal set-up for the spread of illness."

In fact, research Pickering did a few years ago showed children in daycare 30 percent more likely to contract diarrheal illness than children cared for at home.

"There is a real need to provide daycare workers with special training in food and formula handling as well as in the control of infectious disease," said Dr. Susan Aronson, who is working through the American Academy of Pediatrics to improve the quality of daycare nationwide. Dr. Aronson is a clinical professor of pediatrics at the Hahnemann Medical Center, Philadelphia, Penn.

Recognizing that need, national health and social service agencies are moving ahead with commendable speed.

The American Red Cross, with the American Academy of Pediatrics and the National Academy of Sciences, has developed an accredited Child Care Course to train childcare workers in everything from first aid, food handling and preventing infectious disease to communicating with children and parents. The course, divided into seven short training modules which can be taken at the worker's convenience, will help workers pass newly-instituted local requirements. For more information, contact the local chapter of the American Red Cross. In some places, scholarship money can be arranged for qualified applicants.

To improve overall standards for daycare centers, guide licensing boards, and make vital information available to childcare professionals and parents, the American Public Health Association and the American Academy of Pediatrics recently published the comprehensive *National Health and Safety Performance Standards: Guidelines for Out-of-Home Child Care Programs.*

Covering family daycare (where a few children are cared for in someone's home), group daycare (7 to 12 youngsters in someone's home) and child care centers, the directives span all aspects of health and safety. The manual ($50) is available from Publication Sales, APHA, 1015 15th Street, N.W., Washington, D.C. 20005.

Health professionals are designing courses and setting up new licensing standards. What can parents and childcare providers do to protect our pre-school children's wellbeing?

A lot. The [section] "Improving the Health of Daycare" gives general information on how a safe, well-run center should operate. There is also a special section on food handling tips for both parents and daycare workers.

"I like to keep a positive perspective," said Dr. Janet Mohle-Boetani, a CDC epidemiologist who was in Lexington, Ky., last year as a community educator to help stop a shigella outbreak in daycare centers. "Sanitation in daycare can be a real problem. But, from the epidemiological viewpoint, daycare centers can be viewed as 'communities' where infection control practices can be put in place and monitored."

Doubtless that's the key—in daycare, as elsewhere, keeping children healthy depends on knowing the rules and *following* them.

The Pathogen Problem

Experts currently mention six pathogens as important in outbreaks of daycare center illness. Shigella, a bacteria that causes diarrhea and can be transmitted by infected people to food or water, causes "15,000 to 20,000 reported cases of shigellosis per year, mostly in children under 4," according to Dr. Dean Cliver in *Foodborne Diseases*, 1990.

Cryptosporidium, a microscopic parasitic protozoan which causes mild to severe diarrhea, is an emerging problem. When ingested, cysts carrying the protozoan migrate to the small intestine where they cause illness. Infants and AIDS patients are particularly vulnerable.

Hepatitis A, Giardia, E. coli and common viral infections are also showing an upswing in daycare settings. Carried on human hands and in infected stool particulates, water and food, these pathogens demand careful control, especially in daycare situations where there is repeated diaper changing and young children are putting *everything* in their mouths.

Improving the Health of Daycare

These recommendations are based on American Red Cross, American Academy of Pediatrics, Centers for Disease Control (CDC) and U.S. Department of Agriculture guidelines.

In well-run centers, the following health rules should be standard operating procedure:

- There should be adequate refrigeration and reheating facilities for foods and beverages.

- Diaper-changing, potty-training and toilet areas should be kept scrupulously clean and stationed away from food preparation and eating areas.

- Used diapers and wipes should be stored in closed containers that are removed daily.

- Items children touch, particularly things that "go in the mouth," should be sanitized regularly.

- Children should never share Kleenex or washcloths, and their personal belongings—tooth and hair brushes, clothing and pajamas—should be labeled and kept separate.

- Ample space for ventilation should be left between cribs, beds, cots and nap rugs so that children don't pick up each other's "bugs." Staff can alternate the head-to-foot position of beds so children's heads aren't lined up in a row. This reduces the spread of infection.

- The center should be vigilant on vaccination requirements and have a well-defined, professionally verified policy on illness exclusion—when and for what reasons ill or contagious youngsters cannot come in.

For in-depth information, order "Healthy Young Children: A Manual for Programs" ($15), National Association for the Education of Young Children, 1834 Connecticut Ave., N.W., Wash., D.C. 20009-5786, 202-232-8777.

Note: A fine 16-minute video on the importance of handwashing for daycare children and staff ("ABCs of Clean," $10) is available from the Soap & Detergent Association., 475 Park Ave., New York, N.Y. 10016, 212-725-1262.

Food Handling

Parents

- Formula—Pour into bottles labeled with your child's name. Cap and refrigerate. Place in center refrigerator as soon as you arrive.

- Breast milk—Put in labeled bottles or liners. Refrigerate or freeze. Refrigerate on arrival at the center.

- Lunches, snacks—Make sure any perishable snacks for your children are refrigerated at the center.

- Handwashing—As soon as children can understand, stress handwashing after toileting and before eating.

Daycare Workers

- Accept from parents only sealed bottles of formula or breast milk labeled with the child's name. Discard any leftover bottle contents—milk, water or juice—unrefrigerated over 2 hours.

- Serve food sent from home only if properly covered and refrigerated. It should look safe and wholesome. CAUTION: Never taste suspect food. It could make you sick.

- Handwashing—Teachers and children should wash hands after toileting, messy play and before eating.

145

- Meal management—Don't let children share foods or utensils. Discard food left on plates.

—by Mary Ann Parmley

Section 6.6

How Would You Know if the Blue Cheese or Pepperoni Were about to Turn on You?

(Source: *Food News for Consumers*, Spring 1992.)

"How could I tell if my blue cheese went bad?" a caller recently asked USDA's Meat and Poultry Hotline. The Hotline answers questions on the care of perishable foods.

It's a good question. In a "healthy" state blue cheese is veined with mold!

So here are some guidelines on how to judge the fitness and eatability of specialty cheeses, buttermilk, yogurt, sourdough bread, hard sausages, sauerkraut and so forth. The key to the puzzle is that all these foods are *fermented*.

Fermentation. "From time immemorial," said USDA microbiologist Carl Custer, "people have fermented foods both to preserve them and impart distinctive flavors." The problem with most foods, Custer explained, is that they have a nearly neutral pH.

That means they are neither an acid like vinegar nor a base like lye. Unfortunately, the micro-organisms that cause spoilage and foodborne illness thrive at neutral pH levels. So over time people stumbled onto ways to acidify food to extend its usefulness.

Fermentation is one such method. Many kinds of food fermentation, using helpful lactic acid bacteria, make foods more acidic and extend shelf-life.

But fermented foods, like all perishables, must still be properly handled. Because, with longer storage and repeated handling, there is

146

the opportunity for spoilage and food poisoning organisms to reach the food and start growing.

Cheeses. Made from separated milk solids, specialty cheeses are then ripened using bacteria and/or molds chosen to give certain textures and flavors. For example, blue cheese is mold-ripened by *Penicillium roqueforti*, while brie is aged by *Penicillium camembert*.

Normal storage: Firm cheeses keep well several weeks in the refrigerator if protected from mold and drying. A soft brie retains top quality about a week in the refrigerator. Re-wrap cheese after cutting.

Care must also be taken to use cheese properly. Don't leave cheese at room temperature for extended periods (2+ hours). Like all perishables and all opened or sliced fermented foods, cheese can be contaminated by microorganisms on people's hands, by coughs, sneezes and "bugs" in the air. Too-long exposure at room temperature can give these microscopic and therefore invisible food poisoners time to multiply to disease-causing levels.

Check refrigerated cheese before serving it. Discard a soft cheese if you see any signs of mold—it can easily spread through soft tissues. Hard cheeses are past saving if mold growth is extensive or cheese has lost its original color and texture. Discard blue or other blue-veined cheese if you see mold growth different from the normal veining. Invader-molds may appear as white, pink, green, blue, black or grey flecks or furry patches.

Fermented Sausages. Dry and semi-dry fermented sausages are made from ground meat treated with seasoning and curing agents. Starter cultures are also used to shorten fermentation time.

Genoa salami, summer sausage, Lebanon bologna and pepperoni are some common varieties.

Watch the labels on these sausages for handling instructions. Some semi-dry sausages require refrigeration, most dry sausages don't. But all sausages should be refrigerated after you cut into them and expose the moist inner surfaces.

Storage times? Opened whole semi-dry sausage will last 3-6 weeks refrigerated; opened whole dry sausage will last 6-8 weeks. Extremely dry jerky or beef sticks, once opened, last 2-3 months refrigerated. Sealed vacuum-packed slices will last about 2 weeks; once opened, 1 week.

A salty, white film which can form on the skin of these sausages is harmless and can be cut away, but sliminess or discolored spots on casings mean you should discard the meat.

Buttermilk, Yogurt, Sour Cream. Buttermilk, yogurt and sour cream can be puzzling because it's not always as easy to determine when they're no longer useable as it is with ordinary milk. Milk sours with definite smell and flavor changes.

Cultured buttermilk. Cultured buttermilk which some food historians say originated in southern Russia, results from a lactic acid bacteria starter mixture or culture. Best if used the first week, buttermilk normally keeps 2 weeks refrigerated. Beyond that, it can become too bitter to drink. Actual spoilage can appear as off-odors or the separation of greyish liquid on top.

Sour Cream. Pasteurized, homogenized cream treated with lactic starter culture becomes sour cream.

Lasting 2-3 weeks in refrigeration, sour cream should be discarded if you see mold spots, pink or green scum or cloudy liquid that has separated on top.

Yogurt. The "friendly" bacteria *Lactobacillus bulgaricus* and *Streptococcus thermophilus* turn milk into yogurt. Yogurt, with a normal refrigerated lifespan of 1 to 2 weeks, should be discarded at any sign of mold growth—blue, green or pink mold is common—or if it develops a yeasty aroma.

Sourdough bread. Classic sourdough bread draws its flavor from the acidic Lactobacillus sanfrancisco. Wrapped in paper and stored in a bread box, it will stay fresh a day or so. Just beyond that, if it's dried out, you can microwave a serving to soften it. Use the microwaved portion immediately. Like other breads, over-aged sourdough can become moldy.

Sauerkraut. Sauerkraut, made from cabbage salted and fermented in its own juice, can be either canned or fresh at the deli case. While the growth of lactic acid bacteria during fermentation make kraut somewhat spoilage-resistant, its eating quality is another matter. Experts suggest canned kraut should be eaten within 6 months for

The Fermented Foods Storage Chart

Chart assumes items have been opened or cut into.
N/R means not recommended.

	Refrigerator	Freezer
Cheese		
Cheddar	4-8 weeks	6 months
Swiss	4 weeks	6 months
Blue	2-4 weeks	6 months
Brie, ripe	1 week	6 months
Other Dairy Products		
Buttermilk	1 week, top quality	3 months
	2nd week, may turn bitter	
Sour cream	2-3 weeks	N/R
Yogurt	1-2 weeks	1 ½ months
Sausage*		
Salami	1-2 weeks	4 months
Summer sausage	1-2 weeks	4 months
Lebanon bologna	1-2 weeks	4 months
Genoa salami	2-3 weeks	6 months
Pepperoni	2-3 weeks	6 months
Hard salami	2-3 weeks	6 months
Jerky & Beef sticks	2-3 months	1 year
Sauerkraut, fresh	1 week	N/R
Pickles, processed	1-2 months	N/R
Olives	1-2 months	N/R

*These are general, rule-of-thumb guidelines. You should also check package directions and use-by dates on individual products.

Additional information on food storage is available in a Food Marketing Institute pamphlet "The Food Keeper," 50 cents, from FMI, 800 Connecticut Ave., N.W., Wash., D.C. 20006. Send SSAE. Janet Bailey's comprehensive Keeping Food Fresh, Harper & Row, 1989, is also quite helpful.

full flavor, and that fresh kraut retains top quality refrigerated about 1 week.

Spoilage appears as mold growth or surface scum.

Processed Pickles. Processed Pickles, lactic-acid fermented cucumbers in glass jars, may be kept on the cabinet shelf about a year. Once opened, you can keep them refrigerated for 1-2 months. Discard if the liquid turns cloudy or scum forms on the surface. Mushy pickles should also be discarded.

Fermented Olives. Fermented olives that we see on the grocery shelves are stuffed green olives, Spanish green olives and some Greek and Sicilian brand black olives.

Surprisingly, fresh-picked olives are bitter and largely inedible. So olives to be fermented are first treated with lye to remove bitterness, then brined and sometimes processed with lactic acid or lactobacilli bacteria.

The resulting canned olives are shelf-stable up to 1 year. Opened, they can be refrigerated in their own liquid for 1-2 months.

Discard olives when they become soft, spotted or produce a spoiled odor.

—by Mary Ann Parmley

Section 6.7

What to Do about Mold

(Source: *Food News for Consumers*, Winter 1993.)

Mold—Is It Just a Nuisance?

In many cases, yes, particularly in warm, humid weather when food molds quickly. Worldwide, though, mold causes great economic losses, destroying crops and shortening food storage times in the home.

But Certain Molds Can Be Dangerous

Some molds cause allergic reactions and respiratory problems. And a few molds, in the right conditions, produce poisonous substances that can make you sick. These are called mycotoxins.

How Can You Tell If a Mold Is Dangerous?

You can't. That's the problem. Some mold toxins are powerful even in small amounts. Some toxins can survive for a long time in food. Some aren't even destroyed by cooking.

So you can't always safely scrape or cut the mold off food. These guidelines will help you in avoiding mold growth and handling the moldy food you encounter anyway.

How Mold Grows

Mold is a type of fungus. In many molds, the body consists of "root" threads that invade the food it lives on, a stalk that rises above the food and spores that form at the ends of the stalks. The spores give the mold the color you see. When airborne, the spores spread the mold from place to place like dandelion seed.

Once a food shows heavy mold growth, you can bet that the "root" threads have invaded it deeply. In dangerous molds, the mycotoxins are often contained in and around these threads. In some cases, the toxins may have spread throughout the food.

How Can Mold Grow in the Refrigerator?

While most molds prefer warmer temperatures, they can grow in the colder range. Molds also tolerate salt and sugar better than most other food invaders. So you may find mold in refrigerated jams and jelly (high sugar) and on cured, salty meats—ham, bacon, salami.

Minimize Mold Growth in Your Refrigerator and Kitchen

Cleanliness is Vital in Controlling Mold

Mold spores from affected food can build up in your refrigerator, shortening the life of other foods.

Suggestion: Clean the inside of the refrigerator every few months with 1 tbsp. of baking soda dissolved in a quart of water. Rinse with clear water and dry. Scrub visible mold (usually black) on rubber casings with 3 tbsp. of bleach in a quart of water.

Keep dishrags, dish cloths, sponges and mops clean and fresh. A musty smell means they're spreading mold around. Discard items you can't clean or launder.

Don't Unknowingly Buy Moldy Food

Quick shopping sometimes means you don't examine food well before you buy it. But it's important to check food in glass jars and fresh fruits and vegetables for mold growth. Check the stem areas on fresh produce. Notify the store manager about mold on any foods.

Fresh meat and poultry are usually mold-free, but cured meats and smoked turkey may not be. Examine them carefully. Exceptions? Some salamis—San Francisco and Italian types—have a characteristic thin, white mold coating. They shouldn't show any other mold.

Protect Food from Spore "Invaders" When It's Sitting Out

When serving food, keep it covered to prevent exposure to mold spores in the air. Plastic wrap is good for food you want to stay moist— fresh or cut fruits or vegetables, green and mixed salads. Just remember, don't leave any perishables out of the refrigerator over 2 hours.

Don't want moisture buildup? Cake and cheese keepers with their own covers will protect those foods without excess moisture buildup. For breads, use clean paper towels as a cover—this lets bread "breathe."

Empty opened cans of perishable food into clean refrigerator dishes and refrigerate promptly. Reseal boxed food as tightly as possible to keep air that contains mold spores out.

Oh, No... There's Mold On It

Buying smaller amounts and using food quickly can help prevent mold growth. But when you see moldy food...

Don't *sniff* the moldy item. You don't want respiratory trouble. If food is covered with mold, discard it. Put it in a small paper bag or wrap it in plastic for disposal in a covered trash can children and animals can't get into. Clean the refrigerator, if necessary, where the food was sitting. Check nearby items it might have touched. Mold spreads quickly in fruits and vegetables.

If the food shows only a tiny mold spot, follow these guidelines. Generally, we suggest that you can save hard or firm foods with only minor mold problems, but most soft or liquid foods showing mold should be discarded.

- **Cheese.** Some cheese is made with mold, but you may spot mold that shouldn't be there. In hard block cheeses, cut off at least an inch around and below the mold spot. Keep your knife or instrument out of the mold itself. After the "surgery," re-cover the cheese in fresh wrap. Don't try to save individual cheese slices, soft cheese, cottage cheese, cream, sour cream or yogurt.

- **Hard salamis & country ham.** You can cut a small spot of mold off hard salamis using the cheese rule. Again, keep the knife out of the mold.

  You can cut mold off dry-cured country ham if it's only a small, surface spot. You can cut away a small mold spot on the inside of country ham too, following the cheese rule. But if the ham is covered with brown or black mold, discard it.

  Discard moldy bacon, hotdogs, sliced lunch meats, meat pies or opened canned ham.

- **Smoked turkey.** Cut a small mold spot off the surface using the cheese rule. Throw moldy cooked chicken out.

- **Jams, jellies, syrups.** Discard such items showing any mold growth. Experts now feel mold toxins (if present) can spread through this soft material quite rapidly.

- **Fruits and vegetables.** Cut out small mold spots from the surface of firm fruits and vegetables (cabbage, bell peppers, carrots), but discard soft vegetables (tomatoes, cucumbers, lettuce) showing mold.

- **Potatoes.** Note any damaged areas on the surface and cut away tissue that is blackened or discolored. It's best to do this before cooking, but you can also do it after cooking and before eating.

- **Throw away on sight.** Discard visibly moldy bread, cake, buns, pastry, corn-on-the-cob, stored nuts, flour, whole grains, rice, dried peas and beans and peanut butter.

Carefully check any food you've had a while that the store or seller sold as "natural." Processed without preservatives, they are prone to mold growth.

Consumers are not facing the "mold" problem alone

There is continual federal monitoring of crops at high risk for toxic mold growth. These crops include grains, nuts, celery, apples and tomatoes. Government works with farmers and the food industry to ensure that these foods and products made from them are safe when they arrive at the grocery. Your responsibility begins when you take food home.

For more information on mold or the handling of perishable foods, call USDA's Meat and Poultry Hotline, 800-535-4555. Washington, D.C. residents call 202-720-3333.

—by Mary Ann Parmley

Research assistance from Dr. John Richard—USDA Mycotoxin Research, Peoria, Ill., Dr. Charles Lattuada—USDA Food Microbiology, Beltsville, Md., Marilyn Johnston—USDA's Meat Poultry Hotline.

Section 6.8

Is Your Holiday Turkey in Jeopardy?

(Source: *Food News for Consumers*, Holidays 1991.)

Defrosted on the counter, prestuffed, slow-baked, partially cooked, stored whole without carving...? If any of these situations sounds like your usual Thanksgiving dinner preparation plans, you may be putting your turkey in jeopardy.

Over the last six years, USDA's staff on the Meat and Poultry Hotline have faced many challenges trying to save Thanksgiving turkeys that have been prepared in questionable ways. "It's difficult to advise consumers on Thanksgiving Day that the turkey they have worked so hard to serve may not be safe to eat," says Susan Templin Conley, Hotline Manager.

According to Conley, there are six basic problems that Hotline staff members hear every year. Read on to see if you may unknowingly be creating any of these scenarios.

Mistake 1: Defrosting at Room Temperature

"We've always done it that way...There's no room in the refrigerator...We forgot it was in the trunk of the car...It's in a cold basement." While there are many reasons why consumers find themselves with turkeys defrosted at room temperature, some planned and some unplanned, the result is the same—a potentially unsafe turkey. Bacteria grow rapidly at room temperature. Bacteria will begin to grow on the outside portion of the bird that defrosts first. These surface bacteria can multiply to dangerously high levels that cooking may not destroy.

Instead

Plan on 1 day of refrigerator defrost time for every 5 pounds of turkey. A 10-pound turkey will take approximately 2 days to defrost in the refrigerator, a 15-pound turkey 3 days and a 20-pound turkey 4 days.

Some callers worry that a frozen turkey will spoil if left in the refrigerator for 4 days. Don't be concerned. Even after a turkey fully defrosts, it is safe in the refrigerator for an additional 1-2 days.

If you forget to take your turkey out of the freezer early enough, don't panic. You're not in hot water yet, especially if you remember to use the COLD WATER technique. Even a 20 pound frozen turkey can be defrosted in 10 hours using the cold water defrost method. Submerge the wrapped bird in cold water, adding ice or new cold water every 30 minutes.

Mistake 2: Prestuffing a Turkey the Night Before

It's okay to prestuff Christmas stockings, but not Thanksgiving birds! Stuffing a turkey the night before is risky business. The cavity of the bird actually insulates the stuffing from the cold temperatures, and can keep the stuffing in a temperature range that encourages bacterial growth.

Instead

Prepare dry stuffing ingredients the day before. Tightly cover and leave at room temperature. The perishables—butter, or margarine, mushrooms, oysters, cooked celery and onion, broth—should be refrigerated. Combine the dry and wet ingredients and stuff the bird immediately before the turkey goes into the oven.

Mistake 3: Cooking at Low Temperatures Overnight

Every year Hotline staff members worry about "how low consumers will go" when it comes to oven temperature settings. On Thanksgiving Day in 1990, Hotline staff talked with numerous families who calmly slept the night away while bacteria were busily multiplying on their turkeys in 200°F ovens. Cooking below 325°F is unsafe because low temperatures permit the bird (and the stuffing) to remain in the "danger zone" (40°-140° F) too long. While in this "zone" bacteria can grow and some produce heat-resistant toxins.

Instead

Cook perishable foods at an oven temperature no lower than 325°F.

Mistake 4: Partially Cooking a Bird the Day Before

Some time-savers are safer than others. Partially cooking a turkey is not one of them. Interrupted cooking can actually increase the possibility of bacterial growth. The turkey may be heated long enough to activate bacterial growth, but not long enough to kill it.

Instead

Cook the turkey completely in one operation. Several other ideas for SAFE time saving include: 1) Using oven cooking bags, 2) Baking stuffing separately from the turkey, 3) Cooking and carving the turkey 1 to 2 days before the holiday, and storing it in the refrigerator for reheating on the big day.

Mistake 5: Cooking a Turkey Ahead of Time and Leaving It Whole in the Refrigerator

Cooking the turkey a day or two before the holiday is fine, but re-frigerating the bird whole, without carving, is another form of turkey jeopardy. A cooked turkey, stuffed or unstuffed, is too big and dense to cool down quickly and efficiently in a home refrigerator. In addition, reheating the turkey the next day in a slow oven to prevent drying out could allow even more growth of potential food poisoning bacteria.

Instead

Roast the turkey 1 or 2 days before the holiday. Use a meat thermometer to make sure that the bird reaches 180°F. Remove stuffing immediately after taking the bird from the oven. Allow the turkey to sit for 20 to 30 minutes so that the meat juices can settle. Carve the bird into appropriate serving slices. Arrange turkey slices in shallow baking pans. Cover and refrigerate. Reheat Thanksgiving Day in a conventional oven or microwave. Make sure that meat and stuffing are reheated to "steamy hot", 165°F.

Problem 6: Power Failure

The oven broke down, an ice storm downed power lines, there's no gas for the gas grill. You can't keep your bird hot...or you can't keep your bird cold.

These unplanned situations do arise through the fault of no one. Besides causing anxiety and stress, they can also lead to an unsafe bird.

Solution

Time is of the essence. If your bird has been in any of these situations for over 2 hours, your turkey could become risky. After 2 hours the turkey enters the "danger zone" where food poisoning bacteria can multiply rapidly. But to discuss your unique situation, call one of our food experts on the Meat and Poultry Hotline.

USDA's Meat and Poultry Hotline answers questions on the safe storage and handling of meat, poultry and other perishable foods.

Normal hours are 10 a.m.-4 p.m. weekdays, Eastern Time. In Novem-
ber the hours will be extended to 9 a.m. to 5 p.m. The Hotline will also
be open the weekend before Thanksgiving, Nov. 23 and 24, 9 a.m. to 5
p.m. On Thanksgiving Day, the lines will operate 8 a.m. to 2 p.m. Call
1-800-535-4555. Washington, D.C. area residents call 202-447-3333.

—by Pat Moriarty, R.D., and Barbara O'Brien, R.D.

Section 6.9

The Food Science of Freezing

(Source: *Food News for Consumers*, Holidays 1991.)

Foods in the freezer—are they safe? Last year some 5,500 callers
to the USDA Meat and Poultry Hotline weren't sure about the safety
of items stored in their own home freezers.

The confusion seems to be based on the fact that few people understand how freezing protects food. They think the recommended
storage times they see for frozen items relate to safety rather than
quality.

Actually food stored at 0°F will nearly always be safe. Only the
quality suffers with lengthy freezer storage.

Freezing keeps food safe by slowing the movement of molecules,
causing foodborne illness microbes to enter a dormant stage. It's similar to how extreme cold can prevent mechanical equipment from func-
tioning and why a car may not start in sub-zero temperatures.

"Freezing preserves food for extended periods because it prevents
the growth of microorganisms that cause both food spoilage and
foodborne illness," said Brad Berry, research food technologist at
USDA's Agricultural Research Service.

Berry explained that freezing inactivates any microbes—bacteria, yeasts and molds—present in food. Once thawed, however, these
microbes will again become active. Since they will then grow at about
the same rate as microorganisms on fresh food, you must handle
thawed items as you would any perishable food.

How Freezing Affects Food Quality

While freezing may keep food safe almost indefinitely, it does affect quality. Tenderness, flavor, aroma, juiciness and color of frozen foods can all be affected.

How well food emerges from freezing depends on how well you understand and compensate for the following factors.

Freshness and quality at time of freezing affect the condition of frozen foods. Foods frozen at peak quality emerge tasting better than foods frozen near the end of their useful life. So freeze items you won't use quickly sooner rather than later.

Fortunately, the freezing process itself is not destructive of nutrients, and, as to meat and poultry products, there is little change in protein value during freezing.

However, freezing only slows the enzyme activity that takes place in foods. Enzymes present in animals, vegetables and fruit promote chemical reactions, such as ripening, in living things. These reactions also continue after harvesting.

Enzyme activity does not harm frozen meats or fish and is neutralized by the acids in frozen fruits. Most vegetables that freeze well, however, are low acid. They require a brief partial cooking to halt enzyme activity that can lead to their deterioration. This is called "blanching."

For successful freezing, blanch or partially cook vegetables in boiling water or in a microwave oven. Then rapidly chill the vegetables prior to freezing and storage. Consult a cookbook for detailed instructions.

Proper packaging helps prevent "freezer burn" and protects flavors. Freezer burn appears as grayish-brown leathery spots on frozen food. It occurs when air reaches its surface. Although undesirable, freezer burn does not make the food unsafe, merely dry in spots. Cut it away either before or after cooking the food.

Supermarket meat wraps, while safe for freezing, are permeable to air. Over time, this contributes to freezer burn and rancidity, when fats and oils develop an off-taste and odor.

For extended storage, overwrap these packages with airtight heavy-duty foil, plastic wrap and bags, or freezer paper as you would any food to be frozen. Do not rely on waxed paper. Freeze unopened vacuum packages as is.

When freezing food in plastic bags, push all the air out before sealing. Residual air can change into ice crystals and cause fats to become rancid.

Freeze food as fast as possible to maintain its quality. Ideally, a food 2-inches thick should freeze completely in about 2 hours. If your home freezer has a "quick-freeze" shelf, use it. And, regardless, arrange packages in one layer until frozen.

Rapid freezing prevents undesirable large ice crystals from forming because the molecules don't have time to take their positions in the characteristic six-sided snowflake.

Slow freezing creates large disruptive ice crystals. During thawing, they damage the cells and dissolve emulsions. This causes meat to "drip"—lose juiciness. Emulsions such as mayonnaise or cream will separate and curdle.

The lower the storage temperature and briefer the time stored, the better the quality and nutrient retention will be. Store all foods at 0°F or lower to retain vitamin content, color, flavor and texture.

Color changes can occur in frozen foods. The bright red color of meat as purchased may turn dark or pale brown depending on its variety. This may be due to freezer burn or abnormally long storage.

Freezing doesn't usually cause color changes in poultry. However, bones and the meat near them can become dark. Bone darkening results when pigment seeps through the porous bones of young poultry into the surrounding tissues when frozen and thawed.

The dulling of color in frozen vegetables and cooked foods is usually the result of excessive drying due to improper packaging or over-lengthy storage.

Defrosting Frozen Foods

When defrosting frozen foods, it's best to plan ahead for slow, safe thawing in the refrigerator. Never leave foods out on the counter at room temperature.

A large frozen item like a turkey requires at least a day for each 5 pounds of weight to thaw in a refrigerator kept at 40°F. Most foods of any size will require a day. There is no need to cut it close. Once food

160

Freezer Storage Chart at 0° F

Item	Months	Item	Months
Meat, Poultry and Eggs		**Side Dishes**	
Bacon and Sausage	1-2	Cranberries, fresh	12
Egg whites or egg substitutes	12	Pasta, cooked	1-2
Gravy, meat or poultry	2-3	Rice, cooked	1-2
Ham, Hotdogs and Lunchmeat	1-2	Stuffing or dressing	1-2
Meat, roasts uncooked	9	Vegetables	8
Meat, chops or steaks	4-12		
Meat, ground	3-4	**Desserts and Breads**	
Meat, cooked	2-3	Cake	3
Poultry, whole uncooked	12	Cookies	8
Poultry, parts uncooked	9	Bread and rolls, baked	3
Poultry Giblets, uncooked	3-4	Bread dough, unbaked	1
Poultry, ground uncooked	3-4	Fruitcake	12
Poultry, cooked	4-6	Ice cream or sherbet	2
Soups and Stews	2-3	Pies, baked	2
Wild game, uncooked	8-12	Pies, pumpkin unbaked	2
		Pies, fruit unbaked	8
Dairy Products			
Milk	1		
Cheese, hard	4		
Butter	9		

thaws in the refrigerator, it's still safe to store for a day or two before using.

Procrastinators who have failed to allow sufficient time to defrost foods in the refrigerator can fall back on two methods—the cold water method and microwave defrosting.

When using cold water to aid defrosting, be sure the food is in a leak-proof package or put it inside a plastic bag. If water contacts the food itself, harmful bacteria could be introduced into the food. Tissues can also absorb water like a sponge, resulting in a watery product.

Immerse the bag in cold water. Check the water frequently to be sure it stays cold. Bacteria can multiply rapidly at room temperature. After thawing, refrigerate the food until ready to use.

When microwave defrosting food, plan to cook it immediately afterward. Some areas of the food may become warm during microwaving, permitting the growth of bacteria in those areas.

Once food is thawed in the refrigerator, it is safe to refreeze it without cooking although there may be a loss of quality. Foods defrosted in the microwave or by the cold water method should be cooked before refreezing.

To keep your holiday food at top quality, follow the freezer storage times in the [chart on the previous page].

References

Meat Freezing, A Source Book, by Brad W. Berry, USDA's Agricultural Research Service, and Kathleen F. Leddy, USDA's Food Safety and Inspection Service, Elsevier Science Publishing Co., Inc., New York, NY, 1989. International Standard Book Number (ISBN) #0-444-87463-1.

Food Science, by Norman N. Potter, AVI Publishing, Westport, Conn.,1986. ISBN #0-87055-496-4.

The Freezing Preservation of Foods, edited by Tressler, Van Arsdel and Copley, AVI Publishing, Westport, Conn.,1981, ISBN #87055-045-4.

—by CiCi Williamson
Certified Home Economist

Section 6.10

Food Safety and the Weekend Camper

(Source: *Food News for Consumers*, Summer 1992.)

You want to get back to nature—fresh air, exercise and old-fashioned outdoor cooking. But how can you manage without sanitation and refrigeration?

Foodborne bacteria can multiply rapidly in warm outdoor temperatures, and food poisoning is the last thing a happy camper needs.

So here's a "Camper's Checklist" to get you off to a safe start.

Choosing a Cooler. Foam chests are lightweight, low cost, and actually have good "cold retention" power. But they're fragile and may not last through numerous outings.

Plastic, fiberglass or steel coolers are more durable and can take a lot of outdoor wear. They have excellent "cold retention" power but, once filled, larger models may weigh 30 or 40 pounds.

Keeping Cold Foods Cold. A block of ice keeps longer than ice cubes. Use clean, empty milk cartons to prefreeze blocks of ice or use frozen gel-packs.

Fill the cooler with COLD or FROZEN foods.

Pack foods in reverse-use order. First foods packed are last to be used.

Take foods in the smallest size needed (e.g., a small jar of mayonnaise).

In the car, put the ice chest in the passenger section. At the campsite, insulate the cooler with a blanket, tarp or poncho.

Camp Cuisine. Today's camper has many more food choices than the Daniel Boones of yesteryear. Advances in food technology have produced relatively lightweight staples that don't need refrigeration or careful packing.

For example...

- Peanut butter in plastic jars
- Concentrated juice boxes

- Canned tuna, ham, chicken and beef
- Dried noodles and soups
- Beef jerky and other dried meats
- Dehydrated foods
- Dried fruits and nuts
- Powdered milk and fruit drinks

Carry items like rice or noodles in plastic bags and take only the amount you'll use.

Water—Is It Safe? Another tough camping problem is access to reliable tap water. Bring bottled water for drinking or mixing with food. Always assume stream and river waters are not safe to drink. If you camp in remote areas, purchase commercial purification tablets or equipment and learn purification techniques.

The Clean Hands-and-Pots Club. If no safe water supply is available, or your bottled water supply is limited, use disposable wipes to clean your hands when working with food.

Take as few pots as possible. Carry items that fit inside each other. Plan one-pot meals. You can use aluminum foil wrap and pans for cooking, but take garbage bags to carry these items back to appropriate disposal sites.

Many camping areas, particularly national parks, prohibit campfires so assume you'll have to take a stove.

Leftover food should be burned, not dumped. If using soap to clean pots, wash the pots at camp, not at the water's edge. Dump dirty water on dry ground, well away from fresh water.

To Learn More

- Check your local library for advice on choosing a campsite, protecting your food from animals, disposing of garbage, etc.

- Contact sources such as the:

  American Camping Association
  5000 State Road 67 N
  Martinsville, Ind. 46151

and the:

National Campers and Hikers Association
4804 Transit Road Bldg. 2
Depew, N.Y. 14043.

- For more information on summer trekking or other food handling questions, call USDA's Meat and Poultry Hotline, 1-800-535-4555, 10 a.m. to 4 p.m. weekdays Eastern Time. Washington D.C. area residents call 202-720-3333.

—by Patricia Moriarty, Registered Dietitician

Section 6.11

A Boater's Guide to Food Safety

(Source: *Food News for Consumers*, Summer 1992.)

Out on the boat at last, you're looking forward to "catchin' some rays." Fish even. The last thing you want is foodborne illness.

But like a lot of boaters, you could be taking some chances. Too much sun and heat can make perishable food dangerous.

Perishable picnic foods and your catch must be handled with care. Mishandled food can become contaminated with bacteria and cause food poisoning.

Staying Safe. Bessie Berry, with the U.S. Department of Agriculture's Meat and Poultry Hotline, explains how to protect yourself.

- Perishable foods, like lunch meats, cooked chicken, and potato or pasta salads, should be kept in a cooler.
- Pack your cooler with several inches of ice or use frozen gel-packs.
- Store food in water-tight containers to prevent contact with melting ice water.

- Keep the cooler out of the sun, covered, if possible, for further insulation.

Tricks of the trade. Not all foods need refrigeration, and Berry suggests that some good non-perishables for boat trips are fresh fruits and vegetables, nuts, trail-mix, canned meat spreads and, yes, peanut butter and jelly. (Once canned meats are opened, put them in the cooler.)

If you don't have a cooler, try freezing sandwiches for your outing. Use coarse-textured breads that don't get soggy when thawed. Take the mayonnaise, lettuce and tomato with you to add at mealtime.

If you bring a cooler, Berry says keep the lid closed as much as possible. Store soft drinks and non-perishable favorites in another case.

Leftovers? Put perishables back on ice as soon as you finish eating. Don't let food sit out while you swim or fish. **Food sitting at outside temperatures for more than 2 hours is not safe. At 90 degrees or above, food should not sit out over 1 hour.** At high temperatures, food spoils quickly. If you have any doubts, throw it out.

Keeping the Catch

Check first with your fish and game agency or state health department to see where you can fish safely, then follow these guidelines.

Finfish

- Scale, gut and clean fish as soon as they're caught.
- Live fish can be kept on stringers or in live wells, as long as they have enough water and mobility to breathe.
- Wrap both whole and cleaned fish in water-tight plastic and store on ice.
- Keep 3 to 4 inches of ice on the bottom of the cooler. Alternate layers of fish and ice.
- Store the cooler out of the sun and cover with a blanket.
- Once home, eat fresh fish in 1 to 2 days or freeze. For top quality, use frozen fish in 3 to 6 months.

Shellfish

For safety, crabs, lobsters and other shellfish must be kept alive until cooked. Store in live wells or out of water in a bushel or laundry basket under wet burlap.

Crabs and lobsters are best eaten the day they're caught. Live oysters should be cooked in 7-10 days; mussels and clams in 4-5 days.

Caution: Everyone should be aware of the potential dangers of eating raw shellfish. Persons with liver disorders or weakened immune systems should not do so.

—by Dianne Durant

Section 6.12

The FOOD Hotlines—
Where Help Is Only a FREE Call Away

(Source: *Food News for Consumers*, Spring 1992.)

When the instructions say to baste your turkey, do you reach for a needle and thread? Have you ever tossed a package of meat on the counter to thaw as you rush off to work? Maybe you're on a special diet and need to know more about a specific product. Do you need information on safely handling perishable foods?

If so, you can call any of the tollfree numbers listed here for professional help. You'll get the assistance you need, and your call will help the company or agency track what consumers are thinking and what they need to know about food products.

Elizabeth Karmel, spokesperson for the Butterball Turkey Talk-Line, said, "Market research in 1981 suggested that consumers were intimidated by the sheer size of a turkey. So the Talk-Line was set up to provide help and reassurance to consumers as they prepared the holiday meal."

Trained personnel at these companies and organizations are waiting to answer your questions. Just pick up the phone.

The Food Lines

- **USDA's Meat and Poultry Hotline,** Washington, D.C., 1-800-535-4555. Washington, D.C. area callers, dial 202-720-3333. Hotline home economists answer questions on the safe handling and storage of meat and poultry. They can also assist you with basic nutrition questions on meat and poultry products and the nutrition labeling on these items. The Hotline is staffed 10 a.m. to 4 p.m., weekdays, Eastern Time. Food safety messages can be heard during off-hours.

- **Assorted Meats and Poultry, (Canned and Non-Canned).** Hormel, Austin, Minn., 1-800-523-4635. Consumer Affairs staff provide recipes and nutrient composition of Hormel products. They also handle complaints. 8 a.m.- 4 p.m., weekdays, Central Time.

- **Kosher Poultry,** Empire Kosher, Mifflintown, Penn., 1-800-367-4734. Ask for Consumer Relations for answers to questions about kosher processing, poultry handling and preparation. Staff can also provide cooking directions, kosher recipes and nutrition information on their own products. 8 a.m.-5 p.m., Mon.-Thurs., 8 a.m. to 3 p.m., Fri., Eastern Time.

- **Lunch Meats and Sausages.** Armour-Swift-Eckrich, Downers Grove, Ill., 1-800-325-7424. Consumer staff will answer questions on nutrition and storage of Eckrich products. They also provide recipes. 8:30 a.m.-4:30 p.m., weekdays, Central Time.

- **Nutrition.** National Center for Nutrition and Dietetics, sponsored by The American Dietetic Association, Chicago, Ill., 1-800-366-1655. Registered dietitians answer food and nutrition related questions. Taped nutrition messages available 24-hours a day. Callers may also leave name and address to receive free nutrition brochure. 9 a.m.- 4 p.m., weekdays, Central Time.

- **Poultry.** Tyson-Holly Farms-Weaver, Springdale, Ark., 1-800-233-6332. Staff handles inquiries on safe handling, nutritional value and preparation of products. They also handle complaints 8 a.m.-5 p.m., weekdays, Central Time.

- **Seafood.** American Seafood Institute, Wakefield, R.I., 1-800-328-3474. Staff will answer questions about purchase, preparation and nutritional value of seafood products. 9 a.m.-5 p.m., weekdays, Eastern Time.

- **Turkey.** Butterball Turkey Talk-Line, Downers Grove, Ill., 1-800-323-4848. Open from late October through Christmas, the staff can talk you through the preparation of a complete turkey dinner with all the trimmings. 8 a.m.- 8 p.m., weekdays, Central Time. Open 6 a.m.-6 p.m. Thanksgiving Day.

Many major food companies also have 800 numbers to answer questions on their own products. If you have a question about an item, check the label for an 800-number listing or call the AT&T 800 information number (1-800-555-1212) to see if the company is listed.

—*by Liz Lapping and Mary Wenberg*

Section 6.13

The Nations Food Protectors— Who Are They? What Do They Do?

(Source: *Food News for Consumers*, Winter 1990.)

Americans consume mountains of food every day. Behind this enormous food supply is an army of food inspectors and support personnel at all levels of government—federal, state and local— monitoring our food to ensure it is safe and wholesome. This includes not only what we eat at home but what we eat out at fast-food spots and other restaurants.

Who are the players and how does it all work? Read on.

The Federal Level

The Food Safety and Inspection Service (FSIS)

Within the U.S. Department of Agriculture, FSIS is responsible for inspecting meat and poultry products sold in interstate and international commerce. This includes meat and poultry products imported for sale here, which must be produced under inspection systems that meet U.S. standards.

A mandatory program, FSIS inspection works to supply the public with safe, wholesome and accurately labeled products. The agency can also *recall* unsafe or suspect products after they've reached the grocery shelf.

The FSIS inspection staff—over 7,500 meat and poultry inspectors, food technologists and veterinarians working in some 7,000 slaughter and processing plants across the country—constitute the largest food inspection force in the federal government. In fact, meat and poultry products are more intensively inspected than any other foods.

Plus, FSIS works closely with the food industry on product labels for consumer information. And, at the plant level, FSIS monitors facilities and equipment to assure they meet federal sanitation standards.

FSIS also runs a nationwide consumer education program to inform the public about proper care and handling of food. An important part of this effort is our tollfree Meat and Poultry Hotline. For help, callers nationwide have only to dial 1-800-535-4555. For Washington, D.C. area residents, the number is 447-3333.

The Agricultural Marketing Service (AMS)

AMS inspects egg products for both domestic and foreign sale.

AMS inspectors keep certain kinds of restricted or "problem" eggs from being sold in the wholesale market. Thus, food processors like the makers of mayonnaise, egg noodles and ice cream and institutions like hospitals and nursing homes receive acceptable egg supplies.

Currently, AMS is coordinating USDA's public awareness campaign in response to the problem of the existence of salmonella bacteria inside some fresh, unbroken shell eggs. AMS is providing information on the proper storage and cooking of eggs in the home and in institutional settings like hospitals and nursing homes.

Other Federal Agencies

The Food and Drug Administration (FDA)

Part of the U.S. Department of Health and Human Services, FDA ensures the safety and wholesomeness of all foods sold in interstate commerce except meat, poultry and some egg products. The program is based on unannounced inspections and sampling of foods.

FDA also monitors for unsafe pesticide levels in food, and researches and develops standards on the composition, quality. nutrition and safety of food, including the safety of food and color additives.

There are approximately 60,000 food processing plants, warehouses, etc, subject to FDA inspection. Of the agency's some 7,000 full-time employees, 910 are inspectors and investigators whose duties cover domestic and imported food, as well as drugs and medical devices.

National Marine Fisheries Service

Located in the U.S. Department of Commerce, this agency offers a voluntary fee-for-service inspection program for fish products. Some 155 fish processors, brokers, retail and food service operations are now enrolled in the inspection program full time. In addition, some 400 spot inspections are currently carried out each year.

Some 325 Commerce Department and cross-licensed federal and local inspectors provide the service.

Inspection services include vessel and plant sanitation, product evaluation (including inspection, grading and certification for domestic, import and export products), laboratory analyses and review of product labels.

The Environmental Protection Agency (EPA)

EPA regulates the manufacture, labeling and use of all pesticides. Through its Office of Pesticides and Toxic Substances, the agency is responsible for approving or "registering" pesticides to ensure that when used according to label directions they will not pose significant risks to human health or the environment.

EPA also sets tolerance levels, or maximum legal limits, for pesticide residues in foods marketed in the U.S. to ensure that consumers are not exposed to unsafe pesticide residue levels.

In addition, EPA works cooperatively with the states to investigate incidents of potential pesticide misuse and to prevent such occurrences.

EPA sets national drinking water standards for all public drinking water supplies currently numbered at about 200,000. FDA standards for bottled water sold nationwide must be modeled closely on these standards.

State and Local Governments

Adding their muscle to federal efforts, state and local governments put considerable energy into food inspection. Some of this is done cooperatively with federal agencies, both to maximize staff effectiveness and to ensure that state standards meet federal rules.

There are cooperative federal and state programs for fish, dairy and other food product inspection.

Roughly half the states have their own meat and poultry inspection programs. State-inspected meat and poultry products may only be sold within that state's boundaries.

Local governments inspect restaurants, fast food spots and similar outlets. They can close establishments for sanitary violations.

—by Herb Gantz

Chapter 7

Food Advice for Emergencies

Chapter Contents

Section 7.1

Help, Power Outage!

(Source: *Food News for Consumers*, Summer 1989.)

When summer storms cause power outages jeopardizing food, here's what to do.

Keep the Freezer Closed

Keep what cold air you have inside. Don't open the door any more than necessary.

You'll be relieved to know that a full, freestanding freezer will stay at freezing temperatures about 2 days; a half-full freezer about 1 day.

If your freezer is not full, group packages together so they form an "igloo" protecting each other.

And, if you think power will be out for several days, try to find some dry ice. Follow the handling instructions carefully. You don't want to touch the dry ice or breathe the fumes in an enclosed area.

Twenty-five pounds of dry ice should hold a 10-cubic-foot full freezer 3 to 4 days.

Although dry ice can be used in the refrigerator, block ice is better. You can put it in the refrigerator's freezer unit and place your refrigerated perishables there—meat, poultry, dairy items.

Group meat and poultry to one side or on a tray so that if they begin thawing, their juices won't get on other food.

If Food Has Started to Thaw, What Can Safely be Kept?

You will have to evaluate each item separately. See the charts [at the end of this section] for different frozen and refrigerated foods. Generally, be very careful with meat and poultry products or any food containing milk, cream, sour cream or soft cheese. When in doubt, throw them out.

What about How the Food Will Taste?

Raw meats and poultry from the *freezer* can usually be refrozen without too much quality loss.

Prepared foods, vegetables and fruits can normally be refrozen, but there may be some quality loss. Fruits and fruit juices can be refrozen with minimal quality loss.

Refrigerated items should be safe as long as power is out no more than a few hours. After that, you may have to discard them unless block ice was added to the refrigerator or they were transferred to the freezer.

These are rule-of-thumb guides. For the actual handling of specific foods, follow the instructions in the charts [at the end of this section].

Be sure to discard any fully-cooked items in either the freezer or the refrigerator that have come into contact with raw meat juices.

Remember, you can't rely on appearance or odor. Never taste food, either, to determine its safety! Some foods may look and smell fine, but if they've been at room temperature too long, food poisoning bacteria may have multiplied enough to cause illness.

Be Prepared

If you live in an area where loss of electricity from summer storms is a problem, you can plan ahead to be prepared for the worst.

- Stock up on shelf-stable foods—canned goods, juices and the new "no-freeze" dinners in paper cartons that last 6-8 months.

- Plan ahead for ice. Buy some freeze-pak inserts and keep them frozen. Buy a cooler. Freeze water in plastic containers.

- Know in advance where you can buy dry and block ice.

- Develop emergency freezer sharing plans with friends in another part of town or in a nearby area.

For more information, call the Meat and Poultry Hotline toll-free at 1-800-535-4555. In the metropolitan Washington, D.C. area call 447-3333.

—by Herb Gantz and Diane VanLonkhuyzen

	Food still cold, held at 40° F or above under 2 hours	Held above 40° F for over 2 hours
Dairy		
Milk, cream, sour cream, buttermilk, evaporated milk, yogurt	Safe	Discard
Butter, margarine	Safe	Safe
Baby Formula, opened	Safe	Discard
Eggs		
Eggs, fresh Hard-cooked in shell Egg Dishes	Safe	Discard
Custards and puddings	Safe	Discard
Cheese		
Hard cheeses, processed cheeses	Safe	Safe
Soft cheeses, cottage cheese	Safe	Discard
Fruits		
Fruit juices, opened	Safe	Safe
Canned fruits, opened	Safe	Safe
Fresh fruits, coconut, raisins, dried fruits, candied fruits, dates	Safe	Safe
Vegetables		
Vegetables, cooked Vegetable juice, opened	Safe	Discard after 6 hours
Baked potatoes	Safe	Discard
Fresh mushrooms, herbs and spices	Safe	Safe
Garlic, chopped in oil or butter	Safe	Discard
Casseroles, soups, stews	Safe	Discard
Meat, Poultry, Seafood		
Fresh or leftover meat, poultry, fish or seafood	Safe	Discard

Figure 7.1a. *Refrigerator Food—When to Save It When to Throw It Out*

	Food still cold, held at 40° F or above under 2 hours	Held above 40° F for over 2 hours
Meat, Poultry, Seafood (con't)		
Thawing meat or poultry	Safe	Discard if warmer than refrigerator temperatures
Meat, tuna, shrimp, chicken, egg salad	Safe	Discard
Gravy, Stuffing	Safe	Discard
Lunchmeats, hotdogs, bacon, sausage, dried beef	Safe	Discard
Pizza - meat topped	Safe	Discard
Canned meats (NOT labeled "Keep Refrigerated") but refrigerated after opening	Safe	Discard
Canned hams labeled "Keep Refrigerated"	Safe	Discard

Pies, Pastry

Pastries, cream filled	Safe	Discard
Pies - custard, cheese filled or chiffons	Safe	Discard
Pies, fruit	Safe	Safe

Bread, Cakes, Cookies, Pasta

Bread, rolls, cakes, muffins, quick breads	Safe	Safe
Refrigerator biscuits, rolls, cookie dough	Safe	Discard
Cooked pasta, spaghetti	Safe	Discard
Pasta salads with mayonnaise or vinegar base	Safe	Discard

Sauces, Spreads, Jams

Mayonnaise, tartar sauce, horseradish	Safe	Discard if above 50° F for over 8 hours
Peanut butter	Safe	Safe
Opened salad dressing, jelly, relish, taco and barbeque sauce, mustard, catsup, olives	Safe	Safe

Figure 7.1b. *Refrigerator Food—When to Save It When to Throw It Out*

	Still contains ice crystals and feels as cold as if refrigerated	Thawed. Held above 40° F for over 2 Hours
Meat, Poultry, Seafood		
Beef, veal, lamb, pork and ground meats	Refreeze	Discard
Poultry and ground poultry	Refreeze	Discard
Variety meats (liver, kidney, heart, chitterlings)	Refreeze	Discard
Casseroles, stews, soups, convenience foods, pizza	Refreeze	Discard
Fish, shellfish, breaded seafood products	Refreeze. However there will be some texture and flavor loss.	Discard
Dairy		
Milk	Refreeze. May lose some texture.	Discard
Eggs (out of shell) and egg products	Refreeze	Discard
Ice Cream, frozen yogurt	Discard	Discard
Cheese (soft and semi-soft), cream cheese, Ricotta	Refreeze. May lose some texture.	Discard
Hard cheeses (cheddar, Swiss, Parmesan)	Refreeze	Refreeze
Casseroles containing milk, cream, eggs, soft cheeses	Refreeze	Discard
Cheesecake	Refreeze	Discard
Fruits		
Juices	Refreeze	Refreeze. Discard if mold, yeasty smell or sliminess develops.
Home or commercially packaged	Refreeze. Will change in texture and flavor.	Refreeze. Discard if mold, yeasty smell or sliminess develops.

Figure 7.2a. *Freezer Food—When to Save It and When to Throw It Out*

	Still contains ice crystals and feels as cold as if refrigerated	Thawed. Held above 40° F for over 2 Hours
Vegetables		
Juices	Refreeze	Discard after held above 40° F for 6 hours.
Home or commercially packaged or blanched	Refreeze. May suffer texture and flavor loss.	Discard after held above 40° F for 6 hours.
Breads, Pastries		
Breads, rolls, muffins, cakes (without custard fillings)	Refreeze	Refreeze
Cakes, pies, pastries with custard or cheese filling	Refreeze	Discard
Pie crusts	Refreeze	Refreeze
Commercial and homemade bread dough	Refreeze. Some quality loss may occur.	Refreeze. Considerable quality loss.
Other		
Casseroles - pasta, rice based	Refreeze	Discard
Flour, cornmeal, nuts	Refreeze	Refreeze

Figure 7.2b. *Freezer Food—When to Save It and When to Throw It Out*

Section 7.2

Facts about Food and Floods

(Source: Developed by the Food Marketing Institute in cooperation with the U.S. Department of Agriculture.)

Is Food Safe to Eat?

Foods that have come in contact with flood waters, or waters from broken pipes, can be dangerous to use. This [text] is intended to help you judge the safety of your foods after a flood or power outage.

You can save many canned foods if they are not dented or damaged. Follow the cleaning methods recommended in this [section]. Throw away any pantry-type foods or fresh foods that came in direct contact with flood water. Flood water may carry silt, raw sewage, oil, or chemical wastes. Refrigerator/freezer foods will need to be thrown out if your power was out for an extended period of time. See [the previous section and the "POWER OUT" recommendations below].

Water for Drinking, Cooking, or Cleaning

After a flood, consider all water unsafe! Listen for public announcements on the safety of your local water supply before using any water for drinking, cooking, or cleaning. If you must use water from your faucet, bring water to a rolling boil for 1 minute (3 to 5 minutes if you live in a high altitude area). Boiling water will make water safe from bacterial, viral, and parasitic diseases. Contact your local health department for specific recommendations if there has been a chemical contamination of your water.

Discard

- Fresh produce

- All glass/jarred foods, including "never opened" jars such as mayonnaise and salad dressing. Containers with cork-lined, waxed cardboard, pop tops, peel-off tops, or paraffin (waxed) seals are nearly impossible to clean around the lid/opening.

- All foods in cardboard boxes (e.g. juice boxes), paper, foil, cellophane, cloth, or any other kind of flexible container.

- Canned goods that are dented (on lids or seams), leaking, or bulging.

- Canned goods that are rusted **unless** the rust can be easily removed by light rubbing.

- Home canned foods

- Spices, seasonings and extracts

- Opened containers and packages of any kind.

- Flour, sugar, grains, pasta, coffee and other staples stored in canisters.

Save

- Canned goods that are not bulging, leaking or dented. **However, all cans must be thoroughly cleaned and sanitized**.

Cleaning Method for Canned Foods

1. Mark contents on the can with a permanent ink pen.

2. Remove paper labels as they can harbor dangerous bacteria.

3. Wash cans in a strong detergent solution with a scrub brush. Carefully clean areas around lids and seams.

4. Soak cans in a solution of two teaspoons of chlorine bleach per quart of room temperature water for 15 minutes.

5. Air dry cans before opening.

Throw away any cans that may have come in contact with industrial or septic waste. If you are unsure about the safety of any food, throw it out!

Power Out

Food in a refrigerator is generally safe if the power was out for less than 2 or 3 hours. Freezer foods will last longer. Food in a full, free-standing freezer will be safe for about 2 days; a half-full freezer for about 1 day. It is safe to refreeze thawed foods that still contain ice crystals. Do not rely on the appearance or odor of a food to determine if it is safe. Bacteria that cause foodborne illness can multiply rapidly on perishable foods that have been at room temperature for more than 2 hours.

Discard the Following Perishable Foods If Kept Above Refrigerator Temperature (40°F) for More than 2 Hours:

- raw or cooked meat, poultry or seafood
- milk/cream, yogurt, soft cheese
- cooked pasta, pasta salads
- custard, chiffon, or cheese pies
- fresh eggs, egg substitutes
- meat or cheese-topped pizza, luncheon meats
- casseroles, stew or soups
- mayonnaise, tartar sauce, and creamy dressings
- refrigerated cookie doughs
- cream-filled pastries

The Foods Listed Below Are Generally Safe Without Refrigeration for a Few Days.

However, double check each food and discard the food if it turns moldy or has an unusual odor or look. These foods spoil and lose quality much faster at warmer temperatures.

- butter, margarine
- fresh fruits and vegetables
- dried fruits
- opened jars of peanut butter, jelly, relish, taco sauce, barbecue sauce, ketchup, mustard, olives, oil-based salad dressings
- fruit juices
- hard or processed cheeses

Cleaning Up the Kitchen

Remember to clean and sanitize any kitchen areas/items that have come in contact with flood waters.

- Scrub kitchen counters, pantry shelves, refrigerators, stoves with warm soapy water. Rinse and wipe with a solution of two teaspoons of chlorine bleach to one quart of water using a clean cloth.

- Sanitize dishes and glassware the same way. To disinfect metal pans and utensils, boil them in water for 10 minutes.

- Discard wooden spoons, wooden cutting boards, plastic utensils, and baby bottle nipples and pacifiers. These items may absorb or hide bacteria making them difficult to clean and sanitize.

- Wash all kitchen linens in detergent and hot water. Use chlorine bleach to sanitize the linens following directions on the bleach container.

For addional information about the safe handling of food, contact USDA's Meat and Poultry Hotline toll-free at: 1-800-535-4555, 10:00 a.m. to 4:00 p.m., Eastern time, Monday through Friday; or contact your local Cooperative Extension Service Office.

For information on other flood-related safety issues contact your local or state health department, local Cooperative Extension Service, local American Red Cross chapter, or Civil Defense or emergency management office.

Section 7.3

Handling Food After a Fire

(Source: *Food News for Consumers*, Spring 1992.)

Fire! Few words can strike such terror. Nor is a residential fire an uncommon occurrence. Some 2 million American homes were hit last year. In the aftermath of fire, people are left with the unsettling task of salvaging their lives and belongings.

"Whether it's a house fire or just a fire in the refrigerator, people try to save whatever they can—including food," said Bessie Berry of the U.S. Department of Agriculture's Meat and Poultry Hotline.

"But, generally, saving food that's been in a fire is just not a good idea," Berry advised.

Food that's been exposed to fire can be compromised by three factors—the heat of the fire, smoke fumes and chemicals used to fight the fire.

Food in cans or jars may appear to be "okay," but if they've been close to the heat of the fire, they may no longer be edible. Why? Heat from the fire can activate food spoilage bacteria.

One of the most dangerous elements of a fire is sometimes not the fire itself, but toxic fumes released from burning materials. Those fumes can kill. They can also contaminate food.

Any type of food stored in permeable packaging—cardboard, plastic wrap, etc.—should be thrown away. Toxic fumes can penetrate the packaging and contaminate the food.

Also discard any raw foods stored outside the refrigerator, like potatoes or fruit, which could be contaminated by fumes.

Surprisingly, according to Berry, food that's stored in refrigerators or freezers can also become contaminated by fumes.

"We think of the refrigerator seal as air-tight, but it's usually not. Fumes can get inside," she said.

If food from your refrigerator has an off-flavor or smell when it's prepared, throw it away, Berry advised.

Chemicals used to fight fires also contain toxic materials and can contaminate food and cookware.

Foods that are exposed to chemicals should be thrown away. The chemicals cannot be washed off the food. This includes foods stored at room temperature, like fruits and vegetables, as well as foods stored in permeable containers like cardboard and screw-topped jars and bottles.

Canned goods and cookware exposed to chemicals can be decontaminated. Wash in a strong detergent solution and then dip in a bleach solution (2 teaspoons bleach per quart of water) for 15 minutes.

For the factsheet for families and individuals "Are You Ready for a Fire?" contact your local chapter of the American Red Cross."

Call the USDA's Meat and Poultry Hotline (1-800-535-4555), your local American Red Cross chapter, Civil Defense or emergency management office for additional information about handling food in disasters.

Fire Stoppers

The American Red Cross recommends that you

- Make your home fire-safe by installing battery-powered smoke detectors on each floor and in the garage. Test the detectors twice a year and keep a working fire extinguisher in the kitchen.

- Plan two emergency escape routes from each room in the house. Have rope or chain ladders for upstairs rooms. Agree on where to meet after the family "escapes."

- Have your own practice fire drills. Instruct everyone to crawl low under "smoke."

—by Dianne Durant

Chapter 8

Food Irradiation

Chapter Contents

Section 8.1

Facts about Food Irradiation

(Source: International Atomic Energy Agency, (Vienna, Austria), December 1991, Pub. No. 91-05549.)

Status and Trends

Food irradiation is the treatment of food by a certain type of energy. The process involves exposing the food, either packaged or in bulk, to carefully controlled amounts of ionizing radiation for a specific time to achieve certain desirable objectives. The process cannot increase the normal radioactivity level of the food, regardless of how long the food is exposed to the radiation, or how much of an energy "dose" is absorbed. It can prevent the division of living cells, such as bacteria, and cells of higher organisms, by changing their molecular structure. It can also slow down ripening or maturation of certain fruits and vegetables by causing biochemical reactions in physiological processes of plant tissues.

Who Is Interested in the Process?

Alongside traditional methods of processing and preserving food, the technology of food irradiation is gaining more and more attention around the world. In 37 countries, health and safety authorities have approved irradiation of altogether some 40 different foods, ranging from spices to grains to deboned chicken meat to fruits and vegetables. Twenty-four of these countries are actually applying the process for commercial purposes.

Decisions in these and other countries have been influenced by the adoption, in 1983, of a worldwide standard covering irradiated foods. The standard was adopted by the Codex Alimentarius Commission, a joint body of the Food and Agriculture Organization of the United Nations (FAO) and World Health Organization (WHO) representing more than 130 countries. It is based on the findings of a Joint Expert Committee on Food Irradiation (JECFI) convened by the FAO, WHO, and International Atomic Energy Agency (IAEA). JECFI has evaluated available data in 1969, 1976, and 1980. In 1980, it concluded that "the irradiation of any food commodity" up to an overall average dose of 10 kilogray "presents no toxicological hazard" and requires no further testing. It stated that irradiation up to 10 kilogray "introduced no special nutritional or microbiological problems" in foods.

Why Are Countries Interested?

Governmental interest in the process is emerging for many reasons. They are largely related to persistently high food losses from infestation, contamination, and spoilage; mounting concerns over foodborne diseases; and growing international trade in food products that must meet stiff import standards of quality and quarantine—all areas in which food irradiation has demonstrated practical benefits when integrated within an established system for the safe handling and distribution of food.

The FAO has estimated that worldwide about 25% of all food production is lost after harvesting to insects, bacteria and rodents. The use of irradiation alone as a preservation technique will not solve all the problems of post-harvest food losses. But it can play an important role in cutting losses and reducing the dependence on chemical pesticides. Many countries lose huge amounts of grain because of insect infestation, moulds, and premature germination. For roots and tuber, sprouting is the major cause of losses. Several countries, including Belgium, France, Hungary, Japan, Netherlands, and USSR are irradiating grains, potatoes, onions, and other products on an industrial scale. Pilot quantities of potatoes, onions, and garlic have been irradiated in Argentina, Bangladesh, Chile, China, Israel, Philippines, and Thailand.

Foodborne diseases pose a widespread threat to human health and they are an important cause of reduced economic productivity. Studies by the US Center for Disease Control show that even in the highly developed country of the United States, foodborne diseases caused by pathogenic bacteria, such as *Salmonella* and *Campylobacter* and by *Trichinae* and other parasites, claim an estimated 7000 lives annually and cause 24-81 million cases of diarrhoeal disease. Economic losses associated with foodborne diseases are high—estimated between US $5 billion and $17 billion by the US Food and Drug Administration.

The relatively low doses of radiation needed to destroy certain bacteria in food can be useful in controlling foodborne disease. Considerable amounts of frozen seafoods, as well as dry food ingredients, are irradiated for this purpose in Belgium and the Netherlands. Electron beam irradiation of blocks of mechanically deboned, frozen poultry products is carried out industrially in France. Spices are being irradiated in Argentina, Brazil, Denmark, Finland, France, Hungary, Israel, Norway, United States, and Yugoslavia.

Trade in food products is a major factor in regional or international commerce, and markets are growing. The inability of countries to satisfy each other's quarantine and public health regulations is a major barrier to trade. For example, not all countries allow importation of chemically treated fruit. Moreover, some countries, including the USA and Japan, have banned the use of certain fumigants identified as health hazards.

The problem is most acute for developing countries whose economies are still largely based on food and agricultural production. Radiation processing offers these countries an alternative to fumigation and some other treatments.

How Much Food Is Being Commercially Irradiated?

Each year about half a million tonnes of food products and ingredients are irradiated worldwide. This amount is small in comparison to the total volumes of processed foods and not many of these irradiated food products enter international commerce.

One factor influencing the pace of the development of food irradiation is public understanding and acceptance of the process. So far, this has been difficult to achieve, in view of the misconceptions and fears often surrounding nuclear-related technologies and the use of radiation.

To help address concerns and correct myths about food irradiation, a series of fact sheets has been prepared by the International Consultative Group on Food Irradiation (ICGFI). Currently (early 1991) 37 countries are participating in the work of ICGFI. The Group was established under the auspices of the FAO, IAEA, and WHO to advise the organizations and their Member States on the use of irradiation to solve food problems related to international trade, public health, economics, regulations, and public information. Information about ICGFI and the technology of food irradiation may be obtained by writing:

The ICGFI Secretariat
Joint FAO/IAEA Division of Nuclear Techniques
in Food and Agriculture
Wagramerstrasse 5
P.O. Box 100
A-1400 Vienna, Austria

Scientific and Technical Terms

The type of **radiation** used in processing materials is limited to radiations from high energy gamma rays, X-rays and accelerated electrons. These radiations are also referred to as **ionizing radiations** because their energy is high enough to dislodge electrons from atoms and molecules and to convert them to electrically charged particles called ions.

Gamma rays and **X-rays**, like radiowaves, microwaves, ultraviolet and visible light rays, form part of the electromagnetic spectrum, occurring in the short wave length, high energy region of the spectrum. They have the same properties and effects on materials, their origin being the main difference between them. X-rays with varying energies are generated by machines. Gamma rays with specific energies come from the spontaneous disintegration of radionuclides.

Naturally occurring and man-made **radionuclides**, also called **radioactive isotopes** or **radioisotopes**, are unstable, and emit radiation as they spontaneously disintegrate, or decay, to a stable state. The time taken by a radionuclide to decay to half the level of **radioactivity** originally present is known as its **half-life**, and is specific for each radionuclide of a particular element. The **becquerel** (Bq) is the unit of radioactivity and equals one disintegration per second.

Only certain radiation sources can be used in food irradiation. These are the radionuclides **cobalt-60** or **caesium-137**; **X-ray** machines having a maximum energy of five million electron volts (MeV); or **electron** machines having a maximum energy of 10 MeV. Energies from these radiation sources are too low to induce radioactivity in any material, including food.

The radionuclide used almost exclusively for the irradiation of food by gamma rays is cobalt-60. It is produced by neutron bombardment in a nuclear reactor of the metal cobalt-59, then doubly encapsulated in stainless steel "pencils" to prevent any leakage during its use in a radiation plant. Cobalt-60 has a half-life of 5.3 years. Caesium-137 is the only other gamma-emitting radionuclide suitable for industrial processing of materials. It can be obtained by reprocessing spent, or used, nuclear fuel elements and has a half-life of 30 years. However, because there are few reprocessing facilities worldwide, the uncertainty of market supply of commercial quantities of caesium-137 has meant that there is almost no demand for its use in radiation plants. In a report on irradiated foods, the American Council on Science and Health noted that "as of November 1988 all interested parties including the (US) Department of Energy now appear to agree that caesium-137 has no future in gamma processing."

Some **machine sources of radiation** are suitable for irradiating certain materials. High energy **electron beams** can be produced from machines capable of accelerating electrons. Electrons cannot penetrate very far into food, compared with gamma radiation or X-rays. X-rays of various energies are produced when a beam of accelerated electrons bombards a metallic target. Although X-rays have good penetrability into food, the efficiency of conversion from electrons to X-rays is generally less than 10%.

Radiation dose is the quantity of radiation energy absorbed by the food as it passes through the radiation field during processing. It is now generally measured by a unit called the **Gray** (Gy). In early work the unit was the **rad** (1 Gy = 100 rads). International health and safety authorities have endorsed the safety of irradiation for all foods up to a dose level of 10,000 Gy (10 kGy). In terms of energy relationships, one gray equals one joule of energy absorbed per kilogram of food being irradiated.

Food Irradiation and Radioactivity

Does the Irradiation Process Make Food Radioactive?

No. **Irradiation under controlled conditions does not make food radioactive.**

Everything in our environment, including food, contains trace amounts of radioactivity. This means that this trace amount (about 150 to 200 becquerels) of natural radioactivity (from elements such as potassium) is unavoidably in our daily diets.

In countries where food irradiation is permitted, both the sources of radiation and their energy levels are regulated and controlled. The irradiation process involves passing the food through a radiation field at a set speed to control the amount of energy or dose absorbed by the food. The food itself never comes into direct contact with the radiation source. The maximum allowable energies for electrons and X-rays—two machine-generated sources of radiation that can be used—are 10 million electron volts (MeV) and 5 MeV, respectively. Even when foods are exposed to very high doses of radiation from these sources, the maximum level of induced radioactivity would be just one-thousandth of a becquerel per kilogram of food. **This is 200,000 times smaller than the level of radioactivity naturally present in food.**

What Is the Difference Between the Terms "Irradiated Food" and "Radioactive Food?"

Irradiated foods are those that have been deliberately processed with certain types of radiation energy to bring about some desirable properties (for example, to inhibit sprouting or to destroy food-poisoning bacteria). Apart from foodstuffs, many other materials are commercially irradiated during manufacturing. These include cosmetics, wine bottle corks, hospital supplies and medical products, and some types of food packaging.

Radioactive foods, on the other hand, are those that have become accidentally contaminated by radioactive substances from weapons testing or nuclear reactor accidents. This type of contamination is totally unrelated to irradiated food which has been processed for preservation and other purposes.

Scientific and Technical References

"Measurement of induced radioactivity in electron- and photon-irradiated beef," by A. Miller and P.E. Jensen, *International Journal of Applied Radiation and Isotopes*, 38 (1987).

Safety of Irradiated Foods, by J.F. Diehl, Marcel Dekker Inc., New York (1990).

"Report on the Safety and Wholesomeness of Irradiated Foods," UK Advisory Committee on Novel and Irradiated Foods, HMSO, London (1986).

"Ionizing energy in food processing and pest control," Report No. 109, Council for Agricultural Science and Technology, Ames, Iowa (1986).

Chemical Changes in Irradiated Foods

Are Chemical Changes In Irradiated Foods, Such as the Formation of Radiolytic Products, Harmful?

No. In general the irradiation process produces very little chemical change in food. None of the changes known to occur have been found to be harmful or dangerous.

Some of the chemical changes produce so-called "radiolytic" products. These products have proven to be familiar ones, such as glucose, formic acid, acetaldehyde, and carbon dioxide, that are naturally present in foods or are formed by heat processing. The safety of these radiolytic products has been examined very critically, and no evidence of their harmfulness has been found.

Many scientific tests using highly sensitive analytical techniques have been done over the past 30 years in attempts to isolate and identify radiolytic products caused by irradiation. No substances truly unique to irradiated foods have been identified. The same products are always found, albeit in varying amounts, in fruits, vegetables, meats, and fish, for example, and in many other types of processed and unprocessed foods.

The United States Food and Drug Administration has estimated that the total amount of undetected radiolytic products that *might* be formed when food is irradiated at a dose of 1 kilogray would be less than 3 milligrams per kilogram of food—or less than 3 parts per million.

Do the "Free Radicals" Which Are Produced During Irradiation Affect the Safety of the Food?

No. There is no evidence to suggest that free radicals, per se, affect the safety of irradiated food.

Free radicals—which in scientific terms are atoms or molecules with an unpaired electron—can be formed during the irradiation process, as well as by certain other food treatments (such as toasting of bread, frying, and freeze drying) and during normal oxidation processes in food. They are generally very reactive, unstable structures, that continuously react with substances to form stable products.

Free radicals disappear by reacting with each other in the presence of liquids, such as saliva in the mouth. Consequently, their ingestion does not create any toxicological or other harmful effects. This has been confirmed by a long-term laboratory study in which animals were fed a very dry milk powder irradiated at 45 kilogray, more than four times the maximum approved dose for food irradiation. No mutagenic effects were noted and no tumors were formed. No toxic effects were apparent in the animals over nine successive generations. Similarly, a toast of bread (unirradiated), which actually contains more free radicals than very dry foods that have been irradiated, can be expected to be harmless.

Scientific and Technical References:

Recommendations for Evaluating the Safety of Irradiated Foods, by A.P. Brunetti et.al., Final Report prepared for the Director, Bureau of Foods, US Food and Drug Administration, Washington, DC (1980).

"Radiolytic Products-Are They Safe?" by C. Merritt, *Safety Factors Influencing the Acceptance of Food Irradiation Technology*, IAEA TECDOC-490, Vienna (1989).

Safety of Irradiated Foods, by J.F. Diehl, Marcel Dekker, Inc., New York (1990).

Nutritional Quality of Irradiated Foods

Does Irradiation Adversely Affect the Nutritional Value of Food?

No more so than other food processing and preservation methods used to achieve the same purpose.

Extensive research has shown that macronutrients, such as protein, carbohydrates, and fat are relatively stable to radiation doses of up to 10 kilogray. Micronutrients, especially vitamins, may be sensitive to any food processing method, including irradiation. Different types of vitamins have varied sensitivity to irradiation and to some other food processing methods. For example, vitamins C and B-1 (thiamine) are sensitive to irradiation as well as to heat processing. The Joint Expert Committee of the Food and Agriculture Organization (FAO), World Health Organization (WHO), and International Atomic Energy Agency (IAEA), which examined these and other issues, stated in its conclusions in 1980 that irradiation does not induce special nutritional problems in food.

The change in nutritional value caused by irradiation depends on a number of factors. They include the radiation dose to which the food has been exposed, the type of food, packaging, and processing conditions, such as temperature during irradiation and storage time.

Most of these factors are also true for other food preservation technologies. For example, measurement of vitamin C content in three varieties of apples kept in cold storage for up to 1 year showed decreases of between 40% to 70%, depending on the variety of apple. Yet it has never been suggested that cold storage is an inappropriate technology for apples and should not be used.

Reports of high vitamin losses from irradiation of pure vitamin solutions, or by using doses higher than those which would be used at commercial irradiation facilities, have no relevance for predicting the radiation sensitivity of a particular vitamin in food. The complexity of the composition of foods often protects individual vitamins from radiation decomposition.

Seemingly conflicting results of low versus high losses of vitamin C for some foods may be attributed to differences in analytical approaches used by researchers. Some have measured only ascorbic acid, while others have measured total vitamin C, a mixture of ascorbic acid and dehydroascorbic acid. Both acids have vitamin C biological activity and are easily transformed from one to the other. If only ascorbic acid were measured, any apparent reduction in vitamin C level would be exaggerated.

Just as vitamins vary in their sensitivity to heat, so do they vary in their sensitivity to radiation. This sensitivity depends upon the conditions under which food is irradiated. Vitamins A, E, C, K and B-1 (thiamine) in foods are relatively sensitive to radiation, while some other B vitamins such as riboflavin, niacin, and vitamin D are much more stable.

Losses are generally less if oxygen is excluded and if the temperature during irradiation is low. Under optimal conditions, vitamin losses in foods irradiated at doses up to 1 kilogray are considered to be insignificant. At higher doses the effect of irradiation will depend on the specific vitamin, temperature, dose, food, and packaging. Depending on the food, thiamine levels may be reduced further by storage and cooking if the food has been exposed to air during storage, but not necessarily if it has been packaged without oxygen.

Scientific and Technical References:

Safety of Irradiated Foods, by J.F. Diehl, Marcel Dekker Inc., New York (1990).

"Composition of Australian Foods, Apples and Pears," by R.B.H. Wills and El-Ghetany, *Food Technology in Australia*, 38 (1986).

Wholesomeness of Irradiated Food, Report of a Joint FAO/IAEA/WHO Expert Committee, Technical Report Series No. 659, World Health Organization, Geneva (1981).

Status of Food Safety and Inspection Service Irradiation Activities, USDA (September 1988).

Genetic Studies

Some Media Reports Claim that Studies in India Have Shown that Eating Irradiated Food Causes Development of Abnormal Chromosomes—Is This True?

No. The issue of abnormal chromosomes as a result of eating irradiated food has been more sensationalized than any other.

The claims focus on the incidence of "polyploidy," which is alleged to result from consumption of products made from wheat immediately after irradiation. Polyploidy means a multiple set of chromosomes. Human cells normally have 46 chromosomes. If they are polyploid they could have 92 or even 138 chromosomes. The incidence of polyploid cells is naturally occurring and varies among individuals; the significance of polyploidy is not known.

Media reports frequently cite results that were published in the mid-1970s by a group of scientists from the National Institute of Nutrition (NIN) in India. The scientists reported increases in the frequency of polyploid cells in rats, mice, monkeys, and even malnourished children that they attributed to consumption of products made from wheat immediately after irradiation at 0.75 kilogray. No polyploidy at all was seen when wheat was irradiated and stored for 12 weeks before consumption. A number of institutions in India and elsewhere have tried to repeat the studies conducted at NIN based on information made available to them. None of these institutions could come up with results similar to those found at NIN.

Reviews included one done by an independent investigative committee appointed by the Government of India. In 1976, the Committee concluded that the available data failed to demonstrate any mutagenic potential of irradiated wheat. A number of national scientific committees and independent researchers in Australia, Canada, Denmark, France, United Kingdom, and United States also have evaluated the alleged incidence of polyploidy. They all concluded that the reported data from NIN do not support the incidence of increased polyploidy.

In 1988 D. MacPhee and W. Hall, advisers to an Australian Parliamentary Committee Inquiry into the use of ionizing radiation, examined the NIN results. They concluded that the inability of other researchers to replicate the NIN results casts doubts upon the reliability of the NIN conclusions; that polyploidy is a poor measure of genetic damage; and that "major biological implausibilities" exist in the chain of occurrences "which allegedly links the consumption of irradiated food with the occurrence of genetic events."

Besides Feeding Tests Using Animals, Have There Been Any Human Feeding Studies of Irradiated Foods?

Yes. In the early 1980s, eight feeding studies using several irradiated food items, including irradiated wheat, were conducted in China using human volunteers. More than 400 individuals consumed irradiated food under controlled conditions for 7 to 15 weeks.

One focus of the research was the possibility of chromosomal changes. Seven of the eight experiments involved investigation of chromosomal aberrations in 382 individuals. No significant difference between the number of chromosomal aberrations in the control and the test groups could be discovered in any of the experiments. Incidences of polyploidy in those who consumed non-irradiated food and those who consumed irradiated samples were within the normal range of the overall value of polyploid cells in participants.

What Are Some of the Other Studies that Have Been Done in This Area?

Some other studies are occasionally cited as corroborating the NIN research. They include one by D.T. Anderson and colleagues reported in 1981. This study, which looked at dominant lethal mutations in mice that were fed irradiated diets, was among those reported by MacPhee and Hall, advisers to a parliamentary committee in Australia, as failing to replicate the NIN results. Another study sometimes cited as supporting the NIN research examined the level of polyploidy in the bone marrow cells of Chinese hamsters fed freshly irradiated laboratory animal diets. These diets were irradiated at 100 kilogray, a dose at least 125 times higher than that used for the NIN studies, and 10 times the internationally recommended limit for food irradiation. Frequently *not* cited is the author's own conclusion about the significance of his study: *"There is no evidence for any mutagenic effect being produced as a result of testing an irradiated diet."*

Extensive feeding tests have validated this conclusion. Over the last 20 years millions of mice, rats, and other laboratory animals have been bred and reared exclusively on an irradiated diet. The diet, treated at doses between 25 and 50 kilogray, has been fed to laboratory animals at many institutions involved in food, drug, and pharmaceutical research in Austria, Australia, Canada, France, Germany, Japan, Switzerland, United Kingdom, and United States. No transmittable genetic defects—teratogenic or oncogenic—have been observed which could be attributed to the consumption of irradiated diets.

Scientific and Technical References:

"An Analysis of the Safety of Food Irradiation: Genetic Effects," by D. MacPhee and W. Hall, *Use of Ionising Radiation*, Report of the House of Representatives Standing Committee on Environment, Recreation and the Arts, AGPS, Canberra (1988).

"Irradiated Laboratory Animal Diets. Dominant Lethal Studies in the Mouse," by D.T. Anderson et al., *Mutation Research*, 80 (1981).

Safety of Irradiated Foods, by J.F. Diehl, Marcel Dekker Inc., New York (1990).

Microbiological Safety of Irradiated Food

Can Irradiation of Food Increase the Risk of Botulism?

Irradiation at internationally recommended levels of up to 10 kilogray does not increase the risk from botulism any more so than other "substerilizing" food processes, such as pasteurization. Food treated by these methods must be handled, packaged, and stored following good manufacturing practices (GMPs). Doing so prevents the growth and toxin production of *Clostridium botulinum*. Alternatively, high-dose irradiation (30-60 kilogray) can be used to destroy any *Clostridium botulinum* organisms present in the food.

Some types of *Clostridia* cause more concern than others. *Clostridium botulinum Type E*, for example, is found at low levels in fish and seafood caught in some areas. It can grow and produce toxin even when the food is refrigerated at temperatures as low as 4°C. Thus, fish and seafood, including products treated by any of the sub-sterilizing processes including irradiation, must be kept at 3°C or below at all times during marketing. Most other types of *Clostridium botulinum* cannot grow and produce toxin at temperatures below 10°C. GMPs require that raw foods such as fish, meat, and chicken are stored at a specific temperature, whether irradiated or not, to prevent the growth of *Clostridium botulinum*.

Can Irradiation of Food Lead to Increased Microbiological Hazards?

No. The microbiological safety of irradiated foods has been investigated by international scientific bodies. One area that scientists have specifically looked at is the reduction of microorganisms that cause spoilage. These microorganisms warn consumers, through off odours or discoloration, that the food may be bad, or unsafe, to eat. Even if irradiation suppressed microorganisms in spoiled food, it cannot suppress the outward signs of spoilage and thus cannot be used to cover up spoiled food. In addition, scientific evidence indicates that proper irradiation can neither increase virulence of pathogenic microorganisms nor their ability to "grow better" in irradiated food.

In 1982, at the request of the Food and Agriculture Organization (FAO) of the United Nations and the World Health Organization (WHO), the Board of the International Committee on Food Microbiology and Hygiene considered the evidence for the microbiological safety of food irradiation. It concluded that modern food handling technology was adequate to control potential problems created by the suppression of spoilage microorganisms and that food irradiation does not present any increased microbiological hazards to health. Independent national expert committees in Denmark, Sweden, United Kingdom, USA, and Canada have since reaffirmed these conclusions. They essentially endorse the findings of the Joint Expert Committee on the Wholesomeness of Irradiated Foods convened in 1980 by the FAO, WHO, and International Atomic Energy Agency.

Important to note is that irradiation is not the only food processing technique which suppresses microorganisms signalling spoilage. Heat pasteurization, chemical treatments, and certain packaging methods have the same effect. Food processed by pasteurization-type methods must be properly packaged, handled, and stored to ensure safety.

Are Foods in Which Microbial Toxin Or Viruses Are Already Formed Suitable for Irradiation?

No, only foods of good hygienic quality should be irradiated. In this respect, irradiation does not differ from heat pasteurization, freezing, or other food processes. While these processes can destroy bacteria, they may not totally destroy preformed toxins and viruses already in the food. It is very important that foods intended for processing—by whatever method—are of good quality and handled and prepared according to good manufacturing practices (GMPs) established by national or international authorities. In some cases, strict regulations prohibit distribution of some foods. Many countries, for example, do not permit oysters to be harvested from areas known to be contaminated with raw sewage because of the danger of hepatitis viruses. No food processing methods should be used to substitute for GMPs in food production and handling.

Scientific and Technical References:

The Microbiological Safety of Irradiated Food, Codex Alimentarius Commission, CX/FH/83/9, Rome (1983).

"Irradiation in the Production, Processing, and Handling of Food", US Food and Drug Administration, final rule, *Federal Register*, 55 (85) 18538-18544 (2 May 1989).

Safety Factors Influencing the Acceptance of Food Irradiation Technology, IAEA TECDOC-490, Vienna (1988).

Safety of Irradiated Foods, by J.F. Diehl, Marcel Dekker Inc., New York (1990).

Irradiation and Food Safety

Can Irradiation Be Used to Make Spoiled Food Good, Or to Clean Up "Dirty" Food?

No. Neither irradiation nor any other food treatment can reverse the spoilage process and make bad food good. If food already looks, tastes or smells bad—signs of spoilage—before irradiation, it cannot be "saved" by any treatment including irradiation. The bad appearance, taste or smell will remain. Food irradiation is not magic.

Treatments such as heat pasteurization, chemical fumigation, and irradiation, however, are effective in destroying or suppressing microbial contamination of food. Heat pasteurization and fumigation have been effectively used in this way for decades to "clean up" foods, specifically to destroy pathogenic microorganisms in milk and other liquid products, and to destroy spoilage microflora or microorganisms and insects in spices and dry foods. These treatments are done intentionally for public health reasons; for example, to destroy microorganisms such as *Salmonella*, *Shigella*, and *Campylobacter* that are associated with food-borne diseases. Irradiation is especially effective as a control measure for parasitic diseases transmitted through solid food, especially those of animal origin.

Food processes such as heating, freezing, chemical treatment, and irradiation are not intended to serve as substitutes for good hygienic practices. Both at the national and international levels, good manufacturing practices (GMPs) govern the handling of specific foods and food products. They must be followed in the preparation of food, whether the food is intended for further processing by irradiation or any other means.

Scientific and Technical References:

"Food Irradiation," by Geoffrey Campbell-Platt, Professor of Food Technology, Department of Food Science and Technology, University of Reading, United Kingdom, The Food Safety Advisory Centre, London.

Report of the Second FAO/IAEA Research Co-ordination Meeting on the Use of Irradiation to Control Infectivity of Food-Borne Parasites, IAEA (1989).

"Irradiation of Dry Food Ingredients," by J. Farkas, CRC Press, Inc., Boca Raton, Florida (1988).

Irradiation and Food Additives and Residues

Does Irradiating Food that Contains Pesticide Residues Or Additives Present Any Health Hazards?

No. There is no scientific evidence to indicate any health hazard associated with irradiation of food containing pesticide residues and additives.

In the United States, the Food and Drug Administration (FDA) has examined the irradiation of foods containing pesticide residues. It specifically calculated the amount of radiolytic products that would be expected to be formed if foods containing pesticide residues were irradiated at a dose of 1 kilogray. This dose is in the upper range of that expected to be used for fruits, vegetables, and grains for disinfestation purposes. If the pesticide residue level in the food is about 1 part per million (an average level) then the calculated total yield of *all* radiolytic products from the pesticide residue would be about 0.000033 milligrams per kilogram of food, or 1 gram in 3000 tonnes of food. The FDA regards this amount as "virtually nil." It concludes that "the potential toxicity of each radiolytic product from a pesticide chemical residue in foods that are irradiated would be negligible" and that "such pesticide residues do not pose a hazard to health."

Studies have been done on food additives that assume the use of higher doses of radiation. A food additive is defined by the Codex Alimentarius Commission of the Food and Agriculture Organization and World Health Organization as a substance not normally used as a food ingredient but which is deliberately added to the food to produce a technological result. Colourants, man-made antioxidants, preservatives such as potassium sorbate, and polyphosphates are examples of food additives, forming 0.01 to 0.1% of the total food weight.

These studies indicate that at a radiation dose of 10 kilogray, which is the maximum dose allowed for food irradiation, yields of all radiolytic products from food additives range from 3 to 30 parts per billion. For a person with a total annual diet of 500 kilograms of food, these figures correspond to a negligible annual individual intake of radiolytic products—between 0.1 and 1 milligram—from an additive in a processed irradiated food that accounts for 5% of the total diet. The probability of harm occurring from radiolytic product formation from food additives is therefore considered to be extremely low indeed.

Scientific and Technical Reference:

Irradiation in the Production, Processing and Handling of Food; Final Rule, *Federal Register* 51;13376-99, U.S. Food & Drug Aministration (18 April 1986).

Packaging of Irradiated Foods

Is There Any Risk in Irradiating Foods in Contact with Plastic Or Other Packaging Materials?

No. Results of extensive research have shown that almost all commonly used food packaging materials tested are suitable for use at doses up to 10 kilogray, which is the internationally approved limit for irradiating foods.

Various types of packaging materials have been approved for use when food is irradiated. Their suitability for food intended for irradiation has been studied in Canada, the United Kingdom, the United States, and a few other countries. A number of food packaging materials were approved for use in food irradiation by the US Food and Drug Administration more than 20 years ago. More recently, Canada has approved additional materials, including a multilayered polyethylene film, as safe for packaging foods which will be irradiated.

Sophisticated tests have been used to evaluate the effect of radiation on plastic and other types of packaging materials. Researchers look at the material's post-irradiation stability, mechanical strength, and permeability to water and gases, and at the extractability of the plastics, additives, and adhesives.

Are Irradiated Materials Used to Package Foods?

Yes. Laminated plastic films with aluminium foil are routinely sterilized by radiation. They are used for hermetically sealed "bag-in-a-box" products, such as tomato paste, fruit juices, and wines. Other aseptic packaging materials, dairy product packaging, single-serving containers (for example, for cream), and wine bottle corks are also sterilized by irradiation prior to filling and sealing to prevent product contamination.

Other types of materials used to wrap food or other products also are routinely processed by radiation in many countries. The radiation process is used to "crosslink" the material's polymer chains for greater strength and heat resistance, and for producing plastics with special properties (for example, shrink wrap).

Scientific and Technical References:

"Packaging Irradiated Food," by J.J. Killoran, *Preservation of Food by Ionizing Radiation*, E.S. Josephson and M.S. Peterson, editors, CRC Press, Boca Raton, Florida (1983).

"Food Packaging Materials and Radiation Processing of Food: A Brief Overview," by N. Chuaqui-Offermans, *Radiation Physics and Chemistry*, 34 (6) (1989).

Safety of Irradiation Facilities

Have There Been Major Accidents at Industrial Irradiation Facilities?

Yes. Over the past 25 years, there have been a few major accidents at industrial irradiation facilities that caused injury or death to workers because of accidental exposure to a lethal dose of radiation. All of the accidents happened because safety systems had been deliberately bypassed and proper control procedures had not been followed. None of these accidents endangered public health and environmental safety.

In most cases, reports of "accidents" have actually turned out to be operational incidents. Such incidents have caused the irradiator to be shut down but they did not harm anyone or pose a risk to the environment. The distinction between accidents and incidents is used by authorities responsible for safety in all industries. This is the case for many other food technologies, such as canning, fumigation and the agro-chemical industry, which are also potentially hazardous to workers. As at irradiation facilities, controls and formal protocols are required to prevent accidents.

The radiation processing industry is considered to have a very good safety record. Today there are about 160 industrial gamma irradiation facilities operating worldwide, a number of which process food in addition to other types of products. Most irradiation facilities are used for sterilizing disposable medical and pharmaceutical supplies, and for processing other non-food items.

Do Workers at Irradiation Facilities Face Dangers from Long-Term Or Accidental Exposure to Radiation?

Any industrial activity includes certain risks to human beings and the environment. One of the risks at irradiation facilities is associated with the potential hazard of accidental exposure to ionizing radiation. Under normal operating conditions, all exposures of workers to radiation are prevented because the radiation source is shielded. Irradiators are designed with several levels of redundant protection to detect equipment malfunction and to protect personnel from accidental radiation exposure. Potentially hazardous areas are monitored and a system of interlocks prevents unauthorized entry into the radiation cell when the source is exposed. Worker safety further rests upon strict operating procedures and proper training. All radiation plants must be licensed. In most countries, regulations require periodic inspection of facilities to ensure compliance with the terms of operating licenses. In the United Kingdom, the Health and Safety Executive has reported to a parliamentary committee that personnel working in the country's 10 irradiation facilities face no unusual dangers: "...*the risk is kept under effective control by the use of sophisticated safety control systems. The plants are constructed with very heavy radiation shielding and thus the process presents no risk to the general public...We do not expect that the legalisation of foodstuffs irradiation will present any novel health and safety issues within our area of interest.*"

More Radioactive Materials Will Need to be Transported If More Food Irradiators Are Built. What Steps Have Been Taken to Minimize the Danger of Radioactive Spills from Transport Accidents?

Radioactive material required for irradiators is transported in lead-shielded steel casks. These are designed to meet national and international standards modelled upon the *Regulations for Safe Transport of Radioactive Materials* of the International Atomic Energy Agency. Large quantities of radioactive material are safely shipped all over the world to supply some 160 irradiators processing a variety of goods, mainly medical products such as syringes, physician gloves, sutures, and hospital gowns. From 1955 to early 1988, for example, Canada shipped approximately 190 million curies of cobalt-60 in 870 separate shipments without any radiation hazard to the environment or release of radioactive materials. Over the same period, approximately one million shipments of radioisotopes for industrial, hospital, and research use were made in North America without radiation accidents. This excellent safety record far exceeds that of other industries shipping hazardous materials such as toxic chemicals, crude oil, or gasoline. The same procedures used so successfully and safely to transport radioactive materials to existing irradiators will of course be used for transporting radioactive materials to any additional irradiators constructed for food processing.

Can an Accident at a Gamma Irradiation Facility Lead to "Meltdown" of the Irradiator and Release of Radioactivity that Would Contaminate the Environment and Endanger People Living Nearby?

No. It is impossible for a "meltdown" to occur in a gamma irradiator or for the radiation source to explode. The source of radiation energy used at irradiators cannot produce neutrons, substances which can make materials radioactive, so no nuclear "chain reaction" can occur at an irradiator. The walls of the irradiation cell through which the food passes, the machinery inside the cell, and the product being processed cannot become radioactive. No radioactivity is released into the environment.

Do Gamma Irradiators Have Radioactive Waste Disposal Problems?

No. Radioactive waste does not accumulate at irradiation facilities because no radioactivity is produced. The radiation energy used at some irradiators—namely electrons or X-rays—is generated by industrial machines called accelerators. At gamma irradiators, radionuclide sources, typically cobalt-60 or more rarely caesium-137, are used as the sources of radiation energy. These elements decay over time to non-radioactive nickel and non-radioactive barium, respectively. The sources are removed from the irradiator when the radioactivity falls to a low level, usually between 6% and 12% of the initial level (this takes 16 to 21 years for cobalt-60). The elements are then returned in a shipping container to the supplier who has the option of reactivating them in a nuclear reactor or storing them. Canada has calculated that all the cobalt-60 it supplied for use in 1988 (about 100 million curies) would require a storage space of about 1.25 cubic metres, roughly equivalent to the space occupied by a small desk.

Basically the same procedures are followed when an irradiation plant closes down. The sources can be acquired by another user or returned to the supplier, the machinery dismantled, and the building used for other purposes. There is no radiation hazard for the new occupants or the general public.

Scientific and Technical References:

Memorandum to the United Kingdom House of Lords Select committee on the European Communities Irradiation of Foodstuffs by the United Kingdom Health and Safety Executive, HMSO, London (1989).

Safety and radiation protection aspects of gamma and electron irradiation facilities, final draft, International Atomic energy Agency, Vienna (1990).

"Safety considerations in the design of gamma irradiation facilities and the handling of cobalt-60 sources," by R.G. McKinnon, *Radiation Physics and Chemistry*, 31 (1988).

Controlling the Process

Do Measures Exist to Control the Irradiation Process to Ensure that Foods Are Properly Treated?

Yes. Over the past 30 years, laws and regulations have been promulgated to govern operations at irradiators used to process non-food products, such as medical supplies. About 160 such irradiators are operating around the world. The plants, which must be approved by governmental authorities before construction, are subject to regular inspections, audits, and other reviews to ensure that they are safely and properly operated. These types of governmental controls would also be valid for irradiation facilities processing food. For example, the principle of lot traceability is an essential part of process controls, whether the product is a pharmaceutical or a fruit, and irrespective of the technology involved.

At the international level, provisional guidelines for good manufacturing practices (GMPs) and good radiation practices for a number of foods have been prepared by the International Consultative Group on Food Irradiation (ICGFI), a joint group of the Food and Agriculture Organization of the United Nations (FAO), World Health Organization (WHO), and International Atomic Energy Agency (IAEA). They cover all aspects of treatment, handling, and distribution. These guidelines provide a good basis for preparing the detailed protocols needed to implement irradiation on a commercial scale.

The guidelines emphasize that, as with all food technologies, effective quality control systems need to be installed and adequately monitored at critical control points at the irradiation facility. Foods should be handled, stored, and transported according to GMPs before, during, and after irradiation. Only foods meeting microbiological criteria and other quality standards should be accepted for irradiation.

The Codex Alimentarius Commission of FAO and WHO has further issued its recommended standards for the irradiation of food. These standards state that irradiated foods should be accompanied by shipping documents identifying the irradiator, date of treatment, lot identification, dose, and other details of treatment.

ICGFI additionally has established an international registry of irradiators that meet standards for good operations. It also organizes training courses for irradiator operators, plant managers, and supervisors on proper processing with emphasis on GMPs, dosimetry, record-keeping, and lot identification, and for food control officials on proper inspection procedures required for food irradiation processing and trade in irradiated foods.

Besides These Regulatory Controls, Are There Tests to Detect Whether Food Has Been Irradiated?

Yes, to some extent. Some scientific tests are being studied for use in determining whether foods have been irradiated. These include thermoluminescence measurement for detection of irradiated spices and electron spin resonance spectroscopy for determining irradiation of meats, poultry, and seafoods containing any bone or shells, and some specific chemical tests.

No single method, however, has yet been developed that reliably detects irradiation of all types of foods or the radiation dose levels that were used. This is partly because the irradiation process does not physically change the appearance, shape, or temperature of products and causes negligible chemical changes in foods.

The lack of a single test to identify a treated product is not unique to the irradiation process. Organically grown produce cannot be identified analytically, nor can meat slaughtered in accordance with Jewish or Islamic requirements. Additionally, chilled or frozen foods cannot be analyzed for unacceptable temperature fluctuations which might have occurred during distribution, nor can thermally sterilized (canned) foods be analyzed after treatment to assure that the correct time-temperature regime was applied.

Scientific and Technical References:

Codex General Standard for Irradiated Foods and Recommended International Code of Practice for the Operation of Irradiation Facilities Used for the Treatment of Food, The Codex Alimentarius, Vol. XV, (1984).

Manual of Food Irradiation Dosimetry, Technical Report Series No. 178, IAEA, Vienna (1977).

Codes of Good Irradiation Practice for Treatment of Various Food Commodities, International Consultative Group on Food Irradiation (1990).

American Society for Testing and Materials Standards, E1204 (Practice for Application of Dosimetry in the Characterization and Operation of a Gamma Irradiation Facility for Food Processing) and E1261 (for the Selection and Application of Dosimetry Systems for Radiation Processing of Food), American Society for Testing and Materials, Philadelphia, PA (1990).

Food Irradiation Costs

Will Irradiation Increase the Cost of Food?

Any food process will add cost. In most cases, however, food prices would not necessarily rise just because a product has been treated. Many variables affect food costs, and one of them is the cost of processing. Canning, freezing, pasteurization, refrigeration, fumigation, and irradiation will add cost to the product. These treatments will also bring benefits to consumers in terms of availability and quantity, storage life, convenience, and improved hygiene of the food.

Broken down, irradiation costs range from US $10 to $15 per tonne for a low-dose application (for example, to inhibit the growth of sprouts in potatoes and onions) to US $100 to $250 per tonne for a high-dose application (for example, to ensure hygienic quality of spices). These costs are competitive with alternative treatments. In some cases, irradiation can be considerably less expensive. For disinfestation of fruit in Thailand and the United States, for example, it has been estimated that the cost of irradiation would be only 10%-20% of the cost of vapour-heat treatment.

How Much Does a Typical Food Irradiation Facility Cost?

The cost to build a food irradiation plant is in the range of US $1 million to $3 million, depending on its size, processing capacity, and other factors. This is within the range of plant costs for other food technologies. For example, a moderately-sized, ultra-high temperature plant for sterilizing milk, fruit juices, and other liquids costs about US $2 million. A small vapour-heat treatment plant for disinfestation of fruits costs about US $1 million.

Scientific and Technical References:

Morrison, R.M. and Roberts, T., "Cost variables for Food Irradiators in Developing Countries," *Food Irradiation for Developing Countries in Africa*, IAEA TECDOC-576 (1990).

Handbook for Conducting Feasibility Studies, Proceedings of a Workshop on Economic Feasibility of Food Irradiation, ICGFI (1986).

Irradiated Foods and the Consumer

Is It True that Consumers Are Opposed to Buying Irradiated Food?

Opinion polls conducted in several Western countries tend to indicate that the majority of consumers would be unwilling to buy irradiated food. Most of these surveys, however, were made by telephone or through on-the-spot interviews without providing sufficient background information on the safety, benefits, and limitations of food irradiation. Uninformed consumers often do not distinguish irradiated food from radioactive food contaminated with radionuclides.

With regard to food, consumers' attitudes tend to be conservative towards acceptance of any new food and especially new food technology. This was clearly brought out, for example, when pasteurization of milk was introduced.

When consumers are given the opportunity to offer an informed opinion or make an informed choice, the results are different. This is substantiated by opinion polls conducted in connection with the provisions of accurate, factual information which yield more positive results. In market trials of labelled irradiated foods sold alongside the non-irradiated ones, consumers willingly bought irradiated products, and in many cases, expressed a preference for the irradiated product. Marketing trials have been conducted over the past several years in Argentina, Bangladesh, Chile, China, France, Hungary, Indonesia, Israel, Philippines, Poland, Thailand, and the USA—all with results favourable to irradiated food.

What Irradiated Food Products Have Been Commercially Marketed on a Trial Basis?

Many irradiated food products have been sold in a number of marketing trials in countries over the past 10 years. They include apples, potatoes, onions, strawberries, mangoes, papaya, dried fish, and fermented pork sausages. Consumer response to the irradiated products was always positive.

Mangoes. In September 1986, about 3 tons of mangoes were irradiated up to a dose of 1 kilogray in Puerto Rico to eliminate fruitfly infestation and delay spoilage. They were then flown to Miami, Florida, for marketing. They were labelled as having been irradiated and sold (with an accompanying information brochure) alongside nonirradiated mangoes at the Farmers Market in North Miami Beach. The irradiated mangoes, sold at the same or higher price than nonirradiated ones, were bought by shoppers who showed preference for the irradiated ones.

Papaya. In March 1987, a shipment of Hawaiian papaya was flown to Los Angeles, California, and irradiated at a dose of 0.41-0.51 kilogray to satisfy quarantine regulations. The papayas were fully labelled according to US Food and Drug Administration requirements, and then sold alongside papayas that had been hot-water dipped in Hawaii at two supermarkets in Anaheim and Irvine, California. Over 200 consumer questionnaires were completed during sales of the two lots of papaya. At the end of the day's market test, 60 kilograms of irradiated papaya and 5.1 kilograms of hot-water dipped papaya were sold, representing a ratio of more than 11:1 in favour of irradiated papaya. Two of every three participating consumers at Anaheim, and four of five at Irvine, stated that they would buy irradiated papaya again.

Strawberries. In separate marketing trials in 1987 and 1988 in Lyon, France, seven tonnes of strawberries irradiated at 2 kilogray were put on sale by a supermarket chain. The product was labelled with the "Radura" logo plus a statement of "ionization" and was sold at slightly higher cost than nonirradiated strawberries. Consumers said they bought irradiated strawberries because of their better quality.

Fermented pork sausages. In 1986, a popular fermented pork sausage (Nham) in Thailand was irradiated and sold alongside nonirradiated Nham in a few supermarkets in Bangkok. Normally consumed "raw" (without cooking or heating), Nham is often contaminated by microbial pathogens including *Salmonella* and occasionally by a parasite, *Trichinella spiralis*. To control these organisms, Nham was irradiated at a minimum dose of 2 kilogray and labelled as required by the Thai Food and Drug Administration. A survey of 138 consumers in 1986 showed that 34.1% bought irradiated Nham out of curiosity and 65.9% bought it because they believed it was safe from microbes. More than nine out of 10 consumers, 94.9%, indicated that they would buy irradiated Nham again. In the 3 months during which the survey was conducted in 1986, irradiated Nham outsold nonirradiated Nham by a ratio of 10:1.

In these tests and others, the most significant factor favouring irradiated food appears to be superior quality and safety. In none of these tests, which were carried out under actual market conditions, was there evidence to indicate that informed customers will not accept irradiated foods.

Are Irradiated Foods Being Sold on a Regular Basis?

Yes. Most irradiated food currently produced in 23 countries is destined for food processing industries and institutional markets (for example, catering services and restaurants). However, in some countries, such as France, Netherlands, South Africa, and Thailand, commercial quantities of some irradiated food items—including strawberries, mangoes, bananas, shrimp, frog legs, spices, and fermented pork sausages—have been sold on a regular basis. These irradiated food items, labelled to indicate the treatment and its purpose, have been successfully sold alongside their non-irradiated counterparts. Consumers have shown no apparent reluctance to purchase the irradiated food products.

Scientific and Technical References:

"Summary of the Puerto Rico Mango Consumer Test Marketing," by Giddings, G.C., *Food Irradiation Newsletter* 10, (1986).

"Consumer In-Store Response to Irradiated Papayas", by C.M. Bruhn and J.W. Noell, *Food Technology*, (September 1987).

"How to Win Consumer Acceptance in the Marketing of Irradiated Food," by P. Moog, *Factors Affecting Practical Application of Food Irradiation*, IAEA TECDOC-544 (1988).

"Consumer Acceptance of Irradiated Nham (fermented pork sausage)," by Y. Prachasitthisak, U. Pringsulka, and S. Chareon, *Food Irradiation Newsletter* 13, (1989).

Section 8.2

Poultry Irradiation and Preventing Foodborne Illness

(Source: USDA Food Safety and Inspection Service, September 1992.)

The Proposal

On September 21, 1992, the U.S. Department of Agriculture approved a rule to permit irradiation of raw, packaged poultry to control certain common bacteria on raw poultry that can cause illness when poultry is undercooked or otherwise mishandled. The rule permits irradiation of prepackaged fresh or frozen poultry at 1.5 to 3.0 kiloGray, the smallest, most practical *"dose"* of irradiation for bacterial control, with the goal of reducing the potential for foodborne illness.

The Food Safety and Inspection Service (FSIS), which is responsible for ensuring that meat and poultry products are safe, wholesome and accurately labeled, is the USDA agency approving the rule. The Food and Drug Administration (FDA) has confirmed that poultry irradiation is safe. FDA's approval is consistent with the views of the scientific community. Internationally, the Joint Expert Committee on Food Irradiation (which was made up of representatives from the World Health Organization of the United Nations and the International Atomic Energy Agency) is among many groups that endorsed the use of food irradiation.

FSIS wholeheartedly accepts the FDA determination. The role of FSIS is to determine how poultry irradiation could be carried out effectively.

Fresh/Frozen Poultry Only

The USDA rule will permit approved plants to irradiate retail and wholesale packages of fresh or frozen poultry (including such uncooked products as whole or cut-up birds, ground, hand-boned and skinless poultry).

The Problem: Potentially Harmful Bacteria

Salmonella, Campylobacter jejuni, and *Listeria monocytogenes* are found throughout the environment, especially on the farm, and in the intestines and on the skin and feathers of some chickens and turkeys (as well as other animals). If the poultry is mishandled—anywhere from the farm to the dinner table—the bacteria can multiply, and can cause illness in some people who eat the contaminated foods. (Thorough cooking destroys the bacteria and prevents illness.)

Irradiation in the range approved in the rule would eliminate from 99.5 to 99.9 percent of the *Salmonella* organisms on the treated poultry. Recent studies suggest that the sensitivity to irradiation is similar for *Salmonella* and *Listeria monocytogenes.* Therefore doses effective for *Salmonella* would also destroy *Listeria* bacteria. That fact has food safety importance, because *Listeria* contamination is difficult to control. *Listeria* multiply slowly even at refrigeration temperatures.

Irradiation Plus Safe Food Handling

Irradiation at the approved level would not necessarily destroy every single bacterial cell present; it would not sterilize the food. After treatment, any surviving organisms could start to multiply again if conditions are favorable. Open packages of irradiated poultry could also be recontaminated; for example, if a food handler were to omit washing his/her hands after using the bathroom and then were to touch the poultry.

Therefore, food handlers would have to handle irradiated poultry as carefully as all other foods.

Labeling Requirements

The new rule requires packages of irradiated poultry to carry the green, international radiation logo as well as the words *"Treated with Radiation"* or *"Treated by Irradiation."* Those words are to be in letters of the same style, color, and type as the product name and to be no less than one-third the size of the largest letter in the product name.

As is the rule for all fresh poultry, the label is also required to carry a handling statement, *"Keep Refrigerated,"* or *"Keep Frozen,"* as appropriate.

Foods That Can Be Irradiated In The United States

Dose Range	Purposes
Low-dose to 1 kiloGray (100 kilorads)	Control trichina parasite in fresh pork; Inhibit growth, maturation in fruits, vegetables, mushrooms, other fresh foods Control insects, mites, other arthropod pests in food
Medium-dose to 10 kiloGray (1,000 kilorads or 1 megarad)	Control microorganisms in dried enzymes Control bacteria in poultry that cause foodborne illness
High-dose above 10 kiloGray (above 1,000 kilorads or 1 megarad)	Control microorganisms in herbs, spices, teas and other dried vegetable substances

Dose: The international unit for quantifying the amount of radiation absorbed by a substance is the Gray (Gy). However, more people are more familiar with the older unit — kilorad (krad). A kilorad is 1,000 rads, and a Megarad is 1 million rads or 1,000 kilorads. The word "rad" stands for "radiation absorbed dose." 100 rad = 1 Gy.

Under the rule, only accurate and documented labeling claims about irradiation are allowed. For example, the label could say *"Irradiated to Control Foodborne Bacteria;"* but not *"pathogen free,"* or *"extended shelf life."*

Public Health Benefits

Poultry irradiation could play a significant role in preventing foodborne illness. Improper cooking and handling of contaminated poultry has been identified as a significant cause of illness; poultry irradiation has been shown to be a safe and effective treatment for reducing contamination on raw products.

How Poultry Irradiation Could Work

FSIS expects, for the near future, that most poultry irradiation will take place in federally inspected irradiation facilities that only perform that function, rather than in typical inspected poultry plants. Prepackaged poultry will be shipped under refrigeration to the plant, where pallets or containers of individually wrapped packages will be removed from the trucks and placed on a conveyor. The conveyor will pass into the irradiation *"chamber,"* where the poultry will be exposed for a pre-set time to absorb the correct dose of ionizing radiation.

The three types of irradiation FDA approved for poultry are gamma radiation, electron radiation and X-ray. Under FDA's approval and USDA's proposal, the radiation dose absorbed by the poultry and its packaging will be no less than 1.5 kiloGray (kGy) and no more than 3.0 kGy.

The rule requires that irradiation facilities meet safety standards and have quality controls to ensure proper handling and licensing of the radiation source and the safety of employees and the environment. Quality controls must be in place to ensure that poultry is processed correctly (including temperature and irradiation controls, packaging requirements, and steps to keep treated poultry separated from untreated poultry).

Packaging Requirements

Under the rule, only FDA-approved packaging materials—approved for use during irradiation—may be used. Fresh poultry must be packaged *before* it is irradiated, because even irradiated poultry could become contaminated if it is in the open, exposed to bacteria. FSIS inspectors must ensure that poultry plants have provided properly sealed packages to the irradiating facility.

To prevent cross-contamination from occurring, the packaging material must keep out liquids and microorganisms. However, the material must also allow air to enter the package, because airtight packaging may create an environment in which *Clostridium botulinum* bacterial spores that might be present could become active and produce the toxin that causes botulism.

Spoilage Bacteria

After irradiation at the approved dose, FDA determined enough spoilage-producing microbes would survive to provide warning signs of spoilage before any *C. botulinum* present could make the poultry toxic. FDA concluded, therefore, that "...irradiation of poultry at 3 kGy does not result in any additional health hazard from *C. botulinum*."

The Rulemaking Process

Irradiation is a technical process. Nevertheless, sources of radiation are considered *"food additives"* under the Food, Drug, and Cosmetic Act. Thus, poultry irradiation had to be approved first by the FDA. Then, FSIS, under the meat and poultry inspection laws, undertook rulemaking.

FDA Review and Approval of the FSIS Petition. On October 24, 1986, FSIS petitioned FDA to permit irradiation of retail-packaged frozen or fresh, uncooked poultry and mechanically separated poultry product. FDA also received a petition from Radiation Technology, Inc.

In reviewing the merits of the petitions, FDA evaluated toxicity studies on irradiated chicken, reports on the efficacy of the process and on the microbiological safety of irradiated poultry, and studies of the nutritional adequacy of the irradiated product.

FDA Finds Poultry Irradiation Safe and Effective. On May 1, 1990, FDA published its approval of poultry irradiation, concluding that at the absorbed dose of 3 kGy, irradiation does not pose a safety hazard to consumers and is effective in reducing bacterial levels—particularly of such illness-causing bacteria as *Salmonella* and *Campylobacter*. Furthermore, FDA concluded consuming irradiated poultry would not have an adverse impact on the nutritional value of a consumer's diet.

FSIS Develops Proposal to Permit Poultry Irradiation. After FDA approved the process in 1990, FSIS began developing this proposed rule.

FSIS Proposes Irradiation of Poultry. On May 6, 1992, FSIS proposed a rule to permit irradiation of raw, packaged poultry to control foodborne pathogens such as *Salmonella, Campylobacter*, and *Listeria monocytogenes*.

FSIS Approves Irradiation of Poultry. On September 21, 1992, FSIS approved the poultry irradiation rule.

Public Comments

In its May 1992 proposal on poultry irradiation, FSIS invited public comment. The agency received 1,062 comments in the 60-day comment period. Approximately half the comments favored the proposal, and half did not.

Many of the commenters who favored the rule were physicians or other health professionals. They supported the safety and endorsed poultry irradiation as an effective way to reduce foodborne illness.

Those who objected to the rule expressed concerns about worker, environmental and consumer safety. In the final rule, FSIS reviewed these concerns and clarified issues about worker and environmental safety. As the purpose of FDA's review, which culminated in its 1990 rule, was to address the safety question, FSIS focused on how irradiation could be used effectively on fresh poultry.

Marketing Irradiated Poultry

Irradiation facilities must apply for FSIS approvals-including approval of the facility, quality controls, and irradiation label. Only after all those steps are followed may irradiated poultry be marketed. The market demand for the product will determine the extent to which the technology is used. The cost has been estimated at about 1.5¢ per pound.

Permitting irradiated poultry could increase the Nation's exports to countries interested in buying irradiated poultry from the United States.

Protecting FSIS Inspectors

Irradiation plants are responsible for proper controls to prevent FSIS employees from exposure to radiation. For instance, because people cannot be in the chamber with the radiation source, each radiation area would have to be *"conspicuously posted"* with appropriate signs and/or barriers. Under the rule, if a plant violates safe work practices, FSIS will withdraw its inspectors, a step that will immediately halt operations.

FSIS will provide specialized safety and radiological health training for its employees assigned to irradiation facilities. In addition to oversight by other Federal agencies, FSIS also will ensure safe and healthful working conditions for its employees through a variety of other controls—including monitoring and maintaining records of radiation exposure.

Application for Inspection

Under FSIS rules, poultry plants that slaughter, cut up and package poultry for interstate commerce must have a Grant of Inspection. If such plants wish to add irradiation capabilities, however, under the rule the new operations also must meet the new quality control (QC) guidelines.

Irradiation facilities whose only function is to irradiate prepacked poultry must meet the necessary sanitation, facility, and operating requirements of existing regulations and must have an FSIS-approved QC system.

Under the rule, irradiation facilities also must verify to FSIS that they have met the requirements of all appropriate agencies. Several agencies are involved: the Nuclear Regulatory Commission (NRC), the Occupational Safety and Health Administration (OSHA), the National Institute of Standards and Technology (NIST) and the FDA. Also, NRC and OSHA can authorize State agencies to regulate radiation facilities, including compliance and safety inspections.

Quality Control System

Irradiation facilities must develop and follow a FSIS-approved QC system including:

Facility and Licensing Requirements. The plant must document its licensing by NRC, OSHA, or appropriate State authorities. Also, the facility must meet certain poultry inspection regulations. In addition, if the plant has no permanent refrigerated storage capacity, it must ensure adequate refrigeration during poultry irradiation.

Training. The plant must document that its personnel will operate under supervision of a trained person. Training must be sufficient and include: QC, food technology, irradiation process, and radiation health and safety.

Poultry Product and Packaging Material. The QC program must identify criteria to ensure the poultry receives an absorbed dose within the required range. The criteria relate to: the type of product (including its size, thickness, weight, and cut); the bulk density (the mass divided by its total volume); the proper packing configuration within the package; and the proper configuration of the entire packaged product (size, shape, number, and weight of the units on a pallet or container to be transported through the radiation chamber).

A guaranty or statement of assurance must accompany each shipment assuring the packaging material complies with the law and that the material is air-permeable, but excludes moisture and microorganisms from penetrating its barrier.

Dosimetry (Measuring Radiation). The QC system must include the American Society of Testing and Materials procedures and equipment used for measuring the dose of ionizing radiation absorbed by the product. To verify the correct dosage has been absorbed, measurements must be made on at least the first, middle, and last unit in each lot of poultry. The plant must demonstrate the accuracy of its dosimetry (measuring) system. Furthermore, the facility will be expected to show their system is calibrated every twelve months to NIST standards.

The QC system must have a means of ensuring that products do not receive more than the maximum allowed absorbed dose. Irradiation is permitted in more than one treatment as absorbed dose is cumulative, provided treatments are applied within the same day and if documentation is such that it assures the correctness of the total absorbed dose.

Labeling. The QC system must ensure proper labeling, as spelled out in the proposal.

Handling, Storage, and Transportation. The QC system must ensure that packages of poultry are intact; that the poultry is kept at appropriate temperatures throughout radiation processing and shipment; that procedures are spelled out for handling improperly irradiated or packaged poultry; that procedures are spelled out for preventing cross-contamination, re-irradiation, and mixing of irradiated and unirradiated products.

Corrective Action. The QC system must include procedures to correct failures and to prevent problems from reoccurring.

Recordkeeping

Under the proposal, irradiation plants must maintain for two years a written record of the QC system, their monitoring activity, and corrective actions taken.

Food Handling Education

Safe food handling would continue to be necessary for irradiated foods. USDA believes there is no such thing as too much food safety education. FSIS outreach includes information especially to benefit those most vulnerable to foodborne illness—the very young, the elderly, the immunocompromised, and for certain diseases pregnant women and their fetuses. FSIS also operates a nationwide toll-free Meat and Poultry Hotline (1-800-535-4555) that now reaches nearly 100,000 persons every year.

Part Two

Animal and Insect Borne Diseases

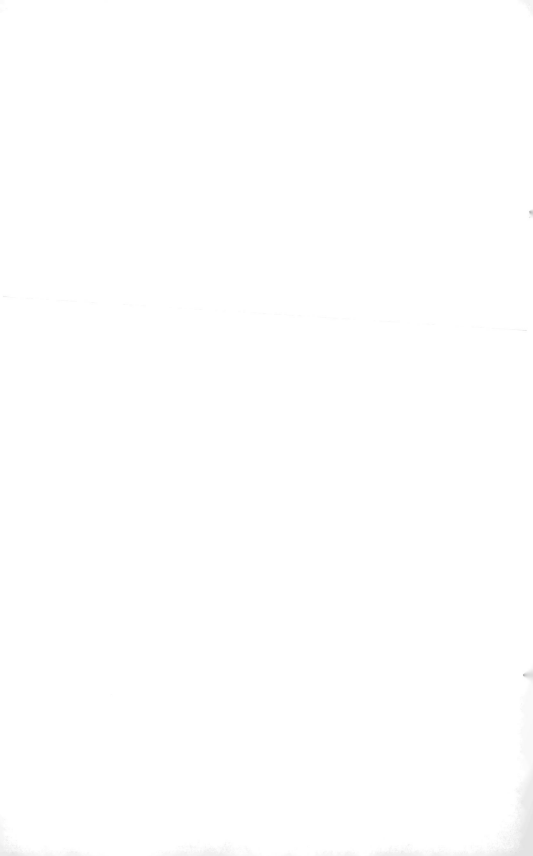

Chapter 9

Hantavirus

Chapter Contents

Section 9.1

Hantavirus Illness in the United States

(Source: CDC Document #310031, October 19, 1994.)

An outbreak of unexplained illness occurred in the Southwestern part of the United States in 1993. Laboratory findings from the Centers for Disease Control and Prevention indicate that the illness is caused by a hantavirus.

The newly recognized hantavirus-associated disease, called Hantavirus Pulmonary Syndrome (HPS), begins with one or more symptoms including fever, severe muscle aches, headache, and cough which progress rapidly to severe lung disease, often requiring intensive care treatment.

Since the hantavirus was discovered in 1993, less than 100 cases of HPS have been identified in 20 states. These states encompass the western half of the United States and most recently a few eastern states as well. Over half the people who get HPS die from the illness. In 1994, about two dozen cases have been confirmed. It is predicted that less than 50 cases will occur this year. So far the earliest known case dates back to 1975. Almost all cases have had evidence of close contact with rodents (deer mice or cotton rats).

Rodents are the primary reservoir host of the recognized hantaviruses. Each hantavirus appears to have a preferred rodent host, but other small mammals can be infected as well. Data strongly suggests that the deer mouse is the primary carrier of the hantavirus seen in all parts of the United States except the Eastern Coast and the Southeast. In the Southeast, the cotton rat has been identified as a carrier for the virus causing HPS. Evidence of infection has also been found in pinon mice, brush mice and western chipmunks. The deer mouse is highly adaptable and is found in different habitats, including human residences in rural and semirural areas, but generally not in urban centers.

Hantaviruses do not cause obvious illness in their rodent hosts. Infected rodents shed virus in saliva, urine, and feces for many weeks, but the duration and period of maximum infectivity are unknown.

Human infection may occur when infective saliva or excreta are inhaled as aerosols produced directly from the animal. Transmission

228

may also occur when fresh or dried materials contaminated by rodent excreta are disturbed, directly introduced into broken skin, introduced into the eyes, or, possibly, ingested in contaminated food or water. Persons have also become infected after being bitten by rodents.

Ticks, fleas, mosquitos and other biting insects are *not* known to have a role in the transmission of hantaviruses. Person-to-person transmission has *not* been associated with any of the previously identified hantaviruses or with the recent outbreak in the Southwest. Cats and dogs are *not* known to be a reservoir host of hantaviruses in the United States. However, these domestic animals may bring infected rodents into contact with humans.

Hantavirus pulmonary syndrome does not appear to be limited to a particular age, race, ethnic group, or gender. The chance of exposure to hantavirus is greatest when individuals work, play or live in closed spaces where there is an active rodent infestation. It is important to be aware of possible rodent exposure, for example, when working in crawl spaces, opening phone line stations or using air condition equipment after winter storage.

Travel to and within all areas where hantavirus infection has been reported is safe. The possibility of exposure to hantavirus for campers, hikers and tourists is very small and reduced even more if steps are taken to reduce rodent contact.

Cleaning of areas with small numbers of rodents should include wearing latex or rubber gloves and wetting down affected areas with general household disinfectant solutions such as Lysol or bleach and water or ammonia. Clearing of areas with large numbers of rodents includes wearing latex or rubber gloves, goggles, HEPA filter mask and wetting the area with disinfectant solutions or bleach and water.

Remember that the chances of getting HPS are very low. However, if you do get the disease, it can be very serious.

Section 9.2

Hantavirus Infection—Southwest United States

(Source: CDC Document #31002, October 21, 1994.)

Summary

This report provides interim recommendations for prevention and control of hantavirus infections associated with rodents in the southwestern United States. It is based on principles of rodent and infection control and contains specific recommendations for reducing rodent shelter and food sources in and around the home, recommendations for eliminating rodents inside the home and preventing them from entering the home, precautions for preventing hantavirus infection while rodent-contaminated areas are being cleaned up, prevention measures for persons who have occupational exposure to wild rodents, and precautions for campers and hikers.

Introduction

The recently recognized hantavirus-associated disease among residents of the southwestern United States and the identification of rodent reservoirs for the virus in the affected areas warrant recommendations to minimize the risk of exposure to rodents for both residents and visitors. While information is being gathered about the causative virus and its epidemiology, provisional recommendations can be made on the basis of knowledge about related hantaviruses. These recommendations are based on current understanding of the epidemiologic features of hantavirus infections in the Southwest; they will be periodically evaluated and modified as more information becomes available.

Rodents are the primary reservoir hosts of recognized hantaviruses. Each hantavirus appears to have preferential rodent hosts, but other small mammals can be infected as well. Available data strongly suggest that the deer mouse (Peromyscus maniculatus) is the primary reservoir of the newly recognized hantavirus in the southwestern United States. Serologic evidence of infection has also been found in pinon mice (P. truei), brush mice (P. boylii), cotton rats

230

(Sigmodon hispidus), and western chipmunks (Tamias spp.). P. maniculatus is highly adaptable and is found in different habitats, including human residences in rural and semirural areas, but generally not in urban centers.

Hantaviruses do not cause apparent illness in their reservoir hosts. Infected rodents shed virus in saliva, urine, and feces for many weeks, but the duration and period of maximum infectivity are unknown. The demonstrated presence of infectious virus in saliva of infected rodents and the marked sensitivity of these animals to hantaviruses following inoculation suggests that biting may be an important mode of transmission among rodents.

Human infection may occur when infective saliva or excreta are inhaled as aerosols produced directly from the animal. Persons visiting laboratories where infected rodents were housed have been infected after only a few minutes of exposure to animal holding areas. Transmission may also occur when dried or fresh materials contaminated by rodent excreta are disturbed, directly introduced into broken skin, introduced onto the conjunctivae, or, possibly, ingested in contaminated food or water. Persons have also become infected after being bitten by rodents.

Arthropod vectors are not known to have a role in the transmission of hantaviruses. Person-to-person transmission has not been associated with any of the previously identified hantaviruses or with the recent outbreak in the Southwest. Cats and dogs are not known to be reservoir hosts of hantaviruses in the United States. However, these domestic animals may bring infected rodents into contact with humans.

Known hantavirus infections of humans occur primarily in adults and are associated with domestic, occupational, or leisure activities that bring humans into contact with infected rodents, usually in a rural setting. Patterns of seasonal occurrence differ, depending on the virus, species of rodent host, and patterns of human behavior, cases have been epidemiologically associated with the following situations:

- planting or harvesting field crops;
- occupying previously vacant cabins or other dwellings;
- cleaning barns and other outbuildings;
- disturbing rodent-infested area while hiking or camping;
- inhabiting dwellings with indoor rodent populations;
- residing in or visiting areas in which the rodent population has shown an increase in density.

Hantaviruses have lipid envelopes that are susceptible to most disinfectants (e.g., dilute hypochlorite solutions, detergents, ethyl alcohol [70%], or most general-purpose household disinfectants). How long those viruses survive after being shed in the environment is uncertain.

The reservoir hosts of the hantavirus in the southwestern United States also act as hosts for the bacterium Yersinia pestis, the etiologic agent of plague. Although fleas and other ectoparasites are not known to play a role in hantavirus epidemiology, rodent fleas transmit plague. Control of rodents without concurrent control of fleas may increase the risk of human plague as the rodent fleas seek an alternative food source.

Eradicating the reservoir hosts of hantaviruses is neither feasible nor desirable. The best currently available approach for disease control and prevention is risk reduction through environmental hygiene practices that deter rodents from colonizing the home and work environment.

General Household Precautions in Affected Areas

Although epidemiologic studies are being conducted to identify specific behaviors that may increase the risk for hantavirus infection in humans in the United States, rodent control in and around the home will continue to be the primary prevention strategy. CDC has issued recommendations for rodent-proofing urban and suburban dwellings and reducing rodent populations through habitat modification and sanitation.

General Precautions for Residents of Affected Areas

Eliminate rodents and reduce the availability of food sources and nesting sites used by rodents inside the home:

- Follow the recommendations in the section on Eliminating Rodents Inside the Home.
- Keep food (including pet food) and water covered and stored in rodent-proof metal or thick plastic containers with tight-fitting lids.
- Store garbage inside homes in rodent-proof metal or thick plastic containers with tight-fitting lids.

- Wash dishes and cooking utensils immediately after use and remove all spilled food.
- Dispose of trash and clutter.
- Use spring-loaded rodent traps in the home continuously.
- As an adjunct to traps, use rodenticide with bait under a plywood or plastic shelter (covered bait station) on an ongoing basis inside the house.

Note: Environmental Protection Agency (EPA)-approved rodenticides are commercially available. Instructions on product use should always be followed. Products that are used outdoors should be specifically approved for exterior use. Any use of a rodenticide should be preceded by use of an insecticide to reduce the risk of plague transmission. Insecticide sprays or powders can be used in place of aerosols if they are appropriately labeled for flea control.

Prevent rodents from entering the home. Specific measures should be adapted to local circumstances:

- Use steel wool or cement to seal, screen, or otherwise cover all openings into the home that have a diameter greater than or equal to 1/4 inch.

- Place metal roof flashing as a rodent barrier around the base of wooden, earthen, or adobe dwellings up to a height of 12 inches and buried in the soil to a depth of 6 inches.

- Place 3 inches of gravel under the base of homes or under mobile homes to discourage rodent burrowing.

Reduce rodent shelter and food sources within 100 feet of the home:

- Use raised cement foundations in new construction of sheds, barns, outbuildings, or woodpiles.
- When possible, place woodpiles 100 feet or more from the house, and elevate wood at least 12 inches off the ground.
- Store grains and animal feed in rodent-proof containers.
- Near buildings, remove food sources that might attract rodents, or store food and water in rodent-proof containers.

- Store hay on pallets, and use traps or rodenticide continuously to keep hay free of rodents.
- Do not leave pet food in feeding dishes.
- Dispose of garbage and trash in rodent-proof containers that are elevated at least 12 inches off the ground.
- Haul away trash, abandoned vehicles, discarded tires, and other items that may serve as rodent nesting sites.
- Cut grass, brush, and dense shrubbery within 100 feet of the home.
- Place spring-loaded rodent traps at likely spots for rodent shelter within 100 feet around the home, and use continuously.
- Use an EPA-registered rodenticide approved for outside use in covered bait stations at places likely to shelter rodents within 100 feet of the home.

Note: Follow the recommendations specified in the section on Cleanup of Rodent-Contaminated Areas if rodent nests are encountered while these measures are being carried out.

Eliminating Rodents Inside the Home and Reducing Rodent Access to the Home

Rodent infestation can be determined by direct observation of animals or inferred from the presence of feces in closets or cabinets or on floors or from evidence that rodents have been gnawing at food. If rodent infestation is detected inside the home or outbuildings, rodent abatement measures should be completed. The directions in the section on Special Precautions should be followed if evidence of heavy rodent infestation (e.g., piles of feces or numerous dead animals) is present or if a structure is associated with a confirmed case of hantavirus disease.

Eliminating Rodent Infestation: Guidance for Residents of Affected Areas

- Before rodent elimination work is begun, ventilate closed buildings or areas inside buildings by opening doors and windows for at least 30 minutes. Use an exhaust fan or cross ventilation if possible. Leave the area until the airing-out period is finished. This airing may help remove any aerosolized virus inside the closed-in structure.

- Second, seal, screen, or otherwise cover all openings into the home that have a diameter of greater than or equal to ¼ inch. Then set rodent traps inside the house, using peanut butter as bait. Use only spring-loaded traps that kill rodents.

- Next, treat the interior of the structure with an insecticide labeled for flea control, follow specific label instructions. Insecticide sprays or powders can be used in place of aerosols if they are appropriately labeled for flea control. Rodenticides may also be used while the interior is being treated, as outlined below.

- Remove captured rodents from the traps. Wear rubber or plastic gloves while handling rodents. Place the carcasses in a plastic bag containing a sufficient amount of a general-purpose household disinfectant to thoroughly wet the carcasses. Seal the bag and then dispose of it by burying in a 2- to 3-foot-deep hole or by burning. If burying or burning are not feasible, contact your local or state health department about other appropriate disposal methods. Rebait and reset all sprung traps.

- Before removing the gloves, wash gloved hands in a general household disinfectant and then in soap and water. A hypochlorite solution prepared by mixing 3 tablespoons of household bleach in 1 gallon of water may be used in place of a commercial disinfectant when using the chlorine solution, avoid spilling the mixture on clothing or other items that may be damaged. Thoroughly wash hands with soap and water after removing the gloves.

- Leave several baited spring-loaded traps inside the house at all times as a further precaution against rodent reinfestation. Examine the traps regularly. Disinfect traps no longer in use by washing in a general household disinfectant or the hypochlorite solution. Disinfect and wash gloves as described above, and wash hands thoroughly with soap and water before beginning other activities.

Note: EPA-approved rodenticides are commercially available. Instructions on product use should always be followed. Products that are used outdoors should be specifically approved for exterior use. Any use of a rodenticide should be preceded by use of an insecticide to reduce the risk of plague transmission. Insecticide sprays or powders can be used in place of aerosols if they are appropriately labeled for flea control.

Clean Up of Rodent Contaminated Areas

Areas with evidence of rodent activity (e.g., dead rodents, rodent excreta) should be thoroughly cleaned to reduce the likelihood of exposure to hantavirus-infected materials. Clean-up procedures must be performed in a manner that limits the potential for aerosolization of dirt or dust from all potentially contaminated surfaces and household goods.

Clean-Up of Rodent-Contaminated Areas: Guidance for Residents of Affected Areas:

- Persons involved in the clean-up should wear rubber or plastic gloves.

- Spray dead rodents, rodent nests, droppings, or foods or other items that have been tainted by rodents with a general-purpose household disinfectant. Soak the material thoroughly and place in a plastic bag. When clean-up is complete (or when the bag is full), seal the bag, then place it into a second plastic bag and seal. Dispose of the bagged material by burying in a 2- to 3-foot-deep hole or by burning If these alternatives are not feasible, contact the local or state health department concerning other appropriate disposal methods.

- After the above items have been removed, mop floors with a solution of water, detergent, and disinfectant. Spray dirt floors with a disinfectant solution. A second mopping or spraying of floors with a general-purpose household disinfectant is optional. Carpets can be effectively disinfected with household disinfectants or by commercial-grade steam cleaning or shampooing. To avoid generating potentially infectious aerosols, do not vacuum or sweep dry surfaces before mopping.

- Disinfect countertops, cabinets, drawers, and other durable surfaces by washing them with a solution of detergent, water, and disinfectant, followed by an optional wiping-down with a general-purpose household disinfectant.

- Rugs and upholstered furniture should be steam cleaned or shampooed. If rodents have nested inside furniture and the nests are not accessible for decontamination the furniture should be removed and burned.

- Launder potentially contaminated bedding and clothing with hot water and detergent. (Use rubber or plastic gloves when handling the dirty laundry; then wash and disinfect gloves as described in the section on Eliminating Rodents Inside the Home.) Machine-dry laundry on a high setting or hang it to air dry in the sun.

Special Precautions for Homes of Persons with Confirmed Hantavirus Infection or Buildings with Heavy Rodent Infestations

Special precautions are indicated in the affected areas for cleaning homes or buildings with heavy rodent infestations. Persons conducting these activities should contact the responsible local, state or federal public health agency for guidance. Those precautions may also apply to vacant dwellings that have attracted numbers of rodents while unoccupied and to dwellings and other structures that have been occupied by persons with confirmed hantavirus infection. Workers who are either hired specifically to perform the clean-up or asked to do so as part of their work activities should receive a thorough orientation from the responsible health agency about hantavirus transmission and should be trained to perform the required activities safely.

Special Precautions for Clean-Up in Homes of Persons with Hantavirus Infection or Buildings with Heavy Rodent Infestation

- A baseline serum sample preferably drawn at the time these activities are initiated, should be available for all persons conducting the clean-up of homes or buildings with heavy rodent infestation. The serum sample should be stored at -20 C.

237

- Persons involved in the clean-up should wear coveralls (disposable if possible), rubber boots or disposable shoe covers, rubber or plastic gloves, protective goggles, and an appropriate respiratory protection device, such as a half-mask air-purifying (or negative-pressure) respirator with a high-efficiency particulate air (HEPA) filter or a powered air-purifying respirator (PAPR) with HEPA filters. Respirators (including positive-pressure types) are not considered protective if facial hair interferes with the face seal, since proper fit cannot be assured. Respirator practices should follow a comprehensive user program and be supervised by a knowledgeable person.

- Personal protective gear should be decontaminated upon removal at the end of the day. If the coveralls are not disposable, they should be laundered on site. If no laundry facilities are available, the coveralls should be immersed in liquid disinfectant until they can be washed.

- All potentially infective waste material (including respirator filters) from clean-up operations that cannot be burned or deep buried on site should be double bagged in appropriate plastic bags. The bagged material should then be labeled as infectious (if it is to be transported) and disposed of in accordance with local requirements for infectious waste.

- Workers who develop symptoms suggestive of HPS within 45 days of the last potential exposure should immediately seek medical attention. The physician should contact local health authorities promptly if hantavirus-associated illness is suspected. A blood sample should be obtained and forwarded with the baseline serum through the state health department to CDC for hantavirus antibody testing.

Precautions for Workers in Affected Areas Who Are Regularly Exposed to Rodents

Persons who frequently handle or are exposed to rodents (e.g. mammalogists, pest-control workers) in the affected area are probably at higher risk for hantavirus infection than the general public because of their frequency of exposure. Therefore, enhanced precautions are warranted to protect them against hantavirus infection.

Precautions for Workers in Affected Areas Who Are Exposed to Rodents

- A baseline serum sample, preferably drawn at the time of employment, should be available for all persons whose occupations involve frequent rodent contact. The serum sample should be stored at -20C.

- Workers in potentially high-risk settings should be informed about the symptoms of the disease and be given detailed guidance on prevention measures.

- Workers who develop a febrile or respiratory illness within 45 days of the last potential exposure should immediately seek medical attention and inform the attending physician of the potential occupational risk of hantavirus infection. The physician should contact local health authorities promptly if hantavirus-associated illness is suspected. A blood sample should be obtained and forwarded with the baseline serum through the state health department to CDC for hantavirus antibody testing.

- Workers should wear a half-face air-purifying (or negative-pressure) respirator or PAPR equipped with HEPA filters when removing rodents from traps or handling rodents In the affected area. Respirators (including positive-pressure types) are not considered protective if facial hair interferes with the face seal, since proper fit cannot be assured, Respirator use practices should be In accord with a comprehensive user program and should be supervised by a knowledgeable person.

- Workers should wear rubber or plastic gloves when handling rodents or handling traps containing rodents. Gloves should be washed and disinfected before removing them, as described above.

- Traps contaminated by rodent urine or feces or in which a rodent was captured should be disinfected with a commercial disinfectant or bleach solution. Dispose of dead rodents as described in the section on Eliminating Rodents Inside the Home.

- Persons removing organs or obtaining blood from rodents in affected areas should contact the Special Pathogens Branch, Division of Viral and Rickettsial Diseases, National Center for Infectious Diseases, Centers for Disease Control and Prevention, [telephone (404) 639-1115] for detailed safety precautions.

Precautions for Other Occupational Groups Who Have Potential Rodent Contact

Insufficient information is available at this time to allow general recommendations regarding risks or precautions for persons in the affected areas who work in occupations with unpredictable or incidental contact with rodents or their habitations. Examples of such occupations include telephone installers, maintenance workers, plumbers, electricians, and certain construction workers. Workers in these jobs may have to enter various buildings, crawl spaces, or other sites that may be rodent infested. Recommendations for such circumstances must be made on a case-by-case basis after the specific working environment has been assessed and state or local health departments have been consulted.

Precautions for Campers and Hikers in the Affected Areas

There is no evidence to suggest that travel into the affected areas should be restricted. Most usual tourist activities pose little or no risk that travelers will be exposed to rodents or their excreta. However, persons engaged in outdoor activities such as camping or hiking should take precautions to reduce the likelihood of their exposure to potentially infectious materials.

Reducing Risk of Hantavirus Infection: Guidance for Hikers and Campers

- Avoid coming into contact with rodents and rodent burrows or disturbing dens (such as pack rat nests).

- Do not use cabins or other enclosed shelters that are rodent infested until they have been appropriately cleaned and disinfected.

- Do not pitch tents or place sleeping bags in areas in proximity to rodent feces or burrows or near possible rodent shelters (e.g., garbage dumps or woodpiles).

- If possible, do not sleep on the bare ground. Use a cot with the sleeping surface at least 12 inches above the ground. Use tents with floors.

- Keep food in rodent-proof containers.

- Promptly bury (or—preferably—burn followed by burying, when in accordance with local requirements) all garbage and trash, or discard in covered trash containers.

- Use only bottled water or water that has been disinfected by filtration, boiling, chlorination, or iodination for drinking, cooking, washing dishes, and brushing teeth.

Conclusion

The control and prevention recommendations in this report represent general measures to minimize the likelihood of human exposure to hantavirus-infected rodents in areas of the southwestern United States affected by the outbreak of hantavirus-associated respiratory illness. Many of the recommendations may not be applicable or necessary in unaffected locales. The impact and utility of the recommendations will be assessed as they are implemented and will be continually reviewed by CDC and the involved state and local health agencies as additional epidemiologic and laboratory data related to the outbreak become available. These recommendations (which were developed in July [1994]) will be supplemented or modified in the future.

To receive additional recommendations for the prevention and control of hantavirus infections associated with rodents in the United States [by fax from the CDC] you will need to call 404-332-4565 and follow the prompts. The following documents on Hantavirus are available 310031, Hantavirus Illness in the United States; 310032, Hantavirus Illness Prevention Information; 310033, Guidelines for Removing Organs or Obtaining Blood from Rodents Potentially Infected with Hantavirus; 310034, Laboratory Management of Agents Associated with Hantavirus Pulmonary Syndrome Interim Biosafety Guidelines; 310035, State Contacts for Hantavirus Information.

Chapter 10

Lyme Disease

Chapter Contents

Section 10.1

Facts about Lyme Disease

(Source: Taken from an undated pamphlet produced by CDC's National Center for Infectious Diseases Division of Vector-Borne Infectious Diseases.)

Lyme disease was first recognized in the United States in 1975, after a mysterious outbreak of arthritis near Lyme, Connecticut. Since then, reports of Lyme disease have increased dramatically, and the disease has become an important public health problem in some areas of the United States.

Lyme disease is an infection caused by *Borrelia burgdorferi*, a member of the family of spirochetes, or corkscrew-shaped bacteria.

How the Disease is Spread

Lyme disease is spread by the bite of ticks of the genus *Ixodes* that are infected with *Borrelia burgdorferi*. The deer (or bear) tick, which normally feeds on the white-footed mouse, the white-tailed deer, other mammals, and birds, is responsible for transmitting Lyme disease bacteria to humans in the northeastern and north-central United States. (In these regions, this tick is also responsible for the spreading of babesiosis, a disease caused by a malaria-like parasite.) On the Pacific Coast, the bacteria are transmitted to humans by the western black-legged tick and in the southeastern states possibly by the black-legged tick.

Ixodes ticks are much smaller than common dog and cattle ticks. In their larval and nymphal stages they are no bigger than a pinhead. Adult ticks are slightly larger. Ticks can attach to any part of the human body but often attach to the more hidden and hairy areas such as the groin, armpits, and scalp.

Research in the eastern United States has indicated that, for the most part, ticks transmit Lyme disease to humans during the nymph stage, probably because nymphs are more likely to feed on a person and are rarely noticed because of their small size (less than 2 mm). Thus, the nymphs typically have ample time to feed and transmit the infection (ticks are most likely to transmit infection after approximately 2 or more days of feeding).

Tick larvae are smaller than the nymphs, but they rarely carry the infection at the time of feeding and are probably not important in the transmission of Lyme disease to humans.

Adult ticks can transmit the disease, but since they are larger and more likely to be removed from a person's body within a few hours, they are less likely than the nymphs to have sufficient time to transmit the infection. Moreover, adult *Ixodes* ticks are most active during the cooler months of the year, when outdoor activity is limited.

Ticks search for host animals from the tips of grasses and shrubs (not from trees) and transfer to animals or persons that brush against vegetation. Ticks only crawl; they do not fly or jump. Ticks found on the scalp usually have crawled there from lower parts of the body. Ticks feed on blood by inserting their mouth parts (not their whole bodies) into the skin of a host animal. They are slow feeders: a complete blood meal can take several days. As they feed, their bodies slowly enlarge.

Although in theory Lyme disease could spread through blood transfusions or other contact with infected blood or urine, no such transmission has been documented. There is no evidence that a person can get Lyme disease from the air, food or water, from sexual contact, or directly from wild or domestic animals. There is no convincing evidence that Lyme disease can be transmitted by insects such as mosquitoes, flies, or fleas.

Campers, hikers, outdoor workers, and others who frequent wooded, brushy, and grassy places are commonly exposed to ticks, and this may be important in the transmission of Lyme disease in some areas. Because new homes are often built in wooded areas, transmission of Lyme disease near homes has become an important problem in some areas of the United States. The risk of exposure to ticks is greatest in the woods and garden fringe areas of properties, but ticks may also be carried by animals into lawns and gardens.

Geographic Distribution

Lyme disease has a wide distribution in northern temperate regions of the world. In the United States, the highest incidence occurs in the

- Northeast, from Massachusetts to Maryland.
- North-central states, especially Wisconsin and Minnesota.
- West Coast, particularly northern California.

For Lyme disease to exist in an area, at least three closely inter-related elements must be present in nature: Lyme disease bacteria, ticks that can transmit them, and mammals (such as mice and deer) to provide food for the ticks in their various life stages. Ticks that transmit Lyme disease can be found in temperate regions that may have periods of very low or high temperature and a constant high relative humidity at ground level.

Life Cycle of Lyme Disease Ticks

Knowing the complex life cycle of the ticks that transmit Lyme disease is important in understanding the risk of acquiring the disease and in finding ways to prevent it.

The life cycle of these ticks requires 2 years to complete. Adult ticks feed and mate on large animals, especially deer, in the fall and early spring. Female ticks then drop off these animals to lay eggs on the ground. By summer, eggs hatch into larvae.

Larvae feed on mice and other small mammals and birds in the summer and early fall and then are inactive until the next spring when they molt into nymphs.

Nymphs feed on small rodents and other small mammals and birds in the late spring and summer and molt into adults in the fall, completing the 2-year life cycle.

Larvae and nymphs typically become infected with Lyme disease bacteria when they feed on infected small animals, particularly the white-footed mouse. The bacteria remain in the tick as it changes from larva to nymph or from nymph to adult. Infected nymphs and adult ticks then bite and transmit Lyme disease bacteria to other small rodents, other animals, and humans, all in the course of their normal feeding behavior.

Lyme Disease in Domestic Animals

Domestic animals may become infected with Lyme disease bacteria and some of these (dogs, for instance) may develop arthritis. Domestic animals can carry infected ticks into areas where humans live, but whether pet owners are more likely than others to get Lyme disease is unknown.

Symptoms and Signs of Lyme Disease

Early Lyme Disease. The early stage of Lyme disease is usually marked by one or more of the following symptoms and signs:

- fatigue
- chills and fever
- headache
- muscle and joint pain
- swollen lymph nodes
- a characteristic skin rash, called erythema migrans

Erythema migrans is a red circular patch that appears usually 3 days to 1 month after the bite of an infected tick at the site of the bite. The patch then expands, often to a large size. Sometimes many patches appear, varying in shape, depending on their location. Common sites are the thigh, groin, trunk, and the armpits. The center of the rash may clear as it enlarges, resulting in a "bulls-eye" appearance. The rash may be warm, but it usually is not painful. Not all rashes that occur at the site of a tick bite are due to Lyme disease, however. For example, an allergic reaction to tick saliva often occurs at the site of a tick bite. The resulting rash can be confused with the rash of Lyme disease. Allergic reactions to tick saliva usually occur within hours to a few days after the tick bite, usually do not expand, and disappear within a few days.

Late Lyme Disease. Some symptoms and signs of Lyme disease may not appear until weeks, months, or years after a tick bite:

- Arthritis is most likely to appear as brief bouts of pain and swelling, usually in one or more large joints, especially the knees.

- Nervous system abnormalities can include numbness, pain, Bell's palsy (paralysis of the facial muscles, usually on one side), and meningitis (fever, stiff neck, and severe headache).

- Less frequently, irregularities of the heart rhythm occur.

- In some persons the rash never forms; in some, the first and only sign of Lyme disease is arthritis, and in others, nervous system problems are the only evidence of Lyme disease.

Lyme Disease and Pregnancy

In rare cases, Lyme disease acquired during pregnancy may lead to infection of the fetus and possibly to stillbirth, but adverse effects to the fetus have not been conclusively documented. The Centers for Disease Control and Prevention (CDC) maintains a registry of pregnant women with Lyme disease to advance the understanding of the effects of Lyme disease on the developing fetus.

Diagnosis

Lyme disease is often difficult to diagnose because its symptoms and signs mimic those of many other diseases. The fever, muscle aches, and fatigue of Lyme disease can easily be mistaken for viral infections, such as influenza or infectious mononucleosis. Joint pain can be mistaken for other types of arthritis, such as rheumatoid arthritis, and neurologic signs can mimic those caused by other conditions, such as multiple sclerosis. At the same time, other types of arthritis or neurologic diseases can be misdiagnosed as Lyme disease.

Diagnosis of Lyme disease should take into account

- History of possible exposure to ticks, especially in areas where Lyme disease is known to occur.

- Symptoms and signs.

- The results of blood tests used to determine whether the patient has antibodies to Lyme disease bacteria. These tests are most useful in later stages of illness, but even then they may give inaccurate results. Laboratory tests for Lyme disease have not yet been standardized nationally.

Treatment and Prognosis

Lyme disease is treated with antibiotics under the supervision of a physician. Several antibiotics are effective. Antibiotics usually are given by mouth but may be given intravenously in more severe cases. Patients treated in the early stages with antibiotics usually recover rapidly and completely. Most patients who are treated in later stages of the disease also respond well to antibiotics. In a few patients who are treated for Lyme disease, symptoms of persisting infection may continue or recur, making additional antibiotic treatment necessary. Varying degrees of permanent damage to joints or the nervous system can develop in patients with late chronic Lyme disease. Typically these are patients in whom Lyme disease was unrecognized in the early stages or for whom the initial treatment was unsuccessful. Rare deaths from Lyme disease have been reported.

Section 10.2

Lyme Disease Prevention

(Source: Taken from NIH Pub. No. 92-3193.)

Avoidance of Ticks

At present, the best way to avoid Lyme disease is to avoid deer ticks. Although generally only about one percent of all deer ticks are infected with the Lyme disease bacterium, in some areas more than half of them harbor the microbe.

Most people with Lyme disease become infected during the summer, when immature ticks are most prevalent. Except in warm climates, few people are bitten by deer ticks during winter months.

Deer ticks are most often found in wooded areas and nearby grasslands, and are especially common where the two areas merge. Because the adult ticks feed on deer, areas where deer are frequently seen are likely to harbor sizable numbers of deer ticks.

To help prevent tick bites, people entering tick-infested areas should walk in the center of trails to avoid picking up ticks from overhanging grass and brush.

To minimize skin exposure to both ticks and insect repellents, people outdoors in tick-infested areas should wear long pants and long-sleeved shirts that fit tightly at the ankles and wrists. As a further safeguard, people should wear a hat, tuck pant legs into socks, and wear shoes that leave no part of the feet exposed. To make it easy to detect ticks, people should wear light-colored clothing.

To repel ticks, people can spray their clothing with the insecticide permethrin, which is commonly found in lawn and garden stores. Insect repellents that contain a chemical called DEET (N,N-diethyl-M-toluamide) can also be applied to clothing or directly onto skin. Although highly effective, these repellents can cause some serious side effects, particularly when high concentrations are used repeatedly on the skin. Infants and children may be especially at risk for adverse reactions to DEET.

Pregnant women should be especially careful to avoid ticks in Lyme disease areas because the infection can be transferred to the unborn child. Such a prenatal infection can make the woman more likely to miscarry or deliver a stillborn baby.

Checking for Ticks

Once indoors, people should check themselves and their children for ticks, particularly in the hairy regions of the body. The immature deer ticks that are most likely to cause Lyme disease are only about the size of a poppy seed, so they are easily mistaken for a freckle or a speck of dirt. All clothing should be washed. Pets should be checked for ticks before entering the house, because they, too, can develop symptoms of Lyme disease. In addition, a pet can carry ticks into the house. These ticks could fall off without biting the animal and subsequently attach to and bite people inside the house.

If a tick is discovered attached to the skin, it should be pulled out gently with tweezers, taking care not to squeeze the tick's body. An antiseptic should then be applied to the bite. Studies by NIH-supported researchers suggest that a tick must be attached for many hours to transmit the Lyme disease bacterium, so prompt tick removal could prevent the disease.

The risk of developing Lyme disease from a tick bite is small, even in heavily infested areas, and most physicians prefer not to treat patients bitten by ticks with antibiotics unless they develop symptoms of Lyme disease.

Tips for Personal Protection

- Avoid tick-infested areas, especially in May, June, and July (local health departments and park or agricultural extension services may have information on the seasonal and geographic distribution of ticks in your area.)

- Wear light-colored clothing so that ticks can be easily spotted.

- Wear long-sleeved shirts and closed shoes and socks.

- Tuck pant legs into socks or boots and tuck shirt into pants.

- Apply insect repellent containing permethrin to pants, socks, and shoes, and compounds containing DEET on exposed skin. Do not overuse these products.

- Walk in the center of trails to avoid overgrown grass and brush.

- After being outdoors in a tick-infested area, remove, wash, and dry clothing.

- Inspect the body thoroughly and remove carefully any attached ticks.

- Check pets for ticks.

How to Remove a Tick

- Tug gently but firmly with blunt tweezers near the "head" of the tick until it releases its hold on the skin.

- To lessen the chance of contact with the bacterium, try not to crush the tick's body or handle the tick with bare fingers.

- Swab the bite area thoroughly with an antiseptic to prevent bacterial infection.

Vaccine Development

Because Lyme disease is difficult to diagnose and sometimes does not respond to treatment, researchers are trying to create a vaccine that will protect people from the disorder. Vaccines work in part by prompting the body to generate antibodies. These custom-shaped molecules lock onto specific proteins made by a virus or bacterium—often those proteins lodged in the microbe's outer coat. Once antibodies attach to an invading microbe, other immune defenses are evoked to destroy it.

Development of an effective vaccine for Lyme disease has been difficult to create for a number of reasons. Scientists need to find out how the immune system protects against the bacterium because people who have been infected once can acquire the infection again. In addition, there are several different strains of the bacterium, each with its own distinct set of proteins, and bacteria within an individual strain may change the shape of their proteins over time so that antibodies can no longer identify and lock onto them.

Tick Eradication

In the meantime, researchers are trying to develop an effective strategy for ridding areas of deer ticks. Studies show that a single fall spraying of pesticide in wooded areas can substantially reduce the number of adult deer ticks residing there for as long as a year. Spraying on a large scale, however, may not be economically feasible and may prompt environmental or health concerns.

Scientists are also pursuing biological control of deer ticks by introducing tiny stingerless wasps, which feed on immature ticks, into tick-infested areas. Researchers are currently assessing the effectiveness of this technique.

Successful control of deer ticks will probably depend on a combination of tactics. More studies are needed before wide-scale tick control strategies can be implemented.

Research—The Key to Progress

Although Lyme disease poses many challenges, they are challenges the medical research community is well equipped to meet. New information on Lyme disease is accumulating at a rapid pace, thanks to the scientific research being conducted around the world.

Section 10.3

Lyme Disease Vaccine Update

(Source: Taken from "Getting Lyme Disease to Take a Hike,"
FDA Consumer, June 1994.)

Vaccines

A vaccine is usually made from a killed microbe, or part of it, that signals the immune system to mount an attack. A Lyme disease vaccine containing a protein from the surface of the spirochete, called Osp A, is being evaluated in humans. It is currently being tested for efficacy in preventing Lyme disease in high-risk northeastern populations.

Vaccine test results in mice published in the June 1992 issue of the *Proceedings of the National Academy of Sciences* suggest that this particular vaccine has a double effect, protecting the mice while also stemming the spread of infection by ticks. In the experiment, uninfected mice were given the vaccine, then exposed to ticks carrying the Lyme bacteria. Vaccinated mice not only remained free of infection, but when the ticks bit them, the antibodies the mice had made after stimulation with the vaccine killed the spirochetes in the ticks too! Mice given a placebo instead of the vaccine became infected. The researchers, from Yale University and Harvard University School of Public Health, hope that Lyme disease may be controlled by adding the vaccine to the plants and water supplies that wild rodents consume. If rodents can no longer harbor the Lyme bacteria, then ticks cannot become infected and spread the disease.

—by Ricki Lewis, Ph.D.

Ricki Lewis, Ph.D., is a writer in Scotia, N. Y., and a biology textbook author.

253

Section 10.4

Lyme Disease—United States, 1993

(Source: *Morbidity and Mortality Weekly Report*, August 12, 1994.)

In 1982, CDC initiated surveillance for Lyme disease (LD), and in 1990, the Council of State and Territorial Epidemiologists adopted a resolution making LD a nationally notifiable disease. This report summarizes surveillance data for LD in the United States during 1993.

LD is defined as the presence of an erythema migrans rash or at least one objective sign of musculoskeletal, neurologic, or cardiovascular disease and laboratory confirmation of infection (*1*). In 1993, 8185 cases of LD were reported to CDC by 44 state health departments, 1492 (15%) fewer cases than were reported in 1992 (9677) (Figure 10.1). Most cases were reported from the northeastern, mid-Atlantic, north-central, and Pacific coastal regions (Figure 10.2). Six states (Alaska, Arizona, Colorado, Mississippi, Montana, and South Dakota) reported no LD cases. The overall incidence rate was 3.3 per 100,000 population. Eight states in established LD-endemic northeastern and upper north-central regions reported rates of more than 3.3 per 100,000 (Connecticut, 41.3; Rhode Island, 27.3; Delaware, 21.0; New York, 15.5; New Jersey, 10.1; Pennsylvania, 8.9; Wisconsin, 8.2; and Maryland, 3.8); these states accounted for 6962 (85%) of the cases reported nationally. Of the total cases, 6132 (75%) were reported from 81 counties that had at least five cases and had rates of at least 10 per 100,000 population.

Most (83%) of the decrease in 1993 resulted from reductions in the numbers of case reports from four states in which LD is endemic (California, Connecticut, New York, and Wisconsin). New York, which reported 34% of the U.S. cases in 1993, accounted for 41% of the decrease (609 cases), and Connecticut accounted for 27% of the decrease (410 cases). Thirteen states reported small increases in the number of cases. New Jersey had the largest increase (786 cases, compared with 681 in 1992).

The age distribution of persons reported with LD was bimodal, with peaks occurring for children aged 5-14 years (1098 cases) and adults aged 30-49 years (2298 cases). Males (51%) and females were nearly equally affected.

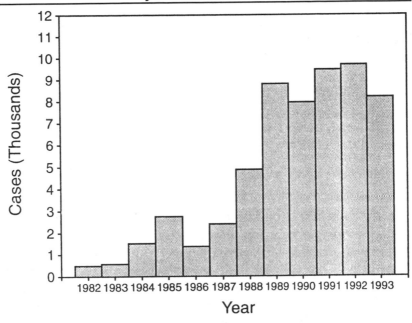

*In 1982, 11 states reported cases, compared with 44 in 1993.

Figure 10.1. *Reported cases of Lyme disease, by year—United States, 1982-1993. in 1982, 11 states reported cases, compared with 44 in 1993.*

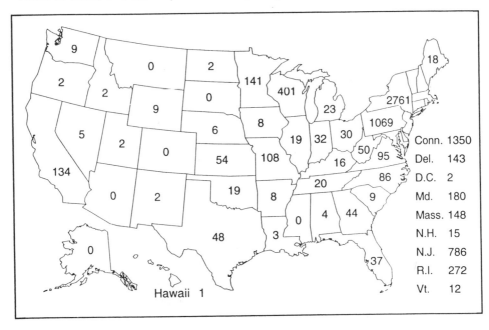

Conn.	1350
Del.	143
D.C.	2
Md.	180
Mass.	148
N.H.	15
N.J.	786
R.I.	272
Vt.	12

Hawaii 1

Figure 10.2. *Reported cases of Lyme disease, by state—United States, 1993.*

Reported by: State health departments. Bacterial Zoonoses Br, Div of Vector-Borne Infectious Diseases, National Center for Infectious Diseases, CDC.

Editorial Note: LD, the most commonly reported vectorborne infectious disease in the United States (2), is caused by the spirochete *Borrelia burgdorferi* and is transmitted by the bite of an infected *Ixodes* tick. In the northeastern and upper north-central regions of the United States, the principal tick vector is *Ixodes scapularis* (black-legged tick), and in Pacific coast states, the principal vector is *Ixodes pacificus* (western black-legged tick).

LD risks are geographically limited; rates vary substantially by town or other geo-political area within counties (3,4), and the distribution of vector ticks varies greatly, even within individual residential properties (5). LD can be prevented by avoiding contact with the tick vector or by applying insect repellents and acaricides as directed, wearing long pants and long-sleeved shirts, tucking pants into socks, checking regularly for ticks, and promptly removing attached ticks.

The decrease in reported cases in 1993 may reflect a combination of three factors: decreased reporting by physicians, decreased case detection (6), and a true decrease in the number of cases. In Connecticut and New York, vector surveillance data suggest that *I. scapularis* population densities were lower in 1993 than in previous years. The decrease in New York also may be attributed to limitations in staffing and decreased reporting by physicians (D. White, Bureau of Communicable Diseases, New York State Department of Health, personal communication, 1994). The increase in New Jersey was attributed to an increase in reported cases from Hunterdon County as a result of improved reporting by physicians and a true increase in disease incidence (CDC, unpublished data, 1993). The actual incidence of LD in the United States is unknown, and estimates are subject to the influences of underreporting, misclassification, and over-diagnosis.

Accurate surveillance data are needed to target populations for LD prevention strategies (e.g., vaccination). In 1993, two U.S. manufacturers received Food and Drug Administration approval to conduct field trials of LD vaccines in humans. One manufacturer is conducting Phase III efficacy trials involving approximately 10,000 participants from endemic areas of the north central, mid-Atlantic, and New England states. The second manufacturer is conducting Phase II safety and immunogenicity trials involving approximately 400 persons residing in New England. Results of Phase I trials conducted in the United States have been published (7), and preliminary results of Phase II safety and efficacy trials (8,9) suggest the vaccine is safe and immunogenic. Both candidate vaccines use a recombinant outer-surface protein as the immunogen. The candidate vaccines stimulate production of antibodies that target *B. burgdorferi* in the midguts of infected ticks while they extract blood from a vaccinated animal (10).

Reliable identification of risks is required for targeting individually applied interventions for LD. LD surveillance data will be needed to determine the effectiveness of control and prevention efforts.

References

1. CDC. Case definitions for public health surveillance. MMWR 1990;39(no. RR-13):19-21.

2. Dennis DT. Epidemiology. In: Coyle PK, ed. Lyme disease. St. Louis:Mosby-Year Book, 1993:27-37.

3. Cartter ML, Mshar P, Hadler JL. The epidemiology of Lyme disease in Connecticut. Conn Med 1989;53:320-3.

4. White DJ, Chang H-G, Benach JL, et al. The geographic spread and temporal increase of the Lyme disease epidemic. JAMA 1991;266:1230-6.

5. Maupin GO, Fish D, Zultowsky J, Campos EG, Piesman J. Landscape ecology of Lyme disease in a residential area of Westchester County, New York. Am J Epidemiol 1991;133:1105-13.

6. CDC. Lyme disease—United States, 1991-1992. MMWR 1993;42:345-8.

7. Keller D, Koster FT, Marks DH, Hosbach P, Erdile LF, Mays JP. Safety and immunogenicity of a recombinant outer surface protein A Lyme vaccine. JAMA 1994;271:1764-8.

8. Hoecke CV, De Grave D, Hauser P, Lebacq E. Evaluation of three formulations of a candidate vaccine against Lyme disease in healthy adult volunteers. In: Proceedings of the VI

International Congress on Lyme Borreliosis. Bologna, Italy: International Congress on Lyme Borreliosis, 1994:123-6.

9. Hosbach P, Koster F, Wormser G, et al. Clinical studies in humans of outer surface protein A (Osp A) vaccine for Lyme disease [Abstractl. In: Proceedings of the VI International Congress on Lyme Borreliosis. Bologna, Italy: International Congress on Lyme Borreliosis, 1994.

10. Fikrig E, Telford SR, Barthold SW, Kantor FS, Spielman A, Flavell RA. Elimination of *Borrelia burgdorferi* from vector ticks feeding on Osp A-immunized mice. Proc Natl Acad Sci 1992;89:5418-21.

Section 10.5

Research on Chronic Lyme Disease

(Source: An unnumbered fact sheet produced by the national institute of Allergy and Infectious Diseases, December 1994.)

In parts of the United States, the most common tick-borne disease is Lyme disease. This emerging infectious disease is caused by a spirochetal (spiral-shaped) bacterium, *Borrelia burgdorferi*. Lyme disease usually is treated successfully in the early stages with antibiotics. Patients who go untreated or who do not respond to antibiotics may develop a chronic multi-system disease with an unpredictable array of symptoms. Many of these symptoms mimic those of other diseases. Diagnostic tests that detect antibodies in the serum of the blood are imperfect, contributing further to the misdiagnosis of this disease.

Chronic Lyme disease most often produces persistent arthritis or nervous system problems, although the heart also can be involved. Lyme arthritis usually affects one or several large joints, often the knee. If the central nervous system is involved, symptoms may include headaches, nausea and vomiting, memory loss and a variety of other cognitive, behavioral and sleep problems. Involvement of the peripheral nerves can result in radiating pain in the limbs, numbness and partial paralysis.

No one knows why in some patients with late Lyme disease symptoms eventually diminish or disappear, whereas in other patients the symptoms persist. Scientists think that in some cases the spirochete may evade the immune system. It then survives in numbers too low to be detected by conventional tests, yet high enough to produce illness. Persistent symptoms also may be the result of an overactive immune response that continues to injure the host's tissues long after the organism has been eradicated.

Continued research is essential to making progress against this disease. Since 1981, when NIAID scientists first isolated the responsible organism, the Institute has supported an active research program on Lyme disease. Much of this research focuses on the pathogenesis, or disease process. This includes the study of the biology of *B. burgdorferi*, how it evades the immune system, how it interacts with its human host, its genetic components that allow the organism to control surface protein expression, and differences in human genes that account for the variations in the immune response among individuals.

In January and again in October 1994, NIAID convened meetings to address the issues surrounding chronic Lyme disease. Attending were scientists involved in Lyme disease at NIH and elsewhere, physicians and patient advocates. The participants acknowledged that determining whether chronic Lyme disease is caused by persistent infection or is a post-infectious disorder is a major research goal. Finding the answer to this question for any individual patient will have an important bearing on his or her treatment. While the participants acknowledged the difficulties in carrying out clinical trials to evaluate chronic Lyme disease, they agreed that clinical trials are necessary to resolve questions about optimal treatment.

Participants agreed that the first trial should focus on a well-defined patient population with probable *B. burgdorferi* infection that might respond to antibiotics. Patients could then be selected on the basis of relapse or non-response following appropriate treatment for early-stage Lyme disease. This would provide common criteria for studying and treating this multi-symptom disease. Such patients might include (1) those with persistent arthritis or persistent fatigue or fibromyalgia; (2) those with cognitive abnormalities, neuroradiculitis, headache or encephalomyelitis; and (3) those with objective evidence of continuing *B. burgdorferi* infection.

The group discussed possible clinical trial designs for a treatment trial for patients with chronic Lyme disease. A Request for Proposals (RFP) reflecting this discussion will be issued in the coming year to solicit proposals for an antibiotic treatment trial.

In the fall of 1994, NIAID staff met with officials of the Centers for Disease Control and Prevention (CDC) to discuss standardization of the Western Blot diagnostic test. Guidelines for laboratories that perform and interpret serologic tests were developed and will be published in the CDC's Morbidity and Mortality Weekly Report (MMWR).

In addition, in fiscal year 1994 NIAID awarded eight new grants to study immune response to Lyme disease infection and vaccination and two contracts to study animal models of Lyme disease. These efforts will ultimately advance our understanding of chronic Lyme disease and lay the groundwork for future clinical trials.

NIAID, a component of the National Institutes of Health, supports research on AIDS, tuberculosis, Lyme disease and other infectious diseases as well as allergies and immunology. NIH is an agency of the U.S. Public Health Service, U.S. Department of Health and Human Services.

Section 10.6

Genetic Susceptibility to Chronic Lyme Arthritis

(Source: *Research Resources Reporter*, July 1991.)

Individuals who suffer the debilitating effects of chronic arthritis associated with Lyme disease may be genetically predisposed to such conditions, according to researchers at New England Medical Center in Boston and New York University Medical School. In a decade-long study involving 130 patients with Lyme disease, Dr. Allen C. Steere and his colleagues found that two hereditary factors, termed HLA-DR2 and HLA-DR4, are associated with chronic Lyme arthritis. In addition, the scientists determined that patients who have HLA-DR4 are less likely to respond to antibiotic therapy.

Dr. Steere, chief of rheumatology at New England Medical Center and professor of medicine at Tufts University School of Medicine, first described Lyme disease in 1977 following an outbreak of the disease around Lyme, Connecticut. Lyme disease is caused by the spirochete *Borrelia burgdorferi*, which is spread by tiny ticks.

According to the investigators, more than 90 percent of those who contract the disease initially show transient influenza-like symptoms such as headache and mild fever. Later, however, approximately 80 percent of patients develop joint problems of varying duration, and some of them have neurologic complications. About 1 in 10 patients develop chronic arthritis that may not respond to antibiotic therapy.

"The question we addressed is simply this: 'Is there anything genetically different about the 10 percent who go on to develop chronic arthritis?'" says Dr. Robert Winchester, professor of medicine at New York University Medical School. "The answer very clearly is that there is something genetically different, and the genes that are related to this difference are the HLA genes."

Human leukocyte antigen (HLA) genes, located on the sixth chromosome, are associated with susceptibility to a number of diseases, including diabetes mellitus, multiple sclerosis, and rheumatoid arthritis. "Each person has a unique collection of these particular genes. They're markers of biologic individuality. They also regulate the immune response and are critical elements in it," says Dr. Winchester.

The HLA genes determine the structure of glycoproteins called HLA antigens that are found on the surface of all cells of the body except red blood cells. These glycoproteins are the same molecules that induce graft rejection when tissues are transplanted from one person to another.

To determine if there is an immunogenetic basis for chronic Lyme arthritis, Dr. Winchester and Dr. Edward Dwyer, an instructor in medicine at New York University Medical School, tested blood samples from 130 patients with various manifestations of Lyme disease and identified the HLA antigens present on the surface of their white blood cells.

"There are six well-characterized HLA designations: A, B, C, DR, DQ, and DP, and all of these are associated with separate genes. But in the entire population individuals differ quite a bit in the detailed structure of these genes-in genetic terminology the variants are called alleles," explains Dr. Dwyer. "To determine HLA type, we have a whole set of antibodies against different HLA types, and we test these against the cells to see which ones interact. This gives us the HLA designation as defined by antibodies."

For comparison, the researchers also performed HLA typing on 86 noninfected subjects. No significant differences in the frequencies of HLA-A, B, or C were noted between control subjects and patients with arthritis.

Of the 130 patients with Lyme disease, 80 had Lyme arthritis. Of the 80 arthritis patients, 22 had arthritis of short duration (1 to 5 months), 30 had arthritis of moderate duration (6 to 11 months), and 28 had chronic arthritis (12 to 48 months' duration).

"Our results showed that 89 percent of patients with chronic arthritis had either the HLA-DR2 or DR4 specificities, and only 27 percent of those who had a transient arthritis had DR2 or DR4," says Dr. Winchester. "This means that if someone is infected by the microorganism the risk for developing chronic arthritis is 22 times greater for a DR2- or DR4-positive patient than for an individual who does not have those types."

HLA-DR4 was the primary marker for susceptibility to chronic arthritis. Fifty-seven percent of patients with chronic conditions expressed HLA-DR4, compared with only 23 percent who had moderate-duration arthritis and 9 percent who had short-duration arthritis. After the HLA-DR4-positive patients were excluded from each group, a secondary association was noted with HLA-DR2.

"This study, in my opinion, really showed that there was an immunogenetic basis behind chronic Lyme arthritis," says Dr. Steere.

In a second part of the study the scientists focused on patients who do not respond to antibiotic therapy. Most people who have Lyme arthritis can be successfully treated with penicillin or doxycycline, among other drugs.

Sixty patients with Lyme arthritis were treated with antibiotics. In 22 patients the arthritis disappeared within 3 months, but 38 patients did not improve. "We found that 53 percent of those who did not respond were DR4-positive, compared with only 9 percent of those who did respond," says Dr. Steere. "One of the two markers that predispose to chronic arthritis therefore also seems to predispose to diminished response to antibiotic therapy."

The researchers suggest two possible mechanisms to explain the onset of chronic Lyme arthritis in genetically susceptible people. One hypothesis is that HLA-DR4 or -DR2 may lead to an autoimmune response that continues even after the spirochete has been killed. An alternate explanation may be that people with HLA-DR2 or -DR4 are selectively immunodeficient. "In other words, they may lack some part of the immune system that's essential for getting rid of the organism with efficiency and dispatch, so the spirochete lingers on in these people," says Dr. Winchester.

"The best way of thinking of this second model is to say that people who have DR2 or DR4 have a 'hole' in their T-cell repertoire, so that in the process of becoming tolerant to themselves, they lose T-cells that are necessary for getting rid of the microorganism," adds Dr. Winchester. T-cells, or T-lymphocytes, are a type of white blood cell that can distinguish a body's own cells from foreign substances. By latching onto the antigens of foreign organisms or cells, T-cells initiate reactions that destroy the foreign matter.

The scientists' findings could have important implications for the development of vaccines for Lyme disease. "I think our study would tend to introduce a little note of caution. If the development of arthritis is an autoimmune process, then one would worry that vaccinating a person might result in an autoimmune disease in those who are genetically susceptible," suggests Dr. Winchester.

In addition to identifying HLA types through serological testing, the researchers also determined genetic variants, or alleles, of HLA-DR4 or -DR2 in five patients with chronic arthritis. "Serological testing is useful, but we've come to realize that there is not a single genetic entity of DR4 but rather a group of related alleles that encode for this type, and the alleles can only be detected by DNA analysis," says Dr. Dwyer.

In the late 1970's, before Lyme arthritis was described as a separate entity, the condition was thought by some scientists to be related to rheumatoid arthritis. However, DNA analysis has highlighted differences between the diseases. "Our studies pointed out that although DR4 is associated with both Lyme arthritis and rheumatoid arthritis (RA), patients with Lyme arthritis did not show the HLA-DR1 type that is associated with RA. And when we did the molecular analysis, we saw that the kind of DR4 allele we found in one of the Lyme patients was not the kind usually seen in RA. We need to do further work on that," Dr. Dwyer explains.

Although the first phase of their study is complete, the collaboration between Drs. Steere and Winchester continues. "We are quite interested in the patients who have chronic neurologic disease, and we are focusing on that right now. Among our other projects, we are looking at the T-cell immune responses that patients with chronic Lyme arthritis have to various parts of the spirochete in an effort to identify particular parts of the organism that seem to be stimulating this response.

"We are continuing to look at patients with arthritis; we do not consider the story closed," says Dr. Steere.

—by Victoria L. Contie

Additional reading:

1. Steere, A.C., Dwyer, E., and Winchester, R., Association of Chronic Lyme arthritis with HLA-DR4 and HLA-DR2 alleles. *New England Journal of Medicine* 323:219-223, 1990.

2. Steere, A.C., Lyme disease. *New England Journal of Medicine* 321:586-596, 1989.

3. Majsky, A., Bojar, M., Jirous, J., Lyme disease and HLA-DR antigens. *Tissue Antigens* 30:188-189, 1987.

The research described in this article was supported by the General Clinical Research Centers program of the National Center for Research Resources, the National Institute of Allergy and Infectious Diseases, and the National Institute of Arthritis and Musculoskeletal and Skin Diseases.

Chapter 11

Plague

Chapter Contents

Section 11.1

General Information

(Source: CDC Document No. 351500, September 27, 1994.)

Plague is caused by a bacterium named *Yersinia pestis* transmitted from rodent to rodent by fleas. Human cases of plague occur in three ways:

1. In most instances by the bite of an infected flea,

2. sometimes through exposure to plague infected animal tissue, and

3. occasionally from inhaling in infected droplets exhaled by animals or humans with plague pneumonia.

Plague is characterized by periodic disease outbreaks within a rodent population. The death rate among rodents is often very high. It is during these outbreaks that hungry infected fleas, having lost their normal hosts, seek other sources of blood thus increasing the risk to humans and other animals.

Epidemics of plague in humans usually involve house rats and their fleas. Rat-borne epidemics continue to occur in some developing countries, particularly in rural areas. The last rat-borne epidemic in the United States occurred in Los Angeles in 1924-25. Since then, all human plague cases in the U.S. have been acquired from wild rodents or their fleas.

Plague in North America is limited to the western states from the Pacific Coast eastward to Texas and Oklahoma. Rock squirrels and their fleas are the most frequent sources of human infection in the southwestern states. For the Pacific states, the California ground squirrel and its fleas are the most common source.

Many other rodent species, for instance, prairie dogs, deer mice, wood rats, chipmunks, and other ground squirrels and their fleas, suffer plague outbreaks and occasionally serve as sources of human infection. Less frequent sources of infection include wild rabbits, wild carnivores, and even antelope, which pick up their infections from wild rodent outbreaks. Domestic cats, and sometimes dogs are readily infected by fleas or from eating infected wild rodents and may serve as a source of infection to persons exposed to them. Pets may also bring plague-infected fleas into the home.

Between outbreaks, the plague bacterium is believed to circulate among certain populations of animals without causing much illness. Such groups of infected animals serve as silent, long-term reservoirs of infection.

Geographical Distribution of Plague

In the United States during the 1980's plague cases averaged about 18 per year. Most of the cases occurred in persons under 20 years of age. About 1 in 7 persons with plague died.

Worldwide there are one to two thousand cases each year. Epidemic plague during the 1980's has occurred at one place or another each year in Africa, Asia, or South America. Epidemic plague is generally associated with domestic rats. Almost all of the cases reported during the decade were rural and occurred among people living in small towns and villages or agricultural areas rather than in larger, more developed, towns and cities.

The following information provides a worldwide distribution pattern:

- There is no plague in Australia.

- There is no plague in western Europe; the last reported cases occurred immediately after World War II.

- In Asia and Eastern Europe, plague is distributed from the Caucasus Mountains in the Soviet Union, through much of the Middle East, eastward through China, and then southward to South. East Asia where it occurs in scattered localized geographic animal populations, called foci. Within these plague foci, there are isolated human cases and occasional outbreaks.

- In Africa plague foci are distributed from the north to the south on the eastern side of the continent, and in southern Africa. Severe outbreaks have occurred in recent years in Kenya, Tanzania, Zaire, and Botswana, with smaller outbreaks in other East African countries. Plague also has been reported in scattered foci in western and northern Africa.

- In North America, plague is found from the Pacific Coast eastward to western Texas and from British Columbia and Alberta, Canada southward to Mexico. Most of the human cases occur in two regions; one in northern New Mexico, northern Arizona, and southern Colorado, another in California, southern Oregon, and far western Nevada.

- In South America active plague foci exist in two regions, the Andean mountain region in parts of Bolivia, Peru, and Ecuador and in Brazil.

How Plague is Transmitted

Plague is transmitted from animal-to-animal and from animal-to-human by the bites of infective fleas. Less frequently, the organism enters through a break in the skin by direct contact with tissue or body fluids of a plague-infected animal, for instance, in the process of skinning a rabbit or other animal.

Primary plague pneumonia is transmitted by inhaling infected droplets expelled by the coughing of a person or animals, especially domestic cats, with pneumonic plague.

Transmission of plague from human-to-human is uncommon and has not been observed in the United States since 1924, but does occur as an important factor in plague epidemics in some developing countries.

Diagnosis

The classic feature of plague introduced through flea bite or a cut or break in the skin is a very painful, usually swollen, and often hot to the touch lymph node, called a bubo. This finding accompanied with fever, extreme exhaustion and a history of possible exposure to rodents, rabbits, or fleas in the *western* United States should lead to suspicion of plague.

Onset of bubonic plague is usually 2 to 6 days after a person is exposed. Initial manifestations include fever headache and general illness, followed by development of painful, swollen regional lymph nodes. Occasionally, buboes cannot be detected for a day or so after the onset of other symptoms. The disease progresses rapidly and invades the blood stream, producing severe illness, called plague septicemia.

Once a human is infected, a progressive illness generally results unless specific antibiotic drug therapy is given. Progression leads to a blood infection, and finally a lung infection. The infection of the lung is termed plague pneumonia, and can be transmitted to others through the inhalation of droplets expelled by the coughing of the plague pneumonia victim.

The incubation period of primary pneumonic plague is 1 to 3 days and is characterized by development of an overwhelming pneumonia with high fever, cough, bloody sputum, and chills. For plague pneumonia victims the death rate is over 60%.

Treatment Information

As soon as a diagnosis of suspected plague is made, the patient should be is isolated, and local and state health departments notified. Confirmatory laboratory work should be initiated, including blood cultures, and lymph node samples if possible. Drug therapy should begin as soon as possible after the laboratory specimens are taken. The best drug is streptomycin, but a number of other antibiotics are also effective.

Those individuals closely associated with the patient, particularly in cases with pneumonia, should be traced, identified, and evaluated. Contacts of pneumonic plague patients should be placed under observation or given preventive antibiotic therapy, depending on the degree and timing of contact.

It is a U.S. Public Health Service requirement that all suspected plague cases be reported to local and state health departments, and the diagnosis confirmed by the CDC. As required by the International Health Regulations, CDC reports all U.S. plague cases to the World Health Organization.

Prevention

Plague will probably continue to exist in its many localized geographic areas around the world and plague outbreaks in wild rodent hosts will continue to occur. Attempts to eliminate wild rodent plague are impractical and futile. Therefore, primary preventive measures are directed toward reducing the threat of infection in humans in high risk areas through three techniques—environmental management, preventive drug therapy, and vaccines.

Environmental

First, the prevention of epidemic plague requires the reduction or elimination of house rat populations in both urban and rural areas. This goal has been reached in the cities, towns, and villages of most developed countries. It has not been achieved in either the rural or urban areas of many developing countries where the threat of epidemic plague continues to exist. Control of plague in such situations requires two things:

1. Close surveillance for human plague cases, and for plague in rodents, and

2. The use of an effective insecticide to control the fleas associated with human plague cases and rodent outbreaks.

In regions such as the American west where plague is widespread in wild rodents the greatest threat is to people living, working, or playing in active infected areas. Plague preventive measures in such areas include:

1. Public health education of citizens and the medical community.

2. Elimination of food and shelter for rodents around homes, work places, and recreation areas by removing brush, rock piles, junk, and food sources (such as pet food), from the site.

3. Surveillance for plague activity in rodent populations in and surrounding high risk areas by public health workers or by citizens reporting rodents found sick or dead to local health departments.

4. The use of appropriate and licensed insecticides can be used to kill fleas during wild animal plague outbreaks to reduce the risk to humans.

5. Treatment of pets (dogs and cats) for flea control once each week.

Preventive Drug Therapy

Secondly, antibiotics may be taken in the event of exposure to the bites of wild rodent fleas during an outbreak or to the tissues or fluids of a plague-infected animal.

Preventive therapy is also recommended in the event of close exposure to another person or to a pet animal with suspected plague pneumonia.

For preventive drug therapy, the preferred antibiotics are the tetracyclines, chloramphenicol, or one of the effective sulfonamides.

Section 11.2

Plague Information for Health Care Workers

(Source: CDC Document No. 351510, November 19, 1992.)

Clinical Types

Human plague has three clinical forms; bubonic, septicemic, and pneumonic. Bubonic plague, the classical disease in humans, is most commonly acquired by the bite of an infected flea, but may also result from direct contact with plague infected tissues or body fluids through a break in the skin. It is characterized by fever, headache, malaise, and by one or more very painful swollen lymph nodes (the bubo) in the region of the body where the organism was inoculated.

Septicemic plague is a direct invasion of the blood stream without lymph node involvement, however, bubonic plague if not treated effectively, may progress to septicemic plague secondarily. Primary septicemic plague is particularly hazardous because the patient's lymphatic defenses have been compromised and it is difficult to correctly diagnose the disease. The presence of plague bacteria in a blood smear is a grave prognostic sign.

Pneumonic plague also is classified as primary or secondary. Plague pneumonia may develop secondarily in the later stages of ineffectively treated or untreated bubonic or septicemic plague. Primary pneumonic plague results from inhalation of infective droplets expelled from another person or an animal with either primary or secondary pneumonic plague. Symptoms include the rapid development of an overwhelming pneumonia characterized by high fever, cough, bloody sputum, chills, and a very high case fatality rate.

Diagnostic Information

Clinical Diagnosis

Once the plague organism is introduced into a human, a progressive infection generally results unless specific antibiotic therapy is given.

The classic feature of bubonic plague introduced percutaneously by flea bite or a break in the skin is an excruciatingly painful, usually swollen lymph node, often hot to the touch, called a bubo. This finding in a patient with fever, prostrations and a history of possible exposure to rodents, rabbits, other animals, or their fleas in the western United States or other endemic areas of the world should lead to suspicion of plague.

The incubation period for bubonic plague is 2 to 6 days. Initial manifestations include fever, headache, and malaise, followed by development of painful, swollen regional lymph nodes. Occasionally, buboes cannot be detected for several days after the onset of symptoms. The disease may progress rapidly to a septicemic phase characterized by toxicity, prostration, shock, and occasionally hemorrhagic phenomena. The presence of plague bacteria in a blood smear is a grave prognostic sign.

The incubation period of primary pneumonic plague is 1 to 3 days and is characterized by development of an overwhelming pneumonia with high fever, cough, bloody sputum, and chills.

The immediate life threatening complications of plague are shock, high fever, convulsions, and interference with proper blood clotting.

Therapy should begin as soon as possible and local and state health departments notified so that epidemiological investigation and control measures can be instituted. Those individuals closely associated with the patient, particularly in cases with pneumonia, should be traced, identified, and evaluated. Contacts of pneumonic plague patients should be placed under self or supervised observation or treated prophylactically, depending on the degree and timing of contact.

In the event of exposure to the bites of wild rodent fleas during an epizootic or to the tissues or exudates of a plague-infected animal preventive therapy may be used to reduce the risk of developing plague.

Preventive therapy is recommended in the event of close exposure to another person (meaning less than 2 meters away) or to a pet animal with suspected plague pneumonia.

The preferred antibiotics for preventive therapy are the tetracyclines, chloramphenicol, or one of the effective sulfonamides.

Laboratory Diagnosis

As soon as plague is suspected, the patient should be isolated and chest x-ray and confirmatory laboratory work should be initiated, including laboratory examination of blood, bubo aspirate, exudates, purulent drainage, and sputum (if appropriate). Optimally, four consecutive blood cultures should be taken at half hour intervals before specific therapy is given, unless the condition of the patient contraindicates. The blood cultures can be completed in one hour and a half and should not cause inordinate delay before specific therapy is begun. Buboes and abscesses may be needle aspirated or swabbed, but should not be excised or incised and drained for diagnostic purposes. Non-fluctuant buboes can be injected with saline before aspiration to improve yield of organisms. Acute and convalescent serum specimens should be obtained from all suspect plague patients to confirm the diagnosis in the event microorganisms cannot be isolated.

When sending specimens to state health laboratories or to CDC, follow these guidelines:

- Identify the patient by giving the patient's age, sex, dates of illness onset and potential exposure, patient's place of residence, and place where exposed (if possible).

- Label each specimen with a unique number, code, or description for identification.

- Give instructions that specimens are to be tested for plague.

- Package the specimens in leak proof containers to be shipped according to directions in "Biosafety in Microbiological and Biomedical Laboratories" 2nd Edition, 1988." CDC and NIH Publication Number HHS-NIH 88-8395.

- Clinical specimens and serum specimens should be refrigerated or frozen; cultures should be held at indoor ambient temperature. It is not necessary to freeze serum specimens if they are shipped and tested immediately.

- Send specimens by the most rapid means available.

Treatment

All patients with bubonic plague should be strictly isolated for a period of at least 48 hours after treatment has been initiated.

The more effective drug against *Y. pestis* is streptomycin, especially with pneumonic plague. However due to its ototoxicity, it should generally be given for only around 5 days. Tetracycline can be given concurrently and used to complete the full 10 days of therapy.

During pregnancy streptomycin or gentamicin should be used. With early therapy in the mother, the pregnancy should not be adversely affected.

Kanamycin, because of safety, is the drug of choice for new-born children.

Chloramphenicol is the drug of choice when treating patients with specific complications of plague in which drug transport to specific tissues is restricted (e.g. plague meningitis and endophthalmitis).

Tetracycline is effective in patients with uncomplicated plague, but is more commonly used as an adjunct to streptomycin or kanamycin for the completion of drug therapy.

The penicillins, including ampicillin and amoxicillin, are not effective in treating plague.

Most, but not all the sulfonamides are effective in treating plague, but their use for primary therapy cannot be recommended if any of the previously mentioned drugs are available.

Public Health Management of Plague Cases

All plague cases represent real or potential public health emergencies that require location and management of case contacts and location and management of the environmental source of the infection.

Plague is one of three internationally reportable diseases. By law, state and local health authorities must be notified of all human plague cases. State authorities in turn notify CDC and CDC notifies the World Health Organization, as required by the International Sanitary Regulations.

Epidemiological investigation, contact tracing, environmental investigations and environmental management of epizootic plaque require specialized skills available to state health departments or CDC.

Human plague cases frequently cause enormous concern to hospital staff and community where a case has occurred. The attending physician should take care to emphasize that plague is readily treatable, that person-to-parson spread is unlikely to occur, and that the disease can be easily prevented in persons with significant exposure to a case of pneumonic plague.

Bubonic and septicemic plague represent no threat to casual contacts, but wound drainage, blood and other body fluids do represent a potential hazard to medical and laboratory personnel.

Plague patients should be isolated until they have received at least 48 hours of specific antibiotic therapy. Medical personnel attending these patients should use gown, gloves, mask, and eye protection. Phlebotomists, laboratorians, radiological personnel, and other technical personnel should be advised to take similar precautions.

Section 11.3

Vaccine Information

(Source: CDC Document No. 351511, September 27, 1994.)

Plague vaccine is unavailable in the United States, and CDC is not aware of any other sources of the vaccine. A candidate vaccine is being reviewed for licensing in the United States, but will probably not be available until 1995. The information given below will be appropriate for the candidate vaccine when it becomes available.

Human risk of plague infection depends on both behavioral and geographic factors. Behavioral high risk situations include:

1. Persons working with the plague bacterium, *Yersinia pestis*, in the laboratory or in the field.

2. Persons working with wild rodents in plague-infected areas or visiting plague infested areas for prolonged periods of time, especially in areas with limited environmental sanitation.

The plague vaccine is an inactivated bacterial vaccine. Reactions may include mild pain, erythema, and swelling at the injection site. With repeated doses, fever, headache, malaise, and reaction at the inoculation site are more common, and tend to be more severe. Sterile abscesses occur rarely.

No fatal or disabling complications have been reported.

The vaccine is given by intramuscular injection, with a primary series of 3 doses requiring 5-7 months to complete. Booster doses may be given at 6 month to 1 year intervals if risk of exposure persists. Consult the package insert for specific dosing amounts and schedule.

Vaccination during pregnancy should be evaluated on a case by case basis, with consideration given to potential behavioral and geographic risks.

Vaccination is not recommended for prevention of plague during outbreak situations because of the considerable length of time required to develop effective immunity.

Chapter 12

Rabies

Chapter Contents

Section 12.1

Rabies Information

(Source: NIH Pub. No. 83-221.)

Rabies—a severe acute viral infection of the central nervous system—is one of the most terrifying diseases known to man. Although only two cases of human rabies were reported in the United States in 1981, the number of documented cases of animal rabies has more than doubled in recent years—from 3,298 in 1978 to 7,211 cases in 1981. As many as 25,000 Americans receive postexposure treatment each year as a result of contact with animals suspected of being rabid. In other parts of the world, many persons and countless wild and domestic animals still die each year of rabies.

In 1980, a new rabies vaccine was licensed that requires fewer injections and is safer and more effective than the previously used duck embryo vaccine (DEV). This new vaccine, developed through research supported by the National Institute of Allergy and Infectious Diseases (NIAID), is produced from viruses grown in cultures of human cells and is called human diploid cell vaccine (HDCV). It is now available from the private medical sector and, in some cases, from state and county health departments.

Epidemiology

Rabies is caused by a virus that is present in the saliva of infected animals, and it is commonly transmitted by bites. All warm-blooded animals are susceptible to rabies, and some may serve as natural reservoirs of the virus.

With the exception of the Scandinavian Peninsula and a few island countries such as Japan, Australia, New Zealand, and Great Britain, rabies is encountered throughout the world. The disease may be absent from large areas for many years and then reappear suddenly or gradually by invasion from bordering countries or by the introduction of an infected animal.

Two principal epidemiologic patterns are recognized: natural or sylvatic rabies of wildlife, and urban rabies of dogs and cats. In the United States, wild animals accounted for 85 percent of reported rabies cases in 1981. Bat rabies was reported from 46 states and accounted for 12 percent of the cases. Skunk rabies occurred in 32 states and accounted for 62 percent of all cases. Rabies in raccoons and foxes is less widely distributed. However. raccoon rabies has become well established and is spreading in areas of northern Virginia, West Virginia, and Maryland. Vaccination of pets and livestock is the most effective control measure in preventing disease and subsequent human exposure.

The disease is usually contracted from the bite of a rabid animal, but on rare occasions, contact of virus-laden saliva with broken skin may be sufficient to transmit infection. Airborne spread can also occur, as has been demonstrated in caves inhabited by infected bats. Skunks have been infected experimentally by being fed infected animals. In recent years, there have been four reported cases of human-to-human rabies transmission by corneal transplants. These cases underscore the importance of not using transplant tissue from anyone who died of a neurologic illness of unknown cause.

Incubation Period

The bite of a rabies-infected animal does not invariably cause disease, but when symptoms do appear it is usually 30 to 50 days following exposure. In dogs, this incubation period is shorter-generally 14 to 60 days. There is a direct relationship between the severity and location of the bite and the length of the incubation period. If the head of an animal or a person is severely bitten, symptoms may appear in as few as 14 days. Under rare circumstances illness may not develop for a year or more.

Rabies in Humans

Rabies in man is suspected if, weeks or months after exposure to the disease, an individual experiences symptoms such as: a short period of mental depression, restlessness, abnormal sensations around the site of exposure, headache, fever, malaise, nausea, sore throat, or loss of appetite. Other early symptoms include unusual sensitivity to sound, light and changes of temperature, muscle stiffness, dilation of pupils and increased salivation. As the disease progresses, the patient usually experiences episodes of irrational excitement alternating with periods of alert calm. Convulsions are common. Most dramatic of all are the severe and extremely painful throat spasms suffered by the victim on attempting to swallow—or even upon viewing—liquids. This fear of water is characteristic of rabies victims and gives the disease its common name, hydrophobia.

Death from cardiac or respiratory failure usually occurs within a week after appearance of rabies symptoms, while the excited state is still predominant. If the patient survives this stage, muscle spasms and agitation cease, only to be replaced by fatal progressive paralysis. In human rabies resulting from the bite of a rabid vampire bat, excitement and hydrophobia are typically absent, and the disease is characterized by paralysis progressing from the legs upward.

Once symptoms appear, the only treatment is vigorous supportive measures to control the respiratory, circulatory, and central nervous system symptoms. Recovery has occurred in a few cases despite the general opinion that rabies in humans is invariably fatal.

Rabies in Animals

Early signs of rabies in animals include altered disposition, fever, loss of appetite, and often, altered phonation, such as a change in tone of a dog's bark. These signs are often slight, however, and may escape notice. After a few days, marked restlessness and agitation may develop, along with trembling. An affected dog may growl and bark constantly and will viciously attack any moving object, person, or animal it encounters. If not restrained, it may leave home and travel great distances, inflicting much damage as it goes. This excited state usually lasts three to seven days and is followed by convulsions and paralysis.

In some instances, signs of excitement and irritability are slight or absent, and paralysis develops within a few days of disease onset. In cases of this type, an early sign is often paralysis of the lower jaw, accompanied by increased salivation. This may cause the animal to appear to be choking on a foreign object, constituting a dangerous trap for humans, who, in attempting to be helpful, may unwittingly expose themselves to infection.

Diagnosis

Clinical diagnosis of rabies in humans is based on the patient's history of exposure and development of characteristic symptoms. To confirm the diagnosis (usually not possible until late in the disease), rabies virus must be demonstrated in saliva or brain tissue. The virus may be identified on the basis of animal inoculation tests or specific staining with fluorescent antibodies. Other useful diagnostic procedures include identification of rabies antibodies in the patient's blood or cerebrospinal fluid and demonstration of characteristic Negri bodies in samples of brain tissue.

Diagnosis of rabies in animals is similar, in most respects, to the procedure in humans, but the disease is easier to confirm at an early stage, since the animal can be killed for detailed brain studies. New methods of diagnosis in living animals are under study. Animals that die after long periods of illness may not have infectious virus in the brain due to the so-called "auto-sterilization" phenomenon. In that event, the tissue or spinal fluid may be tested for antibodies.

Procedure After A Bite

After a person is bitten, a physician should be reached as soon as possible. One valuable preventive measure is to cleanse the wound immediately with soap and water or even water alone to remove saliva from the area. The wound may then be squeezed to promote bleeding, since this will also help to clean it. A physician may cleanse the contaminated area with a 20 percent solution of medicinal soft soap and may use a syringe to apply the solution to the full depth of the wound. These measures will also help to prevent infection by the organism known as *Pasteurella septica*, but the possibility of tetanus may necessitate more specific treatment.

If at all possible, a dog or cat inflicting a bite should be captured alive and kept under surveillance. This may make it possible for the bitten individual to avoid undergoing rabies vaccination unnecessarily. If the animal remains healthy under confinement and veterinary observation for at least seven days, one may assume that it was not infective. If, however, the animal becomes ill or dies, the local health department should be notified immediately and steps taken to ascertain whether the illness is rabies. When the dog or cat cannot be captured alive, but must be killed, damage to the brain should be avoided. The head should be sent to the diagnostic facility indicated by the local health department.

Any wild animal that bites a person without provocation should be killed and the brain examined immediately for rabies. It is not known how long virus is present in the saliva of wild animals prior to their showing clinical signs of rabies.

If the biting animal escapes or is unknown, determination of the probable risk of rabies must be made by a local physician. The degree of risk is judged on the basis of such factors as the prevalence of rabies in the area, the species of the biting animal, the severity of the wound or wounds, and whether the attack was provoked or unprovoked.

Rodents, including squirrels, are rarely infected and unless a bite was entirely unprovoked, the possibility of rabies can ordinarily be discounted.

Antirabies Immunization

If a physician determines that an individual probably has been exposed to rabies, postexposure treatment should begin at once. Treatment includes both passive and active immunization and is effective when appropriately used. Passive immunization provides immediate but transitory protection by the injection of antibody from an outside source. Active immunization stimulates production of one's own antibodies, which requires a period of time but provides longer lasting protection.

The current recommended treatment is passive immunization with one dose of human rabies immune globulin (RIG) and active immunization with killed rabies virus vaccine. Generally, vaccines made with killed viruses can only prevent disease when they are used before exposure. However, rabies has an unusually long incubation period, and there is time for the body to respond to the vaccine and produce protective antibodies. If RIG is not available, antirabies serum (ARS) may be used for passive immunization. However, ARS is a horse serum and may produce more side effects than RIG.

The new rabies vaccine—human diploid cell vaccine (HDCV)—is produced from viruses grown in cultures of human cells. This vaccine is safer and more effective than the previously used duck embryo vaccine (DEV). Until recently, DEV was the only vaccine used in the United States. It was less efficient in producing immunity and required 23 injections into the stomach wall.

Postexposure immunization with HDCV requires only five injections into the muscle of the upper arm over a four-week period. The vaccine schedule calls for five 1-milliliter (ml.) doses on days 0, 3, 7, 14, and 28 after exposure. The incidence of mild systemic reactions, e.g., headache, fever, nausea, muscle aches, and dizziness, is lower with HDCV than with DEV.

Preexposure immunization with HDCV is recommended for persons with special risks of exposure to rabies, such as veterinarians, animal caretakers, laboratory workers, and should be given in three intramuscular injections. The schedule for the vaccine is three 1-ml. doses on days 0, 7, and 21 or 28. People with continuing risk of exposure should receive a booster at least every two years.

In 1982, the Advisory Committee on Immunization Practices (ACIP) recognized that three intradermal (within the skin) injections of 0.01-ml. each of HDCV was an effective preexposure vaccination regimen. Booster vaccinations are still required, however. The Committee stressed that postexposure vaccination should continue to be the larger dose (1-ml.) within the muscle.

Control of Rabies in Animals

Measures necessary for controlling rabies of dogs and cats (urban rabies) have been understood for many years. Stray dogs should be impounded, ownerless ones killed, and all others kept under intelligent restraint. Mass immunization of dogs, and ideally of cats as well, is also essential for adequate rabies control. The live Flury HEP vaccine produces immunity in dogs for three years, at the end of which time the animal should be revaccinated. Nonendemic areas can maintain their disease-free state by quarantining newly arrived dogs and cats.

Whenever a rabid animal is discovered, every effort should be made to locate all animals that were exposed to it so that they may be either destroyed or vaccinated and quarantined for a minimum of four months.

Rabies in wildlife in the past has been combatted by attempts to reduce the animal population in the area. However, this approach is costly, relatively ineffective, and causes serious ecological disturbances.

Scientists at the Public Health Service's Centers for Disease Control, Atlanta, are working with other investigators trying to develop rabies vaccines which would be useful in preventing the disease in wildlife. One of the major problems in the field, of course, is choice of a bait that would pose no harm to nontarget animal species, such as rodents.

An effort has been made in Europe by sprinkling the landscape with chicken heads containing live rabies vaccine as bait for foxes, one of the chief carriers of the disease. After eating the bait, the foxes become immune to rabies, breaking the transmission cycle of the disease.

Research

Although HDCV is a great improvement over previous vaccines, it is not the final answer in rabies protection. It is relatively expensive to produce because it propagates poorly in cell cultures, and needs to be highly concentrated and purified. For this reason, investigators are still seeking improved vaccines and other means of rabies control. NIAID's concern about the rabies problem is demonstrated through its contract program, its grants, and its intramural research.

New technological developments have enabled scientists to identify several different strains of the rabies virus from around the world. The ability to identify distinct strains will be helpful in epidemiologic studies and in improved vaccine production.

NIAID scientists are studying the factors that allow some animals paralyzed from rabies virus infection to recover. These investigations will increase understanding of the protective substances within the central nervous system (CNS). They may also eventually enable scientists to manipulate the immune system in order to enhance recovery from rabies, as well as other viral infections of the CNS.

Investigators are studying two types of mice—one totally susceptible and one totally resistant to the rabies virus. Genetic studies should reveal the reasons for this difference and lead to the development of more effective preventive measures.

Although significant strides have been made in understanding and controlling rabies, it is still a problem throughout the world. As long as this disease remains a threat, NIAID will continue an active role in supporting rabies research.

NIAID is also supporting research to develop methods of producing protective viral antigens by gene engineering and cloning techniques. Once the technology is developed, highly purified vaccines could be produced more economically than at present.

Japanese scientists have developed a killed rabies virus vaccine that is highly efficacious and relatively inexpensive. For this vaccine the virus is propagated in chick embryo cells, which are less expensive to produce than human cells. The Japanese vaccine has already undergone successful field trials in Southeast Asia where rabies is endemic and prevalent.

Many developing countries are still using killed rabies vaccines prepared from baby mouse brains. Although effective, the unpurified vaccines may cause serious side effects as did the original Pasteur vaccine that was prepared from the spinal cord of infected rabbits.

Section 12.2

Rabies Prevention—United States, 1991

(Source: *Morbidity and Mortality Weekly Report*, March 22, 1991.)

Recommendations of the Immunization Practices Advisory Committee (ACIP)

These revised recommendations of the Immunization Practices Advisory Committee (ACIP) on rabies prevention update the previous recommendations (MMWR 1984;33:393-402,407-8) to reflect the current status of rabies and antirabies biologics in the United States. For assistance with problems or questions about rabies prophylaxis, contact your local or state health department. If local or state health department personnel are unavailable, call the Division of Viral and Rickettsial Diseases, Center for Infectious Diseases, CDC (404) 639-1075 during working hours or (404) 639-2888 nights, weekends, and holidays).

Introduction

Following the marked decrease of rabies cases among domestic animals in the United States in the 1940s and 1950s, indigenously acquired rabies among humans decreased to fewer than two cases per year in the 1960s and 1970s and fewer than one case per year during the 1980s (1). In 1950, for example, 4,979 cases of rabies were reported among dogs and 18 were reported among human populations; in 1989, 160 cases were reported among dogs and one was reported among humans. Thus, the likelihood of human exposure to a rabid domestic animal has decreased greatly; however, the many possible exposures that result from frequent contact between domestic dogs and humans continue to be the basis of most antirabies treatments (2).

Rabies among wild animals—especially skunks, raccoons, and bats—has become more prevalent since the 1950s, accounting for >85% of all reported cases of animal rabies every year since 1976 (1). Rabies among animals occurs throughout the continental United States; only Hawaii remains consistently rabies-free. Wild animals now constitute the most important potential source of infection for both humans and domestic animals in the United States. In much of the rest of the world, including most of Asia, Africa, and Latin America, the dog remains the major species with rabies and the major source of rabies among humans. Nine of the 13 human rabies deaths reported to CDC from 1980 through 1990 appear to have been related to exposure to rabid animals outside of the United States (3-9).

Although rabies among humans is rare in the United States, every year approximately 18,000 persons receive rabies preexposure prophylaxis and an additional 10,000 receive postexposure prophylaxis. Appropriate management of persons possibly exposed to rabies depends on the interpretation of the risk of infection. Decisions about management must be made immediately. All available methods of systemic prophylactic treatment are complicated by occasional adverse reactions, but these are rarely severe (10-14).

Data on the efficacy of active and passive rabies immunization have come from both human and animal studies. Evidence from laboratory and field experience in many areas of the world indicates that postexposure prophylaxis combining local wound treatment, passive immunization, and vaccination is uniformly effective when appropriately applied (15-20). However, rabies has occasionally developed among humans when key elements of the rabies postexposure prophylaxis treatment regimens were omitted or incorrectly administered (see Postexposure Treatment Outside the United States).

Rabies Immunizing Products

There are two types of rabies immunizing products.

1. Rabies vaccines induce an active immune response that includes the production of neutralizing antibodies. This antibody response requires approximately 7-10 days to develop and usually persists for ≥2 years.

2. Rabies immune globulins (RIG) provide rapid, passive immune protection that persists for only a short time (half-life of approximately 21 days) (*21,22*).

In almost all postexposure prophylaxis regimens, both products should be used concurrently.

Rabies Immunizing Products, United States, 1991
Human Rabies Vaccine Rabies Vaccine, Human Diploid Cell (HDCV) 　　Intramuscular .... Imovax® Rabies 　　Intradermal .... Imovax® Rabies I.D. Rabies Vaccine Adsorbed (RVA) **Rabies Immune Globulin (RIG)** Rabies Immune Globulin, Human (HRIG):　　　Hyperab® 　　　　　　　　　　　　　　　　　　　　　　　　Imogam® Rabies

Figure 12.1.

Vaccines Licensed for Use in the United States

Two inactivated rabies vaccines are currently licensed for preexposure and postexposure prophylaxis in the United States.

Rabies Vaccine, Human Diploid Cell (HDCV). HDCV is prepared from the Pitman-Moore strain of rabies virus grown in MRC-5 human diploid cell culture and concentrated by ultrafiltration (*23*). The vaccine is inactivated with betapropiolactone (*18*) and is supplied in forms for:

1. Intramuscular (IM) administration, a single-dose vial containing lyophilized vaccine (Pasteur-Merieux Sérum et Vaccins, Imovax® Rabies, distributed by Connaught Laboratories, Inc., Phone: 800-VACCINE) that is reconstituted in the vial with the accompanying diluent to a final volume of 1.0 ml just before administration.

2. Intradermal (ID) administration, a single-dose syringe containing lyophilized vaccine (Pasteur-Merieux Sérum et Vaccins, Imovax® Rabies I.D., distributed by Connaught

Laboratories, Inc.) that is reconstituted in the syringe to a volume of 0.1 ml just before administration (*24*).

A human diploid cell-derived rabies vaccine developed in the United States (Wyeth Laboratories, Wyvac® was recalled by the manufacturer from the market in 1985 and is no longer available (*25*).

Rabies Vaccine, Adsorbed (RVA). RVA (Michigan Department of Public Health) was licensed on March 19,1988; it was developed and is currently distributed by the Biologics Products Program, Michigan Department of Public Health. The vaccine is prepared from the Kissling strain of Challenge Virus Standard (CVS) rabies virus adapted to fetal rhesus lung diploid cell culture (*26-32*). The vaccine virus is inactivated with betapropiolactone and concentrated by adsorption to aluminum phosphate. Because RVA is adsorbed to aluminum phosphate, it is liquid rather than lyophilized. RVA is currently available only from the Biologics Products Program, Michigan Department of Public Health. Phone: (517) 335-8050.

Both types of rabies vaccines are considered equally efficacious and safe when used as indicated The full 1.0-ml dose of either product can be used for both preexposure and postexposure prophylaxis. Only the Imovax® Rabies I.D. vaccine (HDCV) has been evaluated by the ID dose/route for preexposure vaccination (*33-36*); the antibody response and side effects after ID administration of RVA have not been studied (*24*). *Therefore, RVA should not be used intradermally.*

Rabies Immune Globulins Licensed for Use in the United States. HRIG (Cutter Biological [a division of Miles Inc.], Hyperab®; and Pasteur-Merieux Sérum et Vaccins, Imogam® Rabies, distributed by Connaught Laboratories, Inc.) is an antirabies gamma globulin concentrated by cold ethanol fractionation from plasma of hyperimmunized human donors. Rabies neutralizing antibody content, standardized to contain 150 international units (IU) per ml, is supplied in 2-ml (300 IU) and 10-ml (1,500 IU) vials for pediatric and adult use, respectively.

Both HRIG preparations are considered equally efficacious and safe when used as described in this document.

Postexposure Prophylaxis: Rationale for Treatment

Physicians should evaluate each possible exposure to rabies and if necessary consult with local or state public health officials regarding the need for rabies prophylaxis (Figure 12.2). In the United States, the following factors should be considered before specific antirabies treatment is initiated.

Type of Exposure

Rabies is transmitted only when the virus is introduced into open cuts or wounds in skin or mucous membranes. If there has been no exposure (as described in this section), postexposure treatment is not necessary. The likelihood of rabies infection varies with the nature and extent of exposure. Two categories of exposure (bite and nonbite) should be considered.

Bite. Any penetration of the skin by teeth constitutes a bite exposure. Bites to the face and hands carry the highest risk, but the site of the bite should not influence the decision to begin treatment (*17*).

Nonbite. Scratches, abrasions, open wounds, or mucous membranes contaminated with saliva or other potentially infectious material (such as brain tissue) from a rabid animal constitute nonbite exposures. If the material containing the virus is dry, the virus can be considered noninfectious.

Other contact by itself, such as petting a rabid animal and contact with the blood, urine, or feces (e.g., guano) of a rabid animal, does not constitute an exposure and is not an indication for prophylaxis.

Although occasional reports of transmission by nonbite exposure suggest that such exposures constitute sufficient reason to initiate postexposure prophylaxis under some circumstances, nonbite exposures rarely cause rabies (*37*). The nonbite exposures of highest risk appear to be exposures to large amounts of aerosolized rabies virus, organs (i.e., corneas) transplanted from patients who died of rabies, and scratches by rabid animals. Two cases of rabies have been attributed to airborne exposures in laboratories, and two cases of rabies have been attributed to probable airborne exposures in a bat-infested cave in Texas (*38,39*).

The only documented cases of rabies caused by human-to-human transmission occurred among six recipients of transplanted corneas. Investigations revealed each of the donors had died of an illness compatible with or proven to be rabies (*40-43*). The six cases occurred in four countries: Thailand (two cases), India (two cases), the United States (one case), and France (one case). Stringent guidelines for acceptance of donor corneas have reduced this risk.

Apart from corneal transplants, bite and nonbite exposures inflicted by infected humans could theoretically transmit rabies, but no such cases have been documented (*44*). Adherence to respiratory precautions will minimize the risk of airborne exposure (*45*).

Animal Rabies Epidemiology and Evaluation of Involved Species

Wild Animals. Carnivorous wild animals (especially skunks, raccoons, and foxes) and bats are the animals most often infected with rabies and the cause of most indigenous cases of human rabies in the United States since 1960 (*1*). All bites by wild carnivores and bats must be considered possible exposures to the disease. Postexposure prophylaxis should be initiated when patients are exposed to wild carnivores unless 1) the exposure occurred in a part of the continental United States known to be free of terrestrial rabies and the results of immunofluorescence antibody testing will be available within 48 hours or 2) the animal has already been tested and shown not to be rabid. If treatment has been initiated and subsequent immunofluorescence testing shows that the exposing animal was not rabid, treatment can be discontinued.

Signs of rabies among carnivorous wild animals cannot be interpreted reliably; therefore, any such animal that bites or scratches a person should be killed at once (without unnecessary damage to the head) and the brain submitted for rabies testing. If the results of testing are negative by immunofluorescence, the saliva can be assumed to contain no virus, and the person bitten does not require treatment.

If the biting animal is a particularly rare or valuable specimen and the risk of rabies small, public health authorities may choose to administer postexposure treatment to the bite victim in lieu of killing the animal for rabies testing (*46*). Such animals should be quarantined for 30 days.

Rodents (such as squirrels, hamsters, guinea pigs, gerbils, chipmunks, rats, and mice) and lagomorphs (including rabbits and hares) are almost never found to be infected with rabies and have not been

Figure 12.2. *Rabies postexposure prophylaxis guide, United States, 1991.*

Animal type	Evaluation and disposition of animal	Postexposure prophylaxis recommendations
Dogs and cats	Healthy and available for 10 days observation	Should not begin prophylaxis unless animal develops symptoms of rabies*
	Rabid or suspected rabid	Immediate vaccination
	Unknown (escaped)	Consult public health officials
Skunks, raccoons, bats, foxes, and most other carnivores; woodchucks	Regarded as rabid unless geographic area is known to be free of rabies or until animal proven negative by laboratory tests†	Immediate vaccination
Livestock, rodents, and lagomorphs (rabbits and hares)	Consider individually	Consult public health officials. Bites of squirrels, hamsters, guinea pigs, gerbils, chipmunks, rats, mice, other rodents, rabbits, and hares almost never require antirabies treatment

*During the 10-day holding period, begin treatment with HRIG and HDCV or RVA at first sign of rabies in a dog or cat that has bitten someone. The symptomatic animal should be killed immediately and tested.
†The animal should be killed and tested as soon as possible. Holding for observation is not recommended. Discontinue vaccine if immunofluorescence test results of the animal are negative.

291

known to cause rabies among humans in the United States. However, from 1971 through 1988, woodchucks accounted for 70% of the 179 cases of rabies among rodents reported to CDC (*47*). In all cases involving rodents, the state or local health department should be consulted before a decision is made to initiate postexposure antirabies prophylaxis.

Exotic pets (including ferrets) and domestic animals crossbred with wild animals are considered wild animals by the National Association of State Public Health Veterinarians (NASPHV) and the Conference of State and Territorial Epidemiologists (CSTE) because they may be highly susceptible to rabies and could transmit the disease. Because the period of rabies virus shedding in these animals is unknown, these animals should be killed and tested rather than confined and observed when they bite humans (*46*). Wild animals (skunks, raccoons, and bats) and wild animals crossbred with dogs should not be kept as pets (*46*).

Domestic Animals. The likelihood that a domestic animal is infected with rabies varies by region; hence, the need for postexposure prophylaxis also varies. In the continental United States, rabies among dogs is reported most commonly along the U.S.-Mexico border and sporadically from the areas of the United States with enzootic wildlife rabies, especially the Midwest. During most of the 1980s in the United States, more cats than dogs were reported rabid; the majority of these cases were associated with the mid-Atlantic epizootic of rabies among raccoons. The large number of rabies-infected cats may be attributed to fewer cat vaccination laws, fewer leash laws, and the roaming habits of cats. Cattle tend to be most often exposed to rabies via rabid skunks.

In areas where canine rabies is not enzootic (including virtually all of the United States and its territories), a healthy domestic dog or cat that bites a person should be confined and observed for 10 days. Any illness in the animal during confinement or before release should be evaluated by a veterinarian and reported immediately to the local health department. If signs suggestive of rabies develop, the animal should be humanely killed and its head removed and shipped, under refrigeration, for examination by a qualified laboratory. Any stray or unwanted dog or cat that bites a person should be killed immediately and the head submitted as described for rabies examination (*46*).

In most developing countries of Asia, Africa, and Central and South America, dogs are the major vector of rabies; exposures to dogs in such countries represent a special threat. Travelers to these countries should be aware that >50% of the rabies cases among humans in the United States result from exposure to dogs outside the United States. Although dogs are the main reservoir of rabies in these countries, the epizootiology of the disease among animals differs sufficiently by region or country to warrant the evaluation of all animal bites. Exposures to dogs in canine rabies-enzootic areas outside the United States carry a high risk; some authorities therefore recommend that postexposure rabies treatment be initiated immediately after such exposures. Treatment can be discontinued if the dog or cat remains healthy during the 10-day observation period.

Circumstances of Biting Incident and Vaccination Status of Exposing Animal

An unprovoked attack by a domestic animal is more likely than a provoked attack to indicate that the animal is rabid. Bites inflicted on a person attempting to feed or handle an apparently healthy animal should generally be regarded as provoked.

A fully vaccinated dog or cat is unlikely to become infected with rabies, although rare cases have been reported (*48*). In a nationwide study of rabies among dogs and cats in 1988, only one dog and two cats that were vaccinated contracted rabies (*49*). All three of these animals had received only single doses of vaccine; no documented vaccine failures occurred among dogs or cats that had received two vaccinations.

Postexposure Prophylaxis: Local Treatment of Wounds and Vaccination

The essential components of rabies postexposure prophylaxis are local wound treatment and the administration, in most instances, of both HRIG and vaccine (Figure 12.2). Persons who have been bitten by animals suspected or proven rabid should begin treatment within 24 hours. However, there have been instances when the decision to begin treatment was not made until many months after the exposure because of a delay in recognition that an exposure had occurred and awareness that incubation periods of >1 year have been reported.

293

In 1977, the World Health Organization (WHO) recommended a regimen of RIG and six doses of HDCV over a 90-day period. This recommendation was based on studies in Germany and Iran (*16,20*). When used this way, the vaccine was found to be safe and effective in protecting persons bitten by proven rabid animals and induced an excellent antibody response in all recipients (*16*). Studies conducted in the United States by CDC have shown that a regimen of one dose of HRIG and five doses of HDCV over a 28-day period was safe and induced an excellent antibody response in all recipients (*15*).

Local Treatment of Wounds

Immediate and thorough washing of all bite wounds and scratches with soap and water is an important measure for preventing rabies. In studies of animals, simple local wound cleansing has been shown to reduce markedly the likelihood of rabies (*50,51*). Tetanus prophylaxis and measures to control bacterial infection should be given as indicated. The decision to suture large wounds should take into account cosmetic factors and the potential for bacterial infections.

Immunization

Vaccine Usage. Two rabies vaccines are currently available in the United States; either is administered in conjunction with HRIG at the beginning of postexposure therapy. A regimen of five 1-ml doses of HDCV or RVA should be given intramuscularly. The first dose of the five-dose course should be given as soon as possible after exposure. Additional doses should be given on days 3, 7, 14, and 28 after the first vaccination. For adults, the vaccine should always be administered IM in the deltoid area. For children, the anterolateral aspect of the thigh is also acceptable. The gluteal area should never be used for HDCV or RVA injections, since administration in this area results in lower neutralizing antibody titers (*52*).

Postexposure antirabies vaccination should always include administration of both passive antibody and vaccine, with the exception of persons who have previously received complete vaccination regimens (preexposure or postexposure) with a cell culture vaccine, or persons who have been vaccinated with other types of vaccines and have had documented rabies antibody titers. These persons should receive only vaccine (see Postexposure Therapy of Previously Vaccinated Persons). The combination of HRIG (local and systemic) and vaccine is

Figure 12.3. Rabies postexposure prophylaxis schedule, United States, 1991.

Vaccination status	Treatment	Regimen*
Not previously vaccinated	Local wound cleansing	All postexposure treatment should begin with immediate thorough cleansing of all wounds with soap and water.
	HRIG	20 IU/kg body weight. If anatomically feasible, up to one-half the dose should be infiltrated around the wound(s) and the rest should be administered IM in the gluteal area. HRIG should not be administered in the same syringe or into the same anatomical site as vaccine. Because HRIG may partially suppress active production of antibody, no more than the recommended dose should be given.
	Vaccine	HDCV or RVA, 1.0 ml, IM (deltoid area†), one each on days 0, 3, 7, 14 and 28.
Previously vaccinated§	Local wound cleansing	All postexposure treatment should begin with immediate thorough cleansing of all wounds with soap and water.
	HRIG	HRIG should not be administered.
	Vaccine	HDCV or RVA, 1.0 ml, IM (deltoid area†), one each on days 0 and 3.

*These regimens are applicable for all age groups, including children.
†The deltoid area is the only acceptable site of vaccination for adults and older children. For younger children, the outer aspect of the thigh may be used. Vaccine should never be administered in the gluteal area.
§Any person with a history of preexposure vaccination with HDCV or RVA; prior postexposure prophylaxis with HDCV or RVA; or previous vaccination with any other type of rabies vaccine and a documented history of antibody response to the prior vaccination.

recommended for both bite and nonbite exposures (see Postexposure Prophylaxis: Rationale for Treatment), regardless of the interval between exposure and initiation of treatment.

Because the antibody response after the recommended postexposure vaccination regimen with HDCV or RVA has been satisfactory, routine postvaccination serologic testing is not recommended. Serologic testing is only indicated in unusual instances, as when the patient is known to be immunosuppressed. The state health department may be contacted for recommendations on this matter.

HRIG Usage. HRIG is administered only once (i.e., at the beginning of antirabies prophylaxis) to provide immediate antibodies until the patient responds to HDCV or RVA by actively producing antibodies. If HRIG was not given when vaccination was begun, it can be given through the seventh day after administration of the first dose of vaccine. Beyond the seventh day, HRIG is not indicated since an antibody response to cell culture vaccine is presumed to have occurred. The recommended dose of HRIG is 20 IU/kg. This formula is applicable for all age groups, including children. If anatomically feasible, up to one-half the dose of HRIG should be thoroughly infiltrated in the area around the wound and the rest should be administered intramuscularly in the gluteal area. *HRIG should never be administered in the same syringe or into the same anatomical site as vaccine.* Because HRIG may partially suppress active production of antibody, no more than the recommended dose should be given (*53*).

Vaccination and Serologic Testing

The effectiveness of rabies vaccines is primarily measured by their ability to protect persons exposed to rabies. HDCV has been used effectively with HRIG or equine antirabies serum (ARS) worldwide to treat persons bitten by various rabid animals (*15,16*). An estimated one million people worldwide have received rabies postexposure prophylaxis with HDCV since its introduction 12 years ago (*54*).

In studies of animals, antibody titers have been shown to be markers of protection. Antibody titers will vary with time since the last vaccination. Differences among laboratories that test blood samples may also influence the results.

Serologic Response Shortly After Vaccination

All persons tested at CDC 2-4 weeks after completion of preexposure and postexposure rabies prophylaxis according to ACIP guidelines have demonstrated an antibody response to rabies (*15,55,56*). Therefore, it is not necessary to test serum samples from patients completing preexposure or postexposure prophylaxis to document seroconversion unless the person is immunosuppressed (see Precautions and Contraindications). If titers are obtained, specimens collected 2-4 weeks after preexposure or postexposure prophylaxis should completely neutralize challenge virus at a 1:25 serum dilution by the rapid fluorescent focus inhibition test (RFFIT). (This dilution is approximately equivalent to the minimum titer of 0.5 IU recommended by the WHO.)

Serologic Response and Preexposure Booster Doses of Vaccine

Two years after primary preexposure vaccination, a 1:5 serum dilution will fail to neutralize challenge virus completely (by RFFIT) among 2%-7% of persons who received the three-dose preexposure series intramuscularly and 5%-17% of persons who received the three-dose series intradermally (*57*). If the titer falls below 1:5, a preexposure booster dose of vaccine is recommended for a person at continuous or frequent risk (Figure 12.4) of exposure to rabies. The following guidelines are recommended for determining when serum testing should be performed after primary preexposure vaccination:

1. A person in the continuous risk category (Figure 12.4) should have a serum sample tested for rabies antibody every 6 months (*58*).

2. A person in the frequent risk category (Figure 12.4) should have a serum sample tested for rabies antibody every 2 years.

State or local health departments may provide the names and addresses of laboratories performing rabies serologic testing.

Figure 12.4. Rabies Preexposure prophylaxis guide, United States, 1991.

Risk category	Nature of risk	Typical populations	Preexposure recommendations
Continuous	Virus present continuously, often in high concentrations. Aerosol, mucous membrane, bite, or nonbite exposure. Specific exposures may go unrecognized.	Rabies research lab worker;* rabies biologics production workers.	Primary course. Serologic testing every 6 months; booster vaccination when antibody level falls below acceptable level.[†]
Frequent	Exposure usually episodic, with source recognized, but exposure may also be unrecognized. Aerosol, mucous membrane, bite, or nonbite exposure.	Rabies diagnostic lab workers,* spelunkers, veterinarians and staff, and animal-control and wildlife workers in rabies enzootic areas. Travelers visiting foreign areas of enzootic rabies for more than 30 days.	Primary course. Serologic testing or booster vaccination every 2 years.[†]
Infrequent (greater than population at large)	Exposure nearly always episodic with source recognized. Mucous membrane, bite, or nonbite exposure.	Veterinarians and animal-control and wildlife workers in areas of low rabies enzooticity. Veterinary students.	Primary course; no serologic testing or booster vaccination.
Rare (population at large)	Exposures always episodic. Mucous membrane, or bite with source unrecognized.	U.S. population at large, including persons in rabies epizootic areas.	No vaccination necessary.

*Judgment of relative risk and extra monitoring of vaccination status of laboratory workers is the responsibility of the laboratory supervisor (*58*).

[†]Minimum acceptable antibody level is complete virus neutralization at a 1:5 serum dilution by RFFIT. Booster dose should be administered if the titer falls below this level.

Postexposure Treatment Outside the United States

U.S. citizens and residents who are exposed to rabies while traveling outside the United States in countries where rabies is endemic may sometimes receive postexposure therapy with regimens or biologics that are not used in the United States. The following information is provided to familiarize physicians with some of the regimens used more widely abroad. These schedules have not been submitted for approval by the Food and Drug Administration (FDA) for use in the United States. If postexposure treatment is begun outside the United States using one of these regimens or biologics of nerve tissue origin, it may be necessary to provide additional treatment when the patient reaches the United States. State or local health departments should be contacted for specific advice in such cases.

Modifications to the postexposure vaccine regimen approved for use in the United States have been made to reduce the cost of postexposure prophylaxis and hasten the development of active immunity (59). Costs are reduced primarily by substituting various schedules of ID injections (0.1 ml each) of HDCV (or newer tissue culture-derived rabies vaccines for humans) for IM injection of HDCV. Two such regimens are efficacious among persons bitten by rabid animals (60). One of these regimens consists of 0.1-ml ID doses of HDCV given at eight different sites (deltoid, suprascapular, thigh, and abdominal wall) on day 0; four ID 0.1-ml doses given at four sites on day 7 (deltoid, thigh); and one ID 0.1-ml dose given in the deltoid on both day 28 and 91. Another ID regimen shown to be efficacious and now widely used in Thailand employs Purified VERO Cell Rabies Vaccine (Pasteur-Merieux), with 0.1-ml doses given at two different sites on days 0, 3, and 7, followed by one 0.1-ml booster on days 30 and 90 (61).

Strategies designed to hasten the development of active immunity have concentrated on administering more IM or ID doses at the time postexposure prophylaxis is initiated with fewer doses thereafter (62). The most extensively evaluated regimen in this category, developed in Yugoslavia, has been the 2-1-1 regimen (two 1.0-ml IM doses on day 0, and one each on days 7 and 21)(63-65). However, when using HRIG in conjunction with this schedule, there may be some suppression of the neutralizing antibody response (65).

Purified antirabies sera of equine origin (Sclavo; Pasteur-Merieux; Swiss Serum and Vaccine Institute, Bern) have been used effectively in developing countries where HRIG may not be available.

The incidence of adverse reactions has been low (0.8%-6.0%) and most of those that occurred were minor (*66-68*).

Although no postexposure vaccine failures have occurred in the United States during the 10 years that HDCV has been licensed, seven persons have contracted rabies after receiving postexposure treatment with both HRIG and HDCV outside the United States. An additional six persons have contracted the disease after receiving postexposure prophylaxis with other cell culture-derived vaccines and HRIG or ARS. However, in each of these cases, there was some deviation from the recommended postexposure treatment protocol (*69-71*). Specifically, patients who contracted rabies after postexposure prophylaxis did not have their wounds cleansed with soap and water or other antiviral agents, did not receive their rabies vaccine injections in the deltoid area (i.e., vaccine was administered in the gluteal area), or did not receive passive vaccination around the wound site.

Preexposure Vaccination and Postexposure Therapy of Previously Vaccinated Persons

Preexposure vaccination should be offered to persons among high-risk groups, such as veterinarians, animal handlers, certain laboratory workers, and persons spending time (e.g., 1 month) in foreign countries where canine rabies is endemic. Other persons whose activities bring them into frequent contact with rabies virus or potentially rabid dogs, cats, skunks, raccoons, bats, or other species at risk of having rabies should also be considered for preexposure prophylaxis.

Preexposure prophylaxis is given for several reasons. First, it may provide protection to persons with inapparent exposures to rabies. Second, it may protect persons whose postexposure therapy might be delayed. Finally, although preexposure vaccination does not eliminate the need for additional therapy after a rabies exposure, it simplifies therapy by eliminating the need for HRIG and decreasing the number of doses of vaccine needed—a point of particular importance for persons at high risk of being exposed to rabies in areas where immunizing products may not be available or where they may carry a high risk of adverse reactions.

Primary Preexposure Vaccination

Intramuscular Primary Vaccination. Three 1.0-ml injections of HDCV or RVA should be given intramuscularly (deltoid area), one each on days 0, 7, and 21 or 28 (Figure 12.5). In a study in the United States, >1,000 persons received HDCV according to this regimen. Antibody was demonstrated in serum samples of all subjects when tested by the RFFIT. Other studies have produced comparable results (*33,56,72,73*).

Intradermal Primary Vaccination. A regimen of three 0.1-ml doses of HDCV, one each on days 0, 7, and 21 or 28 (*10,33,34,36,72,73*), is also used for preexposure vaccination (Figure 12.5). The ID dose/route has been recommended previously by the ACIP as an alternative to the 1.0-ml IM dose/route for rabies preexposure prophylaxis with HDCV (*24,74*).

Pasteur-Merieux developed a syringe containing a single dose of lyophilized HDCV (Imovax® Rabies I.D.) that is reconstituted in the syringe just before administration. The syringe is designed to deliver 0.1 ml of HDCV reliably and was approved by the FDA in 1986 (*24*). The 0.1-ml ID doses, given in the area over the deltoid (lateral aspect of the upper arm) on days 0, 7, and 21 or 28, are used for primary preexposure vaccination. One 0.1-ml ID dose is used for booster vaccination (see Figure 12.4). The 1.0-ml vial is not approved for multi-dose ID use. RVA should not be given by the ID dose/route (*26*).

Chloroquine phosphate (administered for malaria chemoprophylaxis) interferes with the antibody response to HDCV (*75*). Accordingly, HDCV should not be administered by the ID dose/route to persons traveling to malaria-endemic countries while the person is receiving chloroquine (*76*). The IM dose/route of preexposure prophylaxis provides a sufficient margin of safety in this situation (*76*). For persons who will be receiving both rabies preexposure prophylaxis and chloroquine in preparation for travel to a rabies-enzootic area, the ID dose/route should be initiated at least 1 month before travel to allow for completion of the full three-dose vaccine series before antimalarial prophylaxis begins. If this schedule is not possible, the IM dose/route should be used. Although interference with the immune response to rabies vaccine by other antimalarials structurally related to chloroquine (e.g., mefloquine) has not been evaluated, it would seem prudent to follow similar precautions for persons receiving these drugs.

Type of vaccination	Route	Regimen
Primary	IM	HDCV or RVA, 1.0 ml (deltoid area), one each on days 0, 7, and 21 or 28
	ID	HDCV, 0.1 ml, one each on days 0, 7, and 21 or 28
Booster*	IM	HDCV or RVA, 1.0 ml (deltoid area), day 0 only
	ID	HDCV, 0.1 ml, day 0 only

Figure 12.5. *Rabies preexposure prophylaxis schedule, United States, 1991 (*Administration of routine booster dose of vaccine depends on exposure risk category as noted in Fibure 12.4.)*

Booster Vaccination

Preexposure Booster Doses of Vaccine. Persons who work with live rabies virus in research laboratories or vaccine production facilities (continuous risk category; see Figure 12.4) are at the highest risk of inapparent exposures. Such persons should have a serum sample tested for rabies antibody every 6 months (Figure 12.5). Booster doses (IM or ID) of vaccine should be given to maintain a serum titer corresponding to at least complete neutralization at a 1:5 serum dilution by the RFFIT. The frequent risk category includes other laboratory workers, such as those doing rabies diagnostic testing, spelunkers, veterinarians and staff, animal-control and wildlife officers in areas where animal rabies is epizootic, and international travelers living or visiting (for >30 days) in areas where canine rabies is endemic. Persons among this group should have a serum sample tested for rabies antibody every 2 years and, if the titer is less than complete neutralization at a 1:5 serum dilution by the RFFIT, should have a booster dose of vaccine. Alternatively, a booster can be administered in lieu of a titer determination. Veterinarians and animal control and wildlife officers working in areas of low rabies enzooticity (infrequent exposure group) do not require routine preexposure booster doses of HDCV or RVA after completion of primary preexposure vaccination (Figure 12.4).

Postexposure Therapy of Previously Vaccinated Persons. If exposed to rabies, persons previously vaccinated should receive two IM doses (1.0 ml each) of vaccine, one immediately and one 3 days later. Previously vaccinated refers to persons who have received one of the recommended preexposure or postexposure regimens of HDCV or

RVA, or those who received another vaccine and had a documented rabies antibody titer. HRIG is unnecessary and should not be given in these cases because an anamnestic antibody response will follow the administration of a booster regardless of the prebooster antibody titer (77).

Preexposure Vaccination and Serologic Testing. Because the antibody response after these recommended preexposure prophylaxis vaccine regimens has been satisfactory, serologic testing is not necessary except for persons suspected of being immunosuppressed. Patients who are immunosuppressed by disease or medications should postpone preexposure vaccinations. Immunosuppressed persons who are at risk of rabies exposure should be vaccinated and their antibody titers checked.

Unintentional Inoculation with Modified Life Rabies Virus

Veterinary personnel may be inadvertently exposed to attenuated rabies virus while administering modified live rabies virus (MLV) vaccines to animals. Although there have been no reported rabies cases among humans resulting from exposure to needle sticks or sprays with licensed MLV vaccines, vaccine-induced rabies has occurred among animals given these vaccines. Absolute assurance of a lack of risk for humans, therefore, cannot be given. The best evidence for low risk is the absence of recognized cases of vaccine-associated disease among humans despite frequent inadvertent exposures.

MLV animal vaccines that are currently available are made with one attenuated strain of rabies virus: high egg passage (HEP) Flury strain. The HEP Flury strain has been used in animal vaccines for more than 25 years without evidence of associated disease among humans; therefore, postexposure treatment is not recommended following exposure to this type of vaccine by needle sticks or sprays.

Because the data are insufficient to assess the true risk associated with any of the MLV vaccines, preexposure vaccination and periodic boosters are recommended for all persons whose activities either bring them into contact with potentially rabid animals or who frequently handle attenuated animal rabies vaccine.

Adverse Reactions

Human Diploid Cell Rabies Vaccine and Rabies Vaccine Adsorbed

Reactions after vaccination with HDCV and RVA are less serious and common than with previously available vaccines (*78,79*). In studies using a three-dose postexposure regimen of HDCV, local reactions, such as pain, erythema, and swelling or itching at the injection site, have been reported among 30%-74% of recipients. Systemic reactions, such as headache, nausea, abdominal pain, muscle aches, and dizziness have been reported among 5%-40% of recipients. Three cases of neurologic illness resembling Guillain-Barré syndrome that resolved without sequelae in 12 weeks have been reported (*10,80,81*). In addition, a few other subacute central and peripheral nervous system disorders have been temporally associated with HDCV vaccine, but a causal relationship has not been established (*82*).

An immune complex-like reaction occurs among approximately 6% of persons receiving booster doses of HDCV (*11,12*) 2-21 days after administration of the booster dose. These patients develop a generalized urticaria, sometimes accompanied by arthralgia, arthritis, angioedema, nausea, vomiting, fever, and malaise. In no cases have the illnesses been life-threatening. This reaction occurs much less frequently among persons receiving primary vaccination. The reaction has been associated with the presence of betapropiolactone-altered human serum albumin in the HDCV and the development of immunoglobulin E (IgE) antibodies to this allergen (*83,84*). Among persons who have received their primary vaccination series with HDCV, administration of boosters with a purified HDCV produced in Canada (Connaught Laboratories Ltd., Rabies Vaccine Inactivated [Diploid Cell Origin]-Dried) does not appear to be associated with this reaction (*57*). This vaccine is not yet licensed in the United States.

Vaccines and Immune Globulins Used in Other Countries

Many developing countries use inactivated nerve tissue vaccines made from the brains of adult animals or suckling mice. Nerve tissue vaccine (NTV) is reported to induce neuroparalytic reactions among approximately 1 per 200 to 1 per 2,000 vaccinees; suckling mouse brain vaccine (SMBV) causes reactions in among approximately 1 per 8,000 (*17*).

Human Rabies Immune Globulins

Local pain and low-grade fever may follow receipt of HRIG. Although not reported specifically for HRIG, angioneurotic edema, nephrotic syndrome, and anaphylaxis have been reported after injection of immune globulin (IG). These reactions occur so rarely that a causal relationship between IG and these reactions is not clear.

There is no evidence that hepatitis B virus (HBV), human immunodeficiency virus (HIV, the causative agent of Acquired Immunodeficiency Syndrome [AIDS]), or other viruses have ever been transmitted by commercially available HRIG in the United States.

Management of Adverse Reactions

Once initiated, rabies prophylaxis should not be interrupted or discontinued because of local or mild systemic adverse reactions to rabies vaccine. Usually such reactions can be successfully managed with anti-inflammatory and antipyretic agents (e.g., aspirin).

When a person with a history of serious hypersensitivity to rabies vaccine must be revaccinated, antihistamines may be given. Epinephrine should be readily available to counteract anaphylactic reactions, and the person should be observed carefully immediately after vaccination.

Although serious systemic, anaphylactic, or neuroparalytic reactions are rare during and after the administration of rabies vaccines, such reactions pose a serious dilemma for the attending physician (11). A patient's risk of acquiring rabies must be carefully considered before deciding to discontinue vaccination. Advice and assistance on the management of serious adverse reactions for persons receiving rabies vaccines may be sought from the state health department or CDC.

All serious systemic, neuroparalytic, or anaphylactic reactions to HDCV should be reported immediately to Connaught Laboratories, Inc., Swiftwater, PA 18370. Phone: (800) VACCINE or (717) 839-7187. Serious reactions after the administration of RVA should be reported immediately to Coordinating Physicians, Bureau of Laboratories and Epidemiological Services, Michigan Department of Public Health, P. O. Box 30035, 3500 N. Logan, Lansing, Ml 48909. Phone: (517) 335-8050.

Precautions and Contraindications

Immunosuppression

Corticosteroids, other immunosuppressive agents, antimalarials, and immunosuppressive illnesses can interfere with the development of active immunity after vaccination and may predispose the patient to rabies (*75,85*). Preexposure prophylaxis should be administered to such persons with the awareness that the immune response may be inadequate (see Intradermal Primary Vaccination). Immunosuppressive agents should not be administered during postexposure therapy unless essential for the treatment of other conditions. When rabies postexposure prophylaxis is administered to persons receiving steroids or other immunosuppressive therapy, it is especially important that a serum sample be tested for rabies antibody to ensure that an acceptable antibody response has developed (see Vaccination and Serologic Testing).

Pregnancy

Because of the potential consequences of inadequately treated rabies exposure, and because there is no indication that fetal abnormalities have been associated with rabies vaccination, pregnancy is not considered a contraindication to postexposure prophylaxis (*86*). If there is substantial risk of exposure to rabies, preexposure prophylaxis may also be indicated during pregnancy.

Allergies

Persons who have a history of serious hypersensitivity to rabies vaccine should be revaccinated with caution (see Management of Adverse Reactions).

References

1. Reid-Sanden FL, Dobbins JG, Smith JS, Fishbein DB. Rabies surveillance, United States during 1989. J Am Vet Med Assoc 1990;197:1571-83.

2. Helmick CG. The epidemiology of human rabies postexposure prophylaxis, 1980-1981. JAMA 1983;250:1990-6.

3. CDC. Human rabies diagnosed 2 months postmortem-Texas. MMWR 1985;34:700,705-7

4. CDC. Human rabies acquired outside the United States. MMWR 1985;34:235-6.

5. CDC. Human rabies-California, 1987. MMWR 1988;37:305-8.

6. CDC. Human rabies-Oregon, 1989. MMWR 1989;38:335-7.

7. CDC. Human rabies-Texas. MMWR 1984;33:469-70.

8. CDC. Imported human rabies. MMWR 1983;32:78-80,85-6.

9. CDC. Human rabies acquired outside the United States from a dog bite. MMWR 1981;30:537-40.

10. Bernard KW, Smith PW, Kader FJ, Moran MJ. Neuroparalytic illness and human diploid cell rabies vaccine. JAMA 1982,248:3136-8.

11. CDC. Systemic allergic reactions following immunization with human diploid cell rabies vaccine. MMWR 1984;33:185-7.

12. Dreesen DW, Bernard KW, Parker RA, Deutsch AJ, Brown J. Immune complex-like disease in 23 persons following a booster dose of rabies human diploid cell vaccine. Vaccine 1986;4:45-9.

13. Aoki FY, Tyrrell DA, Hill LE. Immunogenicity and acceptability of a human diploid-cell culture rabies vaccine in volunteers. Lancet 1975;1:660-2.

14. Cox JH, Schneider LG. Prophylactic immunization of humans against rabies by intradermal inoculation of human diploid cell culture vaccine. J Clin Microbiol 1976;3:96-101.

15. Anderson LJ, Sikes RK, Langkop CW, et al. Postexposure trial of a human diploid cell strain rabies vaccine. J Infect Dis 1980;142:133-8.

16. Bahmanyar M, Fayaz A, Nour-Salehi S, Mohammadi M, Koprowski H. Successful protection of humans exposed to rabies infection. Postexposure treatment with the new human diploid cell rabies vaccine and antirabies serum. JAMA 1976;236:2751-4.

17. Hattwick MAW. Human rabies. Public Health Rev 1974;3:229-74.

18. Wiktor TJ, Plotkin SA, Koprowski H. Development and clinical trials of the new human rabies vaccine of tissue culture (human diploid cell) origin. Dev Biol Stand 1978;40:3-9.

19. World Health Organization. WHO expert committee on rabies. WHO Tech Rep Ser 1984;709:1-104.

20. Kuwert EK, Werner J, Marcus I, Cabasso VJ. Immunization against rabies with rabies immune globulin, human (RIGH) and a human diploid cell strain (HDCS) rabies vaccine. J Biol Stand 1978;6:211-9.

21. Winkler WG, Schmidt RC, Sikes RK. Evaluation of human rabies immune globulin and homologous and heterologous antibody. J Immunol 1969;102:1314-21.

22. Cabasso VJ, Loofbourow JC, Roby RE, Anuskiewicz W. Rabies immune globulin of human origin: preparation and dosage determination in non-exposed volunteer subjects. Bull WHO 1971;45:303-15.

23. Wiktor TJ, Sokol F, Kuwert E, Koprowski H. Immunogenicity of concentrated and purified rabies vaccine of tissue culture origin. Proc Soc Exp Biol Med 1969;131:799-805.

24. CDC. Rabies prevention: supplementary statement on the preexposure use of human diploid cell rabies vaccine by the intradermal route. MMWR 1986;35:767-8.

25. CDC. Rabies postexposure prophylaxis with human diploid cell rabies vaccine: lower neutralizing antibody titers with Wyeth vaccine. MMWR 1985;34:90-2.

26. CDC. Rabies vaccine, adsorbed: a new rabies vaccine for use in humans. MMWR 1988;37:217-8,223.

27. Burgoyne GH, Kajiya KD, Brown DW, Mitchell JR. Rhesus diploid rabies vaccine (adsorbed): a new rabies vaccine using FRhL-2 cells. J Infect Dis 1985;152:204-10.

28. Levenbook IS, Elisberg BL, Driscoll BF. Rhesus diploid rabies vaccine (adsorbed): neurological safety in guinea pigs and Lewis rats. Vaccine 1986;4:225-7.

29. Berlin BS, Goswick C. Rapidity of booster response to rabies vaccine produced in cell culture [letter]. J Infect Dis 1984;150:785.

30. Berlin BS, Mitchell JR, Burgoyne GH, Brown WE, Goswick C. Rhesus diploid rabies vaccine (adsorbed), a new rabies vaccine. II. Results of clinical studies simulating prophylactic therapy for rabies exposure. JAMA 1983;249:2663-5.

31. Berlin BS, Mitchell JR, Burgoyne GH, et al. Rhesus diploid rabies vaccine (adsorbed), a new rabies vaccine. Results of initial clinical studies of preexposure vaccination. JAMA 1982;247:1726-8.

32. Berlin BS. Rabies Vaccine Adsorbed: neutralizing antibody titers after three-dose pre-exposure vaccination. Am J Public Health 1990;80:476-7.

33. Nicholson KG Turner GS, Aoki FY. Immunization with a human diploid cell strain of rabies virus vaccine: two-year results. J Infect Dis 1978;137:783-8.

34. Bernard KW, Roberts MA, Sumner; J, et al. Human diploid cell rabies vaccine. Effectiveness of immunization with small intradermal or subcutaneous doses. JAMA 1982;247:1138-42.

35. Bernard KW, Mallonee J, Wright JC, et al. Preexposure immunization with intradermal human diploid cell rabies vaccine. Risks and benefits of primary and booster vaccination. JAMA 1987;257:1059-63.

36. Fishbein DB, Pacer RE, Holmes DF, Ley AB, Yager P, Tong TC. Rabies preexposure prophylaxis with human diploid cell rabies vaccine: a dose-response study. J Infect Dis 1987;156:50-5.

37. Afshar A. A review of non-bite transmission of rabies virus infection. Br Vet J 1979;135:142-8.

38. Winkler WG, Fashinell TR, Leffingwell L, Howard P, Conomy P. Airborne rabies transmission in a laboratory worker. JAMA 1973;226:1219-21.

39. CDC. Rabies in a laboratory worker-New York. MMWR 1977;26:183-4.

40. CDC. Human-to-human transmission of rabies via corneal transplant-Thailand. MMWR 1981;30:473-4.

41. Gode GR, Bhide NK. Two rabies deaths after corneal grafts from one donor [letter]. Lancet 1988;2:791.

42. CDC. Human-to-human transmission of rabies via a corneal transplant-France. MMWR 1980;29:25-6.

43. Houff SA, Burton RC, Wilson RW, et al. Human-to-human transmission of rabies virus by corneal transplant. N Engl J Med 1979;300:603-4.

44. Helmick CG, Tauxe RV, Vernon AA. Is there a risk to contacts of patients with rabies? Rev Infect Dis 1987;9:511-8.

45. Garner JS, Simmons BP. Guidelines for isolation precautions in hospitals. Infect Cont 1983;4(Suppl):245-325.

46. National Association of State Public Health Veterinarians. Compendium of animal rabies control. J Am Vet Med Assoc 1990; 196:36-9.

47. Fishbein DB, Belotto AJ, Pacer RE, et al. Rabies in rodents and lagomorphs in the United States, 1971-1984: increased cases in the woodchuck (Marmota monax) in mid-Atlantic states. J Wildl Dis 1986;22:151-5.

48. CDC. Imported dog and cat rabies-New Hampshire, California. MMWR 1988;37:559-60.

49. Eng TR, Fishbein DB. Epidemiologic factors, clinical findings, and vaccination status of rabies in cats and dogs in the United States in 1988. J Am Vet Med Assoc 1990;197:201-9.

50. Dean DJ, Baer GM. Studies on the local treatment of rabies infected wounds. Bull WHO 1963;28:477-86.

51. Kaplan MM, Cohen D, Koprowski H, Dean D, Ferrigan L. Studies on the local treatment of wounds for the prevention of rabies. Bull WHO 1962;26:765-75.

52. Fishbein DB, Sawyer LA, Reid-Sanden FL, Weir EH. Administration of human diploid-cell rabies vaccine in the gluteal area [letter]. N Engl J Med 1988;318:124-5.

53. Helmick CG, Johnstone C, Sumner J, Winkler WG, Fager S. A clinical study of Merieux human rabies immune globulin. J Biol Stand 1982;10:357-67.

54. Roumiantzeff M. The present status of rabies vaccine development and clinical experience with rabies vaccine. Southeast Asian J Trop Med Public Health 1988;19:549-61.

55. Kuwert EK, Marcus I, Werner J, et al. Post-exposure use of human diploid cell culture rabies vaccine. Dev Biol Stand 1976;37:273-86.

56. CDC. Recommendation of the Immunization Practices Advisory Committee (ACIP). Supplementary statement on pre-exposure rabies prophylaxis by the intradermal route. MMWR 1982;31:279-80,285.

57. Fishbein DB, Dreesen DW, Holmes DF, et al. Human diploid cell rabies vaccine purified by zonal centrifugation: a controlled study of antibody response and side effects following primary and booster pre-exposure immunization. Vaccine 1990;7:437-42.

58. Richardson JH, Barkley WE, eds. Biosafety in Microbioiogical and Biomedical Laboratories. 2nd ed. Washington, DC: U.S. Government Printing Office, 1988. HHS Publication No. (NIH) 88-8395.

59. Nicholson KG. Rabies. Lancet 1990;335:1201-5.

60. Warrell MJ, Nicholson KG, Warrell DA, et al. Economical multiple-site intradermal immunisation with human diploid-cell-strain vaccine is effective for post-exposure rabies prophylaxis. Lancet 1985;1:1059-62.

61. Chutivongse S, Wilde H, Supich C, Baer GM, Fishbein DB. Postexposure prophylaxis for rabies with antiserum and intradermal vaccination. Lancet 1990;335:896-8.

62. Anderson LJ, Baer GM, Smith JS, Winkler WG, Holman RC. Rapid antibody response to human diploid rabies vaccine. Am J Epidemiol 1981;113:270-5.

63. Vodopija I, Sureau P, Lafon M, et al. An evaluation of second generation tissue culture rabies vaccines for use in man: a four-vaccine comparative immunogenicity study using a pre-exposure vaccination schedule and an abbreviated 2-1-1 postexposure schedule. Vaccine 1986;4:245-8.

64. Vodopija I, Sureau P, Smerdel S, et al. Comparative study of two human diploid rabies vaccines administered with anti-rabies globulin. Vaccine 1988;6:489-90.

65. Vodopija I, Sureau P, Smerdel S, et al. Interaction of rabies vaccine with human rabies immunoglobulin and reliability of a 2-1-1 schedule application for postexposure treatment. Vaccine 1988;6:283-6.

66. Wilde H, Chomchey P, Prakongsri S, Punyaratabandhu P. Safety of equine rabies immune globulin [letter]. Lancet 1987;2:1275.

67. Wilde H, Chomchey P, Prakongsri S, Punyaratabandhu P, Chutivongse S. Adverse effects of equine rabies immune globulin. Vaccine 1989;7:10-1.

68. Wilde H, Chomchey P, Punyaratabandhu P. Purified equine rabies immune globulin; a safe and affordable alternative to human rabies immune globulin (experience with 3156 patients). Bull WHO (in press).

69. CDC. Human rabies despite treatment with rabies immune globulin and human diploid cell rabies vaccine- Thailand. MMWR 1987;36:759-60,765.

70. Shill M, Baynes RD, Miller SD. Fatal rabies encephalitis despite appropriate post-exposure prophylaxis. A case report. N Engl J Med 1987;316:1257-8.

71. Wilde H, Choomkasien P, Hemachudha T, Supich C, Chutivongse S. Failure of rabies postexposure treatment in Thailand. Vaccine 1989;7:49-52.

72. Turner GS, Nicholson KG, Tyrrell DA, Aoki FY. Evaluation of a human diploid cell strain rabies vaccine: final report of a three year study of pre-exposure immunization. J Hyg (Lond) 1982;89:101-10.

73. Cabasso VJ, Dobkin MB, Roby RE, Hammar AH. Antibody response to a human diploid cell rabies vaccine Appl Microbiol 1974;27:553-61.

74. CDC. Rabies prevention—United States, 1984. MMWR 1984;33:393-402,407-8.

75. Pappaioanou M, Fishbein DB, Dreesen DW, et al. Antibody response to preexposure human diploid-cell rabies vaccine given concurrently with chloroquine. N Engl J Med 1986;314:280-4.

76. Bernard KW, Fishbein DB, Miller KD, et al. Pre-exposure rabies immunization with human diploid cell vaccine: decreased antibody responses in persons immunized in developing countries. Am J Trop Med Hyg 1985;34:633-47.

77. Fishbein DB, Bernard KW, Miller KD, et al. The early kinetics of the neutralizing antibody response after booster immunizations with human diploid cell rabies vaccine. Am J Trop Med Hyg 1986;35:663-70.

78. Rubin RH, Hattwick MA, Jones S, Gregg MB, Schwartz VD. Adverse reactions to duck embryo rabies vaccine. Range and incidence. Ann Intern Med 1973;78:643-9.

79. Corey L, Hattwick MA, Baer GM, Smith JS. Serum neutralizing antibody after rabies postexposure prophylaxis Ann Intern Med 1976;85:170-6.

80. Boe E, Nylan H. Guillain-Barré syndrome after vaccination with human diploid cell rabies vaccine. Scand J Infect Dis 1980;12:231-2.

81. Knittel T, Ramadori G, Mayet WJ, Löhr H, Meyer zum Buschenfelde KH. Guillain-Barré syndrome and human diploid cell rabies vaccine [Letter]. Lancet 1989;1:1334-5.

82. Tornatore CS, Richert JR. CNS demyelination associated with diploid cell rabies vaccine [Letter]. Lancet 1990;335:1346-7.

83. Anderson MC, Baer H, Frazier DJ, Quinnan GV. The role of specific IgE and beta-propiolactone in reactions resulting from booster doses of human diploid cell rabies vaccine. J Allergy Clin Immunol 1987;80:861-8.

84. Swanson MC, Rosanoff E, Gurwith M, Deitch M, Schnurrenberger P, Reed CE. IgE and IgG antibodies to beta-propiolactone and human serum albumin associated with urticarial reactions to rabies vaccine. J Infect Dis 1987;155:909-13.

85. Enright JB. The effects of corticosteroids on rabies in mice. Can J Microbiol 1974;16:667.

86. Varner MW, McGuinness GA, Galask RP. Rabies vaccination in pregnancy. Am J Obstet Gynecol 1982; 143:717-8.

Chapter 13

Rocky Mountain Spotted Fever

Less than a hundred years ago, Rocky Mountain spotted fever was a mysterious disease that occasionally afflicted Indians and settlers in the northwest United States. The cause was unknown, and the mortality was high.

Today, the disease is no longer mysterious—the cause is known, and a cure is available. After a rapid increase in RMSF cases in the United States in the 1970s, the number of cases stayed approximately the same from 1977 through 1981 and has declined steadily since then.

Diagnosis and Treatment

Spotted fever is caused by one of a group of organisms known as rickettsiae, which are structurally related to bacteria but, in some of their properties, resemble viruses. The spotted fever agent, *Rickettsia rickettsii*, is transmitted by the bite of an infected tick. After an incubation period of three to ten days, the rickettsiae produce an inflammation of the inner lining of the blood vessels. This inflammation is eventually visible in the form of a rash comprising many red spots under the skin.

The appearance of this rash on the wrists and ankles is one of the main clues used by physicians to diagnose spotted fever. However, the

NIH Pub. No. 85-400.

rash is preceded by several days of chills, high fever, headache, and bone pain.

In severe untreated cases, the fever may persist for several weeks. Central nervous system symptoms, such as delirium or coma, usually appear by the end of the first week of fever. During the second week, critical circulatory and pulmonary complications may occur. Full recovery commonly takes several weeks or months in untreated patients.

The outlook for spotted fever patients changed radically in the early 1950s when the antibiotics chloramphenicol and tetracycline were found to be effective treatments. In the majority of patients, when tetracycline is given following prompt diagnosis, the headache and other symptoms abate within 24 to 48 hours, and the fever disappears in three to four days. Treatment is usually continued for 24 to 48 hours after the fever is gone. Relapse may occur in some instances when treatment is initiated very early or is discontinued too soon.

Early diagnosis is especially important since it eliminates the need for heroic treatment and prevents any damage to the brain or heart. Research is in progress to find a rapid and accurate method of laboratory diagnosis of spotted fever. However, at present, most diagnoses must be made on the basis of clinical symptoms and the awareness by both patient and physician of the possibility of tick-borne disease.

Prevention

In most tick-infested areas, the number of rickettsiae-infected ticks varies from less than one percent to about five percent. In addition to the Rocky Mountain wood tick, *Dermacentor andersoni*, other species of hard shell (ixodid) ticks have been found infected and may transmit the disease. Included are the dog tick, *Dermacentor variabilis*, which is the principal vector on the East Coast, and *Amblyomma americanum*, a possible vector in the South.

Generally, ticks are found in mountainous, heavily wooded, or sagebrush areas. The tick season runs from spring through early summer, although ticks may also be encountered in the fall and winter.

Persons entering tick-infested areas should wear proper clothing. Shorts and short-sleeved blouses or shirts should be discouraged. Instead, clothing should be worn that fits tightly at wrists, ankles, and waist. Each outer garment should overlap the one above it, i.e., trouser legs should be covered by high socks or boots, and shirttails should be tucked inside trousers.

Despite these precautions, contact with ticks cannot be prevented. However, a tick seldom attaches to the skin immediately, and it must be attached for several hours before it transmits the disease-causing rickettsiae. Persons living or vacationing in areas where there are ticks should examine themselves and their children at least twice daily. They should thoroughly inspect their bodies, especially the hairy regions, and the inside of their clothing. Household pets should also be examined regularly.

If a tick is found, it should be removed immediately and carefully. This can be done with the fingers or, preferably, with tweezers, being careful not to crush the tick, thus avoiding contamination of the broken skin with any infectious material. The tick should be grasped as close as possible to the point of attachment and should be pulled repeatedly and gently until it is free. A tick should not be jerked loose since this can result in breaking off the mouthparts, which would remain embedded in the skin. The bite wound should be treated with an antiseptic and the hands, which may be contaminated with infectious tick fluids, should be washed thoroughly with soap and water.

Any person who within two weeks after removal of a tick experiences general malaise with fever, headache, and muscle pain should *without delay* consult a physician, describing when and where the tick was found and how it was removed. This will facilitate diagnosis and treatment.

Reducing the tick population in an area is possible, but it is expensive. Chemical pesticides are available, but their toxicity for man and his environment must be considered.

Until about eight years ago, a commercial vaccine was available for the protection of persons living in highly endemic areas. Since this product afforded only limited protection, it has been withdrawn from the market, and at present, no vaccine is commercially available.

Early Investigations of Spotted Fever

Historically, the research on Rocky Mountain spotted fever is closely tied to the establishment and development of the Rocky Mountain Laboratory (RML) of the National Institute of Allergy and Infectious Diseases.

Late in the 19th century, when spotted fever became widespread among settlers of Montana's Bitterroot Valley, the settlers turned to the State and, eventually, to the Federal Government for aid.

It was Dr. Howard Taylor Ricketts who discovered in 1906 that the wood tick was responsible for transmitting the disease. Dr. R.A. Cooley, a Montana entomologist, then made his renowned tick survey in that state and directed studies concerning the life cycle of the wood tick.

In 1921, the United States Public Health Service established a laboratory in an abandoned school building near Hamilton, Montana. This laboratory became the center for studies of spotted fever and other tick-borne diseases, and several early scientists lost their lives to spotted fever. Eventually, a vaccine made from tissues of crushed ticks was developed at RML, and batches of it were shipped out to physicians all over the United States.

Life Cycle of the Tick

Early investigators realized that ticks have a complex life cycle, and it took many years to define how ticks live and how they transmit disease-causing agents.

It is now known that adult ticks feed on large animals, such as horses, cows, sheep, goats, deer, and dogs. When engorged, usually in about 9 days, the females drop to the ground where they lay their eggs—as many as 10,000—and die.

After about 36 days, the eggs hatch into six-legged larvae. These seed ticks then begin a journey in search of small host animals—usually rodents—on which they feed for days. Engorged larvae drop, find cover on the ground, and undergo a transformation that brings them into the eight-legged nymph stage of their biologic development.

Nymphs also seek small animal hosts and, after a feeding period of from three to ten days, drop off, find cover, and change into adult ticks. The entire life cycle requires about two years, since both unfed nymphs and adults pass the winter in hibernation.

If an adult tick fails to find a host on which to feed before the hot dry weather arrives, it goes to the ground again for shade and moisture for the remainder of the summer and a second winter. Unfed adult ticks are said to be able to survive up to two years under optimal conditions.

An infected tick transmits disease only during its feeding periods. Since larvae and nymphs rarely bite man, adult ticks are the main vectors of spotted fever to humans.

Experiments have shown, however, that stage to stage transmission of rickettsiae does take place. In other words, rickettsiae acquired by the tick in one stage of its life are retained through subsequent stages. Adult females transmit these organisms through the ovary to their eggs, from which larvae for the next generation hatch.

Laboratory studies have also shown that many species of animals—particularly rodents—carry spotted fever rickettsiae and are capable of transmitting the organisms to ticks that feed on them.

Research Today

Rocky Mountain spotted fever is still a public health problem, especially in the Southeast and South Central parts of the country. Many basic biological questions about this disease and other infectious diseases are unsolved, and scientists continue to study ticks and tick-borne diseases such as spotted fever.

As long as a vaccine is not available, individuals can protect themselves by taking sensible precautions when entering tick-infested areas. Such efforts will keep spotted fever a disease whose past is far more frightening than its present.

Chapter 14

St. Louis Encephalitis

St. Louis encephalitis (SLE) is a viral disease transmitted by *Culex* mosquitoes. It is a disease of the central nervous system with a broad range of clinical manifestations from asymptomatic to serious disease and death. For every case with symptoms there are up to several hundred infections without symptoms. The severity of illness increases with age with approximately 90 percent of infections in elderly patients resulting in encephalitis. Of symptomatic cases, 5-20 percent are fatal and for those over age 75, the case-fatality rate may be as high as 30 percent. There is no preventive vaccine or curative drug available for the disease.

SLE virus is maintained in a cycle between mosquitoes and birds, the latter serving as host both for the virus and for blood-feeding mosquitoes. Following virus transmission to birds by infectious mosquitoes, the virus appears in the blood of susceptible birds for several days, providing the opportunity for infecting other feeding mosquitoes.

At least 3 *Culex* species may transmit SLE virus. In the western U.S. the virus is transmitted by a mosquito associated with irrigated agriculture. This mosquito develops in a wide variety of flooded ditches and depressions containing vegetation and in vegetated portions of semi-permanent and permanent ponds. Habitat for the transmitting mosquito species in Florida is similar to that in the western U.S. In the central and other eastern states the responsible mosquito

CDC Document No.351901, July 21, 1993.

is associated with urban areas and develops in organically polluted water in ditches or other urban catchments as well as in a wide range of containers, from discarded tires and styrofoam boxes to ignored pet watering dishes. Underground storm water systems in older urban areas may serve as undetected mosquito habitat due to settling of individual sections of the system, thus forming underground pools. This problem may worsen following heavy rains or flooding if sewage contaminated water enters storm water systems. Small streams of slowly moving water with heavy overhanging grass or emergent vegetation along the margins also serve as mosquito habitat.

Culex mosquitoes feed principally at dusk and, to a lesser degree, through the night and at dawn. Proper screening of housing is an important preventative measure. Avoiding out-of-door exposure at dusk and for a couple of hours, reduces exposure to these mosquitoes. Use of repellents containing DEET on clothing and exposed skin is very effective. Repellent with DEET concentrations of 30 percent or less are as effective as those with higher concentrations. Because DEET, in very rare instances, has been associated with seizures in children, it is prudent to use lower concentrations for children and wash treated skin when mosquito exposure is ended.

Part Three

Diseases of Special Concern to International Travelers

Chapter 15

Health Hints for the International Traveler

Introduction

This section includes practical information on how to avoid potential health problems. Some of these recommendations are common-sense precautions; others have been scientifically documented.

Personal and specific preventive measures against certain diseases may require advance planning and advice from a physician concerning immunization and prophylaxis. If more specific information is needed, travelers should contact their local health department or physician.

Travelers who take prescription medications should carry an adequate supply accompanied by a signed and dated statement from a physician; the statement should indicate the major health problems and dosage of such medications, to provide information for medical authorities in case of emergency. The traveler should take an extra pair of glasses or lens prescription, and a card, tag, or bracelet that identifies any physical condition that may require emergency care.

If Medical Care Is Needed Abroad

If medical care is needed abroad, travel agents or the American Embassy or Consulate can usually provide names of hospitals, physi-

Taken From HHS Pub. No. (CDC) 94-8280, *Health Information for International Travel, 1994.*

cians, or emergency medical service agencies. Prior to departure, travelers should contact their own insurance companies concerning their coverage.

WHO Blood Transfusion Guidelines for International Travelers

There is a growing public awareness of the AIDS epidemic, and a resulting concern about acquiring the AIDS virus through blood transfusion. Systematic screening of blood donations is not yet feasible in all developing countries. Requests have been made by persons planning international travels, to have their own blood, or blood from their home country, available to them in case of urgent need. These requests raise logistic, technical and ethical issues which are not easy to resolve. Ultimately, the safety of blood for such persons will depend upon the quality of blood transfusion services in the host country. The strengthening of these services is of the highest priority. While efforts are being made to achieve this end, other approaches are also needed.

Basic Principles:

1. Unexpected, emergency blood transfusion is rarely required. It is needed only in situations of massive hemorrhage like severe trauma, gynecologic and obstetric emergency, or gastrointestinal bleeding.

2. In many cases, resuscitation can be achieved by use of colloid or crystalloid plasma expanders instead of blood.

3. Blood transfusion is not free of risk, even in the best of conditions. In most developing countries, the risk is increased by limited technical resources for screening blood donors for HIV infection and other diseases transmissible by blood.

4. The international shipment of blood for transfusion is practical only when handled by agreement between two responsible organizations, such as national blood transfusion services. This mechanism is not useful for emergency needs of individual patients and should not be attempted by private individuals or organizations not operating recognized blood programs.

Therefore:

1. There are no medical indications for travelers to take blood with them from their home country.

2. The limited storage period of blood and the need for special equipment negate the feasibility of independent blood banking for individual travelers or small groups.

3. Blood should be transfused only when absolutely indicated. This applies even more forcefully in those countries where screening of blood for transmissible diseases is not yet widely performed.

Proposed Options:

1. When urgent resuscitation is necessary, the use of plasma expanders rather than blood should always be considered.

2. In case of emergency need of blood, use of plasma expanders and urgent evacuation home may be the actions of choice.

3. When blood transfusion cannot be avoided, the attending physician should make every effort to ensure that the blood has been screened for transmissible diseases, including HIV.

4. International travelers should: a) take active steps to minimize the risk of injury; b) establish a plan for dealing with medical emergencies; c) support the development within countries of safe and adequate blood supplies.

This information is taken from the WHO publication "World Health Organization Global Programme on AIDS: Blood Transfusion Guidelines for International Travelers."

Motion Sickness

Travelers with a history of motion sickness or sea sickness can attempt to avoid symptoms by taking anti-motion-sickness pills or antihistaminics before departure.

Protection Against Mosquitoes and Other Arthropod Vectors

Although vaccines or chemoprophylactic drugs are available against important vector-borne diseases such as yellow fever and malaria, there are none for most other mosquito-borne diseases such as dengue, and travelers still should avail themselves of repellents and other general protective measures against arthropods. The effectiveness of malaria chemoprophylaxis is variable, depending on patterns of resistance and compliance with medication, and for many vector-borne diseases, no specific preventatives are available.

General Preventative Measures

The principal approach to prevention of vector-borne diseases is avoidance. Tick- and mite-borne infections characteristically are diseases of "place"; whenever possible, known foci of disease transmission should be avoided. Although many vector-borne infections can be prevented by avoiding rural locations, certain mosquito- and midge-borne arboviral and parasitic infections are transmitted around human residences and in urban locations. Most vector-borne infections are transmitted seasonally and simple changes in itinerary may greatly reduce risk for acquiring certain infections.

Exposure to arthropod bites can be minimized by modifying patterns of activity or behavior. Some vector mosquitoes are most active in twilight periods at dawn and dusk or in the evening. Avoidance of outdoor activity during these periods may reduce risk of exposure. Wearing long-sleeved shirts, long pants and hats will minimize areas of exposed skin. Shirts should be tucked in. Repellents applied to clothing, shoes, tents, mosquito nets and other gear will enhance protection.

When exposure to ticks or mites are a possibility, pants should be tucked into socks and boots should be worn; sandals should be avoided. Permethrin-based repellents applied as directed (see below) will enhance protection. During outdoor activity and at the end of the day, travelers should inspect themselves and their clothing for ticks. Ticks are detected more easily on light colored or white clothing. Prompt removal of attached ticks may prevent infection.

When accommodations are not adequately screened or air-conditioned, bednets are essential to provide protection and comfort. Bednets should be tucked under mattresses and can be sprayed with repellent. Aerosol insecticides and mosquito coils may help to clear rooms of mosquitoes; however, some coils contain DDT and should be used with caution.

Repellents

Permethrin-containing repellents (Permanone—use of trade names is for identification only and does not imply endorsement by the Public Health Service or the U.S. Department of Health and Human Services) are recommended for use on clothing, shoes, bednets and camping gear. Permethrin is highly effective as an insecticide/acaricide and as a repellent. Permethrin-treated clothing repels and kills ticks, mosquitoes and other arthropods and retains this effect after repeated laundering. There appears to be little potential for toxicity from permethrin-treated clothing.

Permethrin-containing shampoo (Nix) and cream (Elimite), marketed for use against head lice and scabies infestations, potentially could be extremely effective as repellents when applied on the hair and skin. However, they are approved only to treat existing conditions. Most authorities recommend repellents containing deet (diethylmethylbenzamide) as an active ingredient. Deet repels mosquitoes, ticks, and other arthropods when applied to skin or clothing. Formulations containing <30% deet are recommended because the additional gain in repellent effect with higher concentrations is not significant when weighed against the potential for toxicity. A microencapsulated formulation (Skeedadle) may have a longer period of activity than liquid formulations.

Deet is toxic when ingested. High concentrations applied to skin may cause blistering. Rare cases of encephalopathy in children, some fatal, have been reported after cutaneous exposure. Other neurologic side effects also have been reported. Toxicity did not appear to be dose-related in many cases and these may have been idiosyncratic reactions in predisposed individuals. However, a dose-related effect leading to irritability and impaired concentration and memory has been reported. Recommendations and precautions on the use of repellents are given [below].

Precautions to Minimize Potential for Adverse Reactions from Repellents

- Apply repellent sparingly only to exposed skin or clothing.

- Avoid applying high-concentration (>30% DEET) products to the skin, particularly of children.
- Do not inhale or ingest repellents or get them into the eyes.
- Wear long sleeves and long pants, when possible, and apply repellents (e.g., permethrin) to clothing to reduce cutaneous exposure.
- Avoid applying repellents to portions of children's hands that are likely to have contact with eyes or mouth.
- Pregnant and nursing women should minimize use of repellents.
- Never use repellents on wounds or irritated skin.
- Use repellent sparingly; one application will last approximately 4 hours. Saturation does not increase efficacy.
- Wash repellent-treated skin after coming indoors.
- If a suspected reaction to insect repellents occurs, wash treated skin, and call a physician. Take the repellent container to the physician.

Pregnant Women Traveling Abroad

The problems that a pregnant woman might encounter during international travel are basically the same problems that other international travelers have. These have to do with exposure to infectious diseases and availability of good medical care. There is the additional potential problem that air travel late in pregnancy might precipitate labor.

Information on vaccination and malaria prophylaxis during pregnancy may be found in each disease section.

Potential health problems vary from country to country; therefore, if the traveler has specific questions, she should be advised to check with the embassy or local consulate general's office of the country in question before traveling.

Disabled Travelers

The United States (U.S.) Architectural and Transportation Barriers Compliance Board (Access Board) produces or distributes a variety of publications, at no cost. U.S. air carriers must comply with the U.S. laws or regulations regarding access. Up-to-date information regarding access abroad is more difficult to ascertain. A booklet, *Access*

Travel: Airports, is available free from the Consumer Information Center in Pueblo, Colorado 81009. It lists accessibility features at 553 airports worldwide. U.S. companies or entities conducting programs or tours on cruise ships also have some obligations for access, even if the ship itself is foreign flagged. Write or call, Access Board, Suite 1000, 1331 F Street, N.W., Washington, D.C. 20004-1111, 1-800- USA-ABLE (voice/TDD) for a list of its publications.

Risks from Food and Drink

Contaminated food and drink are common sources for the introduction of infection into the body. Among the more common infections that travelers may acquire from contaminated food and drink are *Escherichia coli* infections, shigellosis or bacillary dysentery, giardiasis, cryptosporidiosis, and hepatitis A. Other less common infectious disease risks for travelers include typhoid fever and other salmonelloses, cholera, infections caused by rotaviruses and Norwalk-like viruses, and a variety of protozoan and helminth parasites (other than those that cause giardiasis and cryptosporidiosis). Many of the infectious diseases transmitted in food and water can also be acquired directly through the fecal-oral route.

Water

Water that has been adequately chlorinated, using minimum recommended waterworks standards as practiced in the United States, will afford significant protection against viral and bacterial waterborne diseases. However, chlorine treatment alone, as used in the routine disinfection of water, may not kill some enteric viruses and the parasitic organisms that cause giardiasis and amebiasis. In areas where chlorinated tap water is not available, or where hygiene and sanitation are poor, travelers should be advised that only the following may be safe to drink:

1. Beverages, such as tea and coffee, made with boiled water

2. Canned or bottled *carbonated* beverages, including *carbonated* bottled water and soft drinks

3. Beer and wine

Where water may be contaminated, ice (or containers for drinking) also should be considered contaminated. Thus, in these areas ice should not be used in beverages. If ice has been in contact with containers used for drinking, the containers should be thoroughly cleaned, preferably with soap and hot water, after the ice has been discarded.

It is safer to drink directly from a can or bottle of a beverage than from a questionable container. However, water on the outside of cans or bottles of beverages might be contaminated. Therefore, wet cans or bottles should be dried before being opened, and surfaces which are contacted directly by the mouth in drinking should first be wiped clean. Where water may be contaminated, travelers should avoid brushing their teeth with tap water.

Treatment of Water

Boiling is by far the most reliable method to make water of uncertain purity safe for drinking. Water should be brought to a vigorous boil and allowed to cool to room temperature—do not add ice. At very high altitudes, for an extra margin of safety, boil for several minutes or use chemical disinfection. Adding a pinch of salt to each quart, or pouring the water several times from one container to another will improve the taste.

Chemical disinfection with iodine is an alternative method of water treatment when it is not feasible to boil water. Two well-tested methods for disinfection with iodine are the use of tincture of iodine (Figure 15.1), and the use of tetraglycine hydroperiodide tablets (Globaline, Potable-Agua, Coghlan's, etc.). The tablets are available from pharmacies and sporting goods stores. The manufacturer's instructions should be followed. If water is cloudy, the number of tablets should be doubled; if water is extremely cold, an attempt should be made to warm the water, and the recommended contact time should be increased to achieve reliable disinfection. Cloudy water should be strained through a clean cloth into a container to remove any sediment or floating matter, and then the water should be treated with heat or iodine. Chlorine, in various forms, has also been used for chemical disinfection. However, its germicidal activity varies greatly with pH, temperature, and organic content of the water to be purified, and is less reliable than iodine.

There are a variety of portable filters currently on the market which according to the manufacturers' data will provide safe drinking water. Although the iodide-impregnated resins and the microstrainer type filters will kill and/or remove many microorganisms, very few published reports in the scientific literature deal both with the methods used and the results of the tests employed to evaluate the efficacy of these filters against water-borne pathogens. Until there is sufficient independent verification of the efficacy of these filters, CDC makes no recommendation regarding their use.

As a last resort, if no source of safe drinking water is available or can be obtained, tap water that is uncomfortably hot to touch may be safer than cold tap water. however proper disinfection or boiling is still advised.

Tincture of iodine (from medicine chest or first aid kit)	Drops* to be added per quart or liter	
	Clear water	Cold or cloudy water†
2%	5	10

*1 drop = 0.05 ml
Let stand for 30 minutes.
Water is safe to use.
†Very turbid or very cold water may require prolonged contact time; let stand up to several hours prior to use, if possible.

Figure 15.1. Treatment of Water with Tincture of Iodine

Food

To avoid illness, food should be selected with care. All raw food is subject to contamination. Particularly in areas where hygiene and sanitation are inadequate, the traveler should be advised to avoid salads, uncooked vegetables, unpasteurized milk and milk products such as cheese, and to eat only food that has been cooked and is still hot, or fruit that has been peeled by the traveler. Undercooked and raw meat, fish, and shellfish may carry various intestinal pathogens. Cooked food that has been allowed to stand for several hours at ambient temperature may provide a fertile medium for bacterial growth and should be thoroughly reheated before serving.

The easiest way to guarantee a safe food source for an infant less than 6 months of age is to have the child breast-feed. If the infant has already been weaned from the breast, formula prepared from commercial powder and boiled water is the safest and most practical food.

Some species of fish and shellfish can contain poisonous biotoxins, even when well cooked. The most common type of fish poisoning in travelers is ciguatera fish poisoning. Barracuda is the most toxic fish and should always be avoided. Red snapper, grouper, amberjack, sea bass, and a wide range of tropical reef fish contain the toxin at unpredictable times. The potential for ciguatera poisoning exists in all subtropical and tropical insular areas of the West Indies, Pacific and Indian Oceans where the implicated fish species are consumed.

Recently, cholera cases have occurred among persons who ate crab brought back from Latin America by travelers. Travelers should not bring perishable seafoods with them when they return.

Cruise Ship Sanitation

The Centers for Disease Control and Prevention (CDC) established the Vessel Sanitation Program (VSP) in 1975 as a cooperative activity with the cruise ship industry as a result of several major disease outbreaks on cruise vessels. This joint program strives to achieve and maintain a level of sanitation on passenger vessels that will lower the risk of gastrointestinal disease outbreaks and provide a healthful environment. The program goals are addressed through encouraging industry to establish and maintain a comprehensive sanitation program and oversight of its success through an inspections process. Every vessel with a foreign itinerary that carries 13 or more passengers is subject to twice yearly inspections and when necessary reinspection. Inspections are only conducted at those ports under U.S. control and cover such environmental aspects as:

1. Water supply, storage, distribution, backflow protection and disinfection.

2. Food preparation during storage, preparation, and service and product temperature control.

3. Potential contamination of food, water, and ice.

4. Employee practices and personal hygiene.

5. General cleanliness, facility repair, and vector control.

A score of 86 or higher at the time of the inspection indicates that the ship is providing an accepted standard of sanitation. In general, the lower the score the lower the level of sanitation; however, a low score does not necessarily imply an imminent risk of an outbreak of gastrointestinal disease. CDC reserves the right to recommend that a ship not sail when circumstances so dictate. This may include but is not restricted to, contamination of the potable water supply, inadequate treatment of the potable water supply, or food temperature violations. A copy of the most recent sanitation inspection report on an individual vessel or a copy of *The Summary of Sanitation Inspections of International Cruise Ships* may be obtained by writing to: Chief, Vessel Sanitation Program, National Center for Environmental Health, 1015 North America Way, Suite 107, Miami, Florida 33132.

Disinsection of Aircraft

International travelers should be aware that some countries require disinsection of certain passenger aircraft in order to prevent the importation of insects such as mosquitos. Disinsection procedures may include the spraying of the aircraft passenger compartment with insecticide while passengers are present. While the recommended disinsection procedures have been determined to be safe by the World Health Organization, they may aggravate certain health conditions (i.e, allergies). Travelers with such conditions or who are otherwise interested in determining what disinsection procedures may be performed on a particular flight should contact their travel agent or airline.

Environmental Effects

International travelers may be subject to certain stresses that may lower resistance to disease, such as crowding, disruption of usual eating and drinking habits, and time changes with "jet lag" contributing to a disturbed pattern of the sleep and wakefulness cycle. These conditions of stress can lead to nausea, indigestion, fatigue, or insomnia. Complete adaptation depends on the number of time zones crossed but may take a week or more.

Heat and cold can be directly or indirectly responsible for some diseases and can give rise to serious skin conditions. Dermatophytoses such as athlete's foot are often made worse by warm, humid conditions.

Excessive heat and humidity alone, or immoderate activity under those conditions, may lead to heat exhaustion due to salt and water deficiency and to the more serious heat stroke or hyperthermia. The ultraviolet rays of the sun can cause severe and very debilitating sunburn in lighter-skinned persons.

Excessive cold affects persons who may be inadequately dressed and particularly the elderly; it can lead to hypothermia and to frostbite of exposed parts of the body.

Breathing and swallowing dust when traveling on unpaved roads or in arid areas may be followed by nausea and malaise, and may cause increased susceptibility to infections of the upper respiratory tract.

Traveling in high altitudes may lead to insomnia, headache, nausea, and altitude sickness, even in young and healthy persons, and can cause distress to those with cardiac or pulmonary conditions. Individual susceptibility to acute mountain sickness is highly variable. Travelers who are at greatest risk are those who ascend rapidly to tourist sites in the Andes and the Himalayas. Acetazolamide has been shown, under both simulated and actual climbing conditions, to hasten the process of acclimatization to high altitudes. The recommended dosage to prevent acute mountain sickness is 250 mg every 8-12 hours, with medication initiated 24-48 hours before, and continued during ascent. Acetazolamide should not be taken by individuals who are allergic to sulfonamides.

Chernobyl

Effects of the Radiological Release At Chernobyl

The Chernobyl Nuclear Power station, located in the Ukraine Republic about 100 kilometers (62 miles) north-west of Kiev and 310 kilometers (193 miles) south-east of Minsk (in Belarus), experienced an uncontrolled release of radioactive material in April, 1986. This event seems to have resulted in the largest short term release of radioactive materials to the atmosphere ever recorded. The radiological contamination primarily affected three Republics: the Ukraine, Belarus, and Russia. The highest areas of radioactive ground contamination occurred within 30 km (19 miles) of Chernobyl.

Area Considerations

Short term international travelers to the republics of Ukraine, Belarus, and Russia (i.e., those who plan to stay in the region less than a few months) should not be concerned about residing in areas that are not controlled (i.e., marked with signs or fenced). However, we do caution longer term visitors that there are some non-controlled areas where an individual could receive a radiation dose from the radioactive ground contamination in excess of the international radiological health standards recommended for most members of the public. Long term visitors should investigate the local conditions prior to choosing a long-term residence. (For example, ground contamination that exceeds 5 curies per square kilometer (5 Ci/km^2) of cesium-137 could result in a radiation dose greater than the recommended standards.)

Food and Water Considerations

Officials of the three republics attempt to monitor all food stuffs sold in the public markets for levels of radioactivity. Radioactive concentration limits have been established for various classes of food, e.g., milk, meat, and vegetables. These limits are comparable to standards used by many western nations including the European Economic Community. Food with contamination levels in excess of these limits is not allowed to be sold in the market. Private farmers regularly make food available for sale outside the official market system. This food is not monitored for radioactivity and it is recommended that travelers not consume this food. Likewise, it is recommended that travelers not consume any wild berries, wild mushrooms or wild game from these regions. And, it is also recommended that travelers drink only bottled water.

Age and Health Considerations

Young children, unborn babies, and nursing infants are potentially at greater risk from exposure to radiation than adults. Pregnant or nursing mothers should pay extra attention in acquiring and consuming food from reliable well-monitored sources.

Injuries

The major causes of serious disability or loss of life are not infectious. Trauma caused by injuries, principally that suffered in motor vehicle crashes, is the leading cause of death and disability in both developed and developing countries worldwide. Motor vehicle crashes result from a variety of factors, including inadequate roadway design, hazardous poor vehicle conditions, lack of appropriate vehicles and vehicle maintenance, unskilled or inexperienced drivers, inattention to pedestrians and pedal-cyclists, or impairment due to alcohol or drug use; all these factors are preventable or can be abated. Defensive driving is an important preventive measure. When driving or riding, insist on a vehicle equipped with safety belts and where available, use them. When available, also insist on a vehicle equipped with airbags and anti-lock brakes. As a high proportion of crashes occur at night when returning from "social events," avoid non-essential night driving, alcohol, and riding with persons who are under the influence of alcohol or drugs. Pedestrian, bicycle, and motorcycle travel are often dangerous, and helmet use is imperative for bicycle and motorcycle travel.

Fire injuries are also a significant cause of injuries and death—inquire about whether hotels have smoke detectors and sprinkler systems, and do not smoke in bed. Travelers may wish to bring their own smoke detectors with them. Always look for a primary and alternate escape route in rooms in which you are meeting or staying. Look for improperly vented heating devices which may cause carbon monoxide poisoning. Remember to escape a fire by crawling low under smoke.

Other major causes of injury trauma include drowning (see swimming precautions [below]) and drug reactions. Protection against potentially hazardous drugs is nonexistent in some countries. Do not buy medications "over the counter" unless you are familiar with the product.

Travelers should also be aware of the potential for violence-related injuries. Risk for assault or terrorist attack varies from country to country; heed advice from residents and tour guides about areas to be avoided, going out at night, and going out alone. Do not fight attackers. If confronted, give up your valuables. For more information, contact the U.S. Department of State, Overseas Citizens Emergency Center, at (202) 647-5225.

Animal-Associated Hazards

Animals in general tend to avoid human beings, but they can attack, particularly if they are with young. In areas of endemic rabies, domestic dogs, cats, or other animals should not be petted. Wild animals should be avoided.

The bites, stings, and contact of some insects cause unpleasant reactions. Medical attention should be sought if an insect bite or sting causes redness, swelling, bruising, or persistent pain. Many insects also transmit communicable diseases. Some insects can bite and transmit disease without the person being aware of the bite, particularly when camping or staying in rustic or primitive accommodations. Insect repellents, protective clothing, and mosquito netting are advisable in many parts of the world (See Protection Against Mosquitoes and Other Arthropod Vectors).

Poisonous snakes are hazards in many parts of the world, although deaths from snake bites are relatively rare. The Australian brown snake, Russell's viper and cobras in southern Asia, carpet vipers in the Middle East, and coral and rattlesnakes in the Americas are particularly dangerous. Most snakebites are the direct result of handling or harassing snakes, which bite as a defensive reaction. Attempts to kill snakes are dangerous, often leading to bites on the fingers. The venom of a small or immature snakes may be even more concentrated than that of a larger individual, therefore all snakes should be left strictly alone.

Less than half of all snake bite wounds actually contain venom, but medical attention should be sought anytime a bite wound breaks the skin. A pressure bandage, ice (if available), and immobilization of the affected limb are recommended first aid measures while the victim is moved as quickly as possible to a medical facility. Specific therapy for snakebite is controversial, and should be left to the judgement of local emergency medical personnel. Snakes tend to be active at night and in warm weather. As a precaution, boots and long pants may be worn when walking outdoors at night in snake-infested regions. Bites from scorpions may be painful but seldom are dangerous except possibly in infants. In general, exposure to bites can be avoided by sleeping under mosquito nets and by shaking clothing and shoes before putting them on, particularly in the morning. Snakes and scorpions tend to rest in shoes and clothing.

Anthrax-Contaminated Goatskin Handicrafts

Anthrax is a disease caused by a bacterial organism that produces spores that are highly resistant to disinfection. These infectious spores may persist on a contaminated item for many years. Anthrax spores have been found on goatskin handicrafts from Haiti.

Travelers to Caribbean countries are advised not to purchase Haitian goatskin handicrafts. Because of the risk, importation of goatskin handicrafts from Haiti will not be permitted at U.S. ports of entry; they will be confiscated and destroyed.

Swimming Precautions

Swimming in contaminated water may result in skin, eye, ear, and certain intestinal infections, particularly if the swimmer's head is submerged. Generally only pools that contain chlorinated water can be considered safe places to swim. In certain areas, fatal primary amebic meningoencephalitis has occurred following swimming in warm dirty water. Swimmers should avoid beaches that might be contaminated with human sewage, or with dog feces. Wading or swimming should be avoided in freshwater streams, canals, and lakes liable to be infested with the snail hosts of schistosomiasis (bilharziasis) or contaminated with urine from animals infected with *Leptospira*. Biting and stinging fish and corals and jelly fish may provide a hazard to the swimmer. Never swim alone or when under the influence of alcohol or drugs, and never dive head first into an unfamiliar body of water.

The Post-Travel Period

Some diseases may not manifest themselves immediately. If travelers become ill after they return home, they should tell their physician where they have traveled.

Most persons who acquire viral, bacterial, or parasitic infections abroad become ill within 6 weeks after returning from international travel. However, some diseases may not manifest themselves immediately, e.g., malaria may not cause symptoms for as long as 6 months to a year after the traveler returns to the United States. It is recommended that a traveler always advise a physician of the countries visited within the 12 months preceding onset of illness. Knowledge of such travel and the possibility the patient may be ill with a disease the physician rarely encounters will help the physician arrive at a correct diagnosis.

Importation or Exportation of Human Remains

There are no federal restrictions on the importation of human remains unless the death was the result of one of the following communicable diseases: cholera or suspected cholera, diphtheria, infectious tuberculosis, plague, suspected smallpox, yellow fever, suspected viral hemorrhagic fevers (Lassa, Marburg, Ebola, Congo-Crimean, and others not yet isolated or named). If the death was the result of one of these diseases, the remains must be cremated or properly embalmed and placed in a hermetically sealed casket, and be accompanied by a death certificate, translated into English, which states the cause of death. Following importation, the local mortician will be subject to the regulations of the State and local health authorities for interstate or intrastate shipment.

The United States has no requirements for the exportation of human remains; however, the requirements of the country of destination must be met. Information regarding these requirements may be obtained from the appropriate embassy or local consulate general.

Importation or Reentry of Pets

Pets which are transported internationally should be free of communicable diseases that may be transmissible to humans. U.S. Public Health Service regulations place the following restrictions on the importation of dogs, cats, nonhuman primates and turtles:

Dogs

Dogs older than 3 months presented for importation from countries where rabies is known to occur, must be accompanied by a valid rabies vaccination certificate which includes the following information:

1. The breed, sex, age, color, markings, and other identifying information,

2. Vaccination date at least 30 days prior to importation (See below)

3. Vaccination expiration date. If not shown, the date of vaccination must be within 12 months prior to the importation, and

4. Signature of a licensed veterinarian.

Dogs not accompanied by the above described certificate may be admitted, provided the importer completes a confinement agreement.

Such dogs must be kept in confinement during transit to, and be vaccinated within 4 days after arrival at, the U.S. destination. Such dogs must remain in confinement for at least 30 days after the date of vaccination.

Dogs less than 3 months of age may be admitted, provided the importer completes a confinement agreement. Such dogs must be kept in confinement during transit and at the U.S. destination until vaccinated at 3 months of age and for at least 30 days after vaccination.

Routine rabies vaccination of dogs is recommended in the U.S. and is required by most State and local health authorities.

Cats

While proof of rabies vaccination is not required for cats, routine rabies vaccination of cats is recommended in the U.S. and is required by most State and local health authorities.

Turtles

Turtles may transmit salmonellosis to humans, and because small turtles are often kept as pets, restrictions apply to their importation. Live turtles with a carapace (shell) length of less than 4 inches and viable turtle eggs may be imported into the United States if the importation is not for commercial purposes. The Public Health Service has no restrictions on the importation of live turtles with a carapace length of more than 4 inches.

Monkeys and Other Nonhuman Primates

Nonhuman primates may transmit a variety of serious diseases to humans. Live monkeys and other nonhuman primates may be imported into the United States only by importers registered with CDC and only for scientific, educational, or exhibition purposes. Monkeys and other nonhuman primates may not be imported for use as pets.

Measures At Port of Entry

U.S. Public Health Service regulations provide for the examination of admissible dogs, cats, nonhuman primates and turtles presented for importation into the U.S. Animals with evidence of disease that may be transmissible to humans may be subject to additional disease control measures.

General

For additional information regarding importation of these animals, contact the Centers for Disease Control and Prevention, Attention: National Center for Prevention Services, Division of Quarantine, Mailstop E03. Atlanta, Georgia 30333, Telephone (404) 639-8107.

Persons planning to import horses, ruminants, swine, poultry, birds, and dogs used in handling livestock should contact the U.S. Department of Agriculture regarding additional requirements, Telephone (301) 436-8170.

Persons planning to import fish, reptiles, spiders, wild birds, rabbits, bears, wild members of the cat family, or other wild or endangered animals should contact the U.S. Department of the Interior, Fish and Wildlife Service, Telephone (202) 342-9242.

Travelers planning to take a pet to a foreign country are advised to meet entry requirements of the country of destination. To obtain this information write to or call the country's embassy in Washington, D.C. or to the consulate nearest you.

Chapter 16

Travelers' Diarrhea

Introduction

Diarrhea is by far the most frequent health problem of travelers to developing counties. Of the estimated 300 million international travelers who will cross the world's frontiers this year, at least 16 million persons from industrialized countries, including more than 8 million U.S. residents, will travel to developing countries. Approximately one-third of these travelers to developing countries will get diarrhea. The economic impact of travelers' diarrhea (TD) is substantial, because fear of sickness is one of the major deterrents to tourism. International tourists worldwide spend over $100 billion annually, and the economies of many nations depend on this travel. For educational, recreational, political, and financial reasons, this international exchange should be fostered.

The incidence of TD varies markedly by destination and may depend in part on the number of dietary indiscretions made by the traveler and on the style of travel. TD is caused by a variety of infectious agents, and the spectrum of clinical illness varies considerably. However, this illness in travelers is usually not severe; high fever, vomiting, or bloody stools occur in only a minority of cases.

Dietary prudence and hygienic measures are safe and simple preventive techniques, but they do not eliminate entirely the risk of diar-

National Institutes of Health, Consensus Development Conference Statement, Volume 5, Number 8.

rhea. Prophylactic measures such as antidiarrheal drugs and oral antimicrobial agents have been used. TD is treated with a variety of regimens, including oral electrolyte solutions, antidiarrheal compounds, and antimicrobial drugs, prescribed either singly or in combination.

There continues to be a debate concerning whether the risk of antimicrobial agents is worth the benefit; whether early therapy of ill travelers is preferable to daily prophylaxis of all travelers; whether all currently employed treatment strategies are useful; and whether given groups of travelers, such as vacationers, students, or business travelers, should be selectively advised to follow special regimens.

To resolve some of these questions, the NIH Office of Medical Applications of Research and the National Institute of Allergy and Infectious Diseases convened a Consensus Development Conference on Travelers' Diarrhea on January 28-30, 1985. After 1 1/2 days of expert presentation of the available data, a consensus panel of epidemiologists, biostatisticians, microbiologists, pediatricians, internists, infectious diseases specialists, travel experts, and lay representatives considered the evidence and agreed on answers to the following questions:

- What is the epidemiology of travelers' diarrhea, and why is it important?
- What causes travelers' diarrhea?
- What prevention measures are effective for travelers' diarrhea?
- What treatment measures are effective for travelers' diarrhea?
- What should be the direction of future research?

What Is the Epidemiology of Traveler's Diarrhea and Why Is It Important?

Travelers' diarrhea is a syndrome characterized by a twofold or greater increase in the frequency of unformed bowel movements. Commonly associated symptoms include abdominal cramps, nausea, bloating, urgency, fever, and malaise. Episodes of TD usually begin abruptly, occur during travel or soon after returning home, and are generally self-limited. Within this context, travelers at risk are defined as individuals from industrialized countries visiting for a period of up to 1 month a region or country where there is an increased risk of developing diarrhea. The public health and medical importance of TD is related to the large numbers of travelers who place themselves at risk each year. Furthermore, TD is but a mild reflection of the severe underlying problem of diarrhea among children in the tropics.

The most important determinant of risk is the destination of the traveler. Attack rates in the range of 20 to 50 percent are commonly reported, but recent data are available from relatively few countries. The best available estimates of country-specific attack rates have been reported for Swiss travelers. Examples of high-risk destinations include most of the developing countries of Latin America, Africa, the Middle East, and Asia. Intermediate risk destinations include most of the Southern European countries and a few Caribbean islands. Low risk destinations include Canada, Northern Europe, Australia, New Zealand, the United States and a number of the Caribbean islands.

TD is slightly more common in young adults than in older people. The reasons for this difference are unclear, but may include a lack of acquired immunity, more adventurous travel styles, and different eating habits. Attack rates are similar in men and women. The most common onset of TD is usually within the first week. but onset may occur at any time during the visit, and even after returning home.

TD is acquired through ingestion of fecally contaminated food and/or water. Both cooked and uncooked foods may be implicated if improperly handled. Especially risky foods include raw vegetables, raw meat, and raw seafood. Tap water ice, unpasteurized milk and dairy products, and unpeeled fruits are associated with increased risk of TD; bottled carbonated beverages (especially flavored beverages), beer, wine, hot coffee or tea, or water boiled or appropriately treated with iodine or chlorine are safe.

The eating place appears to be an important variable, with private homes, restaurants, and street vendors listed in order of increasing risk.

TD typically results in four to five loose or watery stools per day. The median duration of diarrhea is 3 to 4 days. Ten percent of the cases persist longer than 1 week, approximately 2 percent longer than 1 month, and less than 1 percent longer than 3 months. Persistent diarrhea is thus quite uncommon and may differ considerably from acute TD with respect to etiology and risk factors. Travelers may experience more than one attack of TD during a single trip. Approximately 15 percent experience vomiting, and 2 to 10 percent may have diarrhea accompanied by fever or bloody stools, or both. Rarely is TD life-threatening. In an extensive survey of several hundred thousand Swiss travelers, no deaths could be attributed to TD.

What Causes Travelers' Diarrhea?

Infectious agents are the primary cause of TD. This statement is based on investigations designed to isolate known infectious organisms from diarrheal stools of tourists and on studies that demonstrated the efficacy of antibacterial agents. In addition, induced disease in volunteers has confirmed the causal role of the putative bacterial and viral agents in producing TD.

All travelers from industrialized countries going to developing countries quickly develop a rapid, dramatic change in their intestinal flora. These new organisms often include the potential enteric pathogens. Those who develop diarrhea have ingested an inoculum of virulent organisms sufficiently large to overcome individual defense mechanisms, resulting in symptoms.

Enteric Bacterial Pathogens

Enterotoxigenic *Escherichia coli* (ETEC) are the most common causative agents of TD in all countries where surveys have been conducted. The discovery and understanding of the mechanisms of action of cholera enterotoxin led to investigations that demonstrated enterotoxins in *E. coli* and other bacteria. These organisms adhere in the small intestine, where they multiply and produce an enterotoxin (either heat stable or heat labile) that causes fluid secretion and diarrhea.

Identification of the ETEC is a difficult task, requiring sophisticated techniques that remain somewhat insensitive.

Other *E. coli* have different virulence traits. These have been termed enteroadherent, enteroinvasive, and enteropathogenic *E. coli*. No systematic search for these other *E. coli* has been conducted in patients with TD. Limited data suggest that they are a minor cause of TD.

Salmonella gastroenteritis is a well-known disease that occurs throughout the world. In the industrialized nations, this large group of organisms is the most common cause of outbreaks of food-associated diarrhea. In the developing countries, the proportion of cases of TD caused by salmonellae varies but is not high. Salmonellae also can cause dysentery characterized by bloody mucus-containing small-volume stools.

Shigellae are well known as the cause of bacillary dysentery. They cause TD in about 5 to 15 percent of travelers in a few countries.

Few of the infected travelers had dysentery, but most had watery diarrhea.

Campylobacter jejuni is a common cause of diarrhea throughout the world. Recent, limited data have shown that *C. jejuni* is responsible for a small percentage of the reported cases of TD, some with bloody diarrhea. Additional studies are needed to determine how frequent it causes TD.

Vibrio parahaemolyticus is associated with the ingestion of raw or poorly cooked seafood and has caused TD in Japanese people traveling in Asia. How frequently it causes disease in other areas of the world is unknown.

Other potential bacterial pathogens, including *Aeromonas hydrophila, Yersinia enterocolitica, Pleisiomonas shigelloides, Vibrio cholerae* (non-01), and *Vibrio fluvialis*, are known to cause diarrhea in children and adults. In Thailand, *Aeromonas* and *Pleisiomonas* have been isolated from stools of Peace Corps volunteers who had TD. A better appreciation of the importance of each of these bacteria as causative agents of TD requires a more intensive search for them, using appropriate selective isolation media or rapid diagnostic techniques.

Viral Enteric Pathogens—Rotavirus and Norwalk-Like Virus

Along with the newly acquired bacterial flora, many viruses also are acquired. In six studies, for example, 0 to 36 percent of diarrheal illnesses (median 22 percent) were associated with rotaviruses in the stools. However, a comparable number of asymptomatic travelers also had rotaviruses, and up to 50 percent of symptomatic rotavirus infections were associated with nonviral pathogens. Ten to fifteen percent of travelers develop a serologic conversion to Norwalk-like viruses. The roles of adenoviruses, astroviruses, coronaviruses, enteroviruses, or other viral agents in causing TD are even less clear. Although viruses are commonly acquired by travelers, they do not appear to be frequent causes of TD in adults.

Parasitic Enteric Pathogens

The few studies that have included an examination for parasites reveal that 0 to 9 percent have *Giardia lamblia* or *Entamoeba histolytica. Cryptosporidium* has recently been recognized in sporadic cases of TD.

Dientamoeba fragilis, Isospora belli, Balantidium coli, or *Strongyloides stercoralis* may cause occasional cases of TD. While not major causes of acute TD, these parasites should be sought in persisting, unexplained cases.

Unknown Causes

No data have been presented to support noninfectious causes of TD such as changes in diet, jet lag, altitude, and fatigue. Current evidence indicates that in all but a few instances (e.g., drug-induced or preexisting gastrointestinal disorders) an infectious agent or agents cause diarrhea in tourists.

Even with the application of the best current methods for detecting bacteria, viruses, and parasites, in various studies 20 to 50 percent remain without recognized etiologies. The unrecognized causes may be attributed to:

- Recognized pathogens that were not uniformly sought in every study (such as *Campylobacter, Aeromonas, Yersinia, Pleisiomonas, Vibrios*, viruses, and parasites like *Cryptosporidium*).

- Unrecognized pathogens.

- Known bacterial pathogens that were not detected. Our best methods for detecting enterotoxigenic *E. coli* and Shigella, for example, are insensitive and miss 30 to 40 percent of cases in outbreak or volunteer studies.

What Prevention Measures Are Effective for Travelers' Diarrhea?

There are four possible approaches to prevention of TD. They include instruction regarding food and beverage preparation, immunization, use of nonantimicrobial medications, and prophylactic antimicrobial drugs.

Data indicate that meticulous attention to food and beverage preparation, as mentioned above, can decrease the likelihood of developing TD. Most travelers, however, encounter great difficulty in observing the requisite dietary restrictions.

No available vaccines and none that are expected to be available in the next 5 years are effective against TD.

Several nonantimicrobial agents have been advocated for prevention of TD. Available controlled studies indicate that prophylactic use of difenoxine, the active metabolite of diphenoxylate (Lomotil), actually increases the incidence of TD in addition to producing other undesirable side effects. No antiperistaltic agents (e.g., Lomotil and Imodium) are effective in preventing TD. No data support the prophylactic use of activated charcoal.

Bismuth subsalicylate, taken in liquid form as the active ingredient of Pepto-Bismol (2 oz four times daily), has decreased the incidence of diarrhea by 60 percent in one study.

Available data are not extensive enough to exclude a risk to the traveler from the use of such large doses of bismuth subsalicylate over a period of several weeks. In patients already taking salicylates for arthritis, large concurrent doses of bismuth subsalicylate can produce toxic serum concentrations of salicylate. On the basis of its modest potential benefit achieved with large doses, together with its uncertain risks, bismuth subsalicylate is not recommended for prophylaxis of TD.

Controlled data are available on the prophylactic value of several antimicrobial drugs. Entero-vioform and related halogenated hydroxyquinoline derivatives (e.g., clioquinol, iodoquinol, Mexaform, Intestopan, and others) are not helpful in preventing TD, may have serious neurological side effects, and should never be used for prophylaxis of TD.

Carefully controlled studies have indicated that two agents, doxycycline and trimethoprim/sulfamethoxazole (TMP/SMX), when taken prophylactically, are consistently effective in reducing the incidence of TD by 50 to 86 percent in various areas of the developing world. One study shows that trimethoprim alone is also effective.

The benefits of widespread prophylactic use of doxycycline or TMP/SMX or TMP alone in several million travelers must be weighed against the potential drawbacks. The known risks include allergic and other side effects (such as common skin rashes, photosensitivity of the skin, blood disorders, Stevens-Johnson syndrome, and staining of the teeth in children) as well as other infections that may be induced by antimicrobial therapy (such as antibiotic-associated colitis, Candida vaginitis, and possibly salmonella enteritis). Because of the uncertain risk of widespread administration of these antimicrobial agents, their prophylactic use is not recommended. Nor is there any basis for recommending their use prophylactically for special groups of travelers. For example, the physician should not recommend an agent for prophylactic use by a business traveler and deny such use by a honeymoon couple. Furthermore, there is no documented evidence that there are any groups of disease entities that are worsened sufficiently by an episode of TD to risk the rare undesirable side effects of prophylactic antimicrobial drugs.

The selective pressure of prophylactic use of antimicrobial agents on the genetic pool of antimicrobial resistance is of concern, but may be insignificant in light of the widespread use of over-the-counter antimicrobial agents in many developing countries. The increasing frequency of resistance to multiple antimicrobial agents (including both doxycycline and TMP/SMX) will limit the effectiveness of these agents in many areas.

Available data support only the instruction of travelers in regard to sensible dietary practices as a prophylactic measure. On the basis of apparent risk/benefit ratios, prophylactic antimicrobial agents are not recommended for travelers. This recommendation is justified by the excellent results of early treatment of TD as outlined below. By avoiding prophylactic antimicrobial agents, only those people traveling to high-risk areas who develop moderate to severe TD (less than 30 percent of travelers at risk) will be exposed to the side effects of antimicrobial agents, and the exposure will be restricted to 3 days or fewer in those individuals. Some travelers may wish to consult with their physician and may elect to use prophylactic antimicrobial agents for travel under special circumstances, once the risks and benefits are clearly understood.

What Treatment Measures Are Effective for Traveler's Diarrhea?

The individuals with TD have two major complaints for which they desire relief—abdominal cramps and diarrhea. Many agents have been proposed to control these symptoms, but few have been demonstrated to be effective by rigorous clinical trials.

Nonspecific Agents

A variety of "adsorbents" have been used in the treatment of diarrhea. For example, activated charcoal has been found ineffective in the treatment of diarrhea. Kaolin and pectin have been widely used for diarrhea. The combination appears to give the stools more consistency but has not been shown to decrease cramps and frequency of stools nor to shorten the course of infectious diarrhea.

Lactobacillus preparations and yogurt have also been advocated, but no evidence supports these treatments for TD.

Bismuth subsalicylate preparation (1 oz every 30 minutes for eight doses) decreased the rate of stooling by one-half in a study of travelers with diarrhea when compared with a placebo group. However, there was no difference between the two groups in stool output in the first 4 hours of the study. There is concern about taking, without supervision, large amounts of bismuth and salicylate, especially in individuals who may be intolerant to salicylates, who have renal insufficiency, or who take salicylates for other reasons.

Antimotility Agents

Antimotility agents are widely used in the treatment of diarrhea of all types. Natural opiates (paregoric, deodorized tincture of opium, and codeine) have long been used to control diarrhea and cramps. Synthetic agents, diphenoxylate and loperamide, come in convenient dosage forms and provide prompt symptomatic but temporary relief. However, they should not be used in patients with high fever or with blood in the stool. These drugs should be discontinued if symptoms persist beyond 48 hours. Diphenoxylate and loperamide should not be used in children under the age of 2.

Oral Fluids

Most individuals with TD do not develop serious dehydration. Fluid and electrolyte balance can be maintained by potable fruit juices, caffeine-free soft drinks, and salted crackers. The individual with TD should avoid alcohol and caffeine-containing beverages. Dairy products aggravate diarrhea in some people and should be avoided. Individuals with severe dehydration may require special fluid and electrolyte replacement in the form of oral replacement solutions such as those recommended by the World Health Organization.

Antimicrobial Treatment

Travelers who develop diarrhea with three or more loose stools in an 8-hour period, especially if associated with nausea, vomiting, abdominal cramps, fever, or blood in the stools, may benefit from antimicrobial treatment. A typical 3- to 5-day illness con be shortened to 1 to 1½ days by effective antimicrobial agents. Those best studied to date are TMP/SMX, 160 mg TMP and 800 mg SMX, or TMP alone, 200 mg taken twice daily. Preliminary evidence suggests that doxycycline, taken 100 mg twice daily, is also effective. Three days of treatment is recommended, although 2 days or fewer may be sufficient. Nausea and vomiting without diarrhea should not be treated with antimicrobial drugs.

Precautions in Children and Pregnant Women

Although children do not make up a large proportion of travelers to high-risk areas, some children do accompany their families. Teenagers should follow the advice given to adults, with possible adjustment of doses of medication. Physicians should be aware of the risks of tetracyclines to children under 12 years. There is a paucity of data available about usage of antidiarrheal drugs in children. Drugs should be prescribed with caution for pregnant women and nursing mothers.

Summary Recommendation for Treatment

TD is usually a mild, self-limited disorder, with complete recovery even in the absence of therapy; hence, therapy should be considered optional.

1. Fluids should be taken as described above.

2. If rapid relief of symptoms is desired after one or two unformed stools accompanied by cramps, nausea, or malaise, diphenoxylate or loperamide may be taken. An alternative is to start bismuth subsalicylate (1 oz every 30 minutes for eight doses). Although this regimen decreases the number of stools and increases their consistency, the beneficial activity of bismuth subsalicylate is somewhat slower than that of antimotility drugs.

3. If it is important to shorten the course or decrease the severity of moderate to severe TD, antimicrobial agents may be taken. After three or more loose stools with symptoms, consideration can be given to a short course of TMP/SMX or TMP alone or doxycycline.

4. A small percentage of travelers have persisting diarrhea with serious fluid loss, fever, and blood or mucus in the stools. This suggests that a more serious illness is involved, and such individuals should seek medical attention.

In conclusion, travelers to areas of high risk should obtain an antimotility drug or bismuth subsalicylate for milder forms of TD, and an antimicrobial agent (TMP/SMX or TMP alone or doxycycline) for more severe TD. Advice concerning side effects of these drugs and various aspects of hygiene and dietary precautions should be obtained. By obtaining the proper drugs in advance, the beleaguered traveler might avoid buying over-the-counter drugs abroad with potentially dangerous ingredients.

What Should Be the Direction of Future Research?

Although much has been learned about TD over the past 25 years, there is considerable need for additional research on this important syndrome.

Epidemiology

1. Epidemiologic data are needed from well-designed surveys and prospective studies, especially among travelers to countries and regions not previously examined. These investigations should be expanded to include young and elderly travelers, for whom few data exist.

2. Case-control studies should be designed to identify independent risk factors and specific etiologic agents. Such studies should apply all available microbiologic techniques to determine systematically the risk of TD attributable to specific microorganisms in various countries.

Etiology

1. The development of rapid diagnostic techniques (e.g., hybridization techniques and use of monoclonal antibodies) would facilitate all clinical and epidemiologic research.

2. Additional information should be sought regarding the pathogenesis of TD, which should lead to more specific therapeutic interventions.

3. There is a need for careful monitoring of increasing resistance to antimicrobial drugs, especially among the enterotoxigenic *E. coli*, in different intermediate and high-risk destinations.

4. There is a particular need to assess the frequency, risk factors, and microbiology of persistent diarrhea following travel. Better approaches to diagnosis in these patients are needed.

Prevention and Treatment

1. Newer approaches to vaccine development should be applied to the causal microorganisms of TD.

2. Randomized prospective studies or carefully controlled observational studies should be conducted to determine the true efficacy of dietary restrictions.

3. All agents effective in prevention and treatment of TD should be investigated in larger populations traveling to as-yet-unstudied destinations. Such populations should include children and elderly travelers.

4. Large-scale drug surveillance studies are required to identify important but uncommon toxicities or side effects of various drugs.

5. Minimal effective doses and duration for preventing and treating TD remain to be determined for general therapeutic agents.

6. The active agents and mode of action of bismuth subsalicylate remain to be elucidated, and the tablet form of the drug requires further evaluation.

7. A better understanding of the neurohumoral control of intestinal secretion and its potential interaction with micro-

bial enterotoxins may help in the design of more rational therapeutic strategies for TD. Further study of antisecretory and absorption-enhancing agents may improve pharmacologic therapy and enhance the efficacy and acceptability of oral replacement solutions. Improved understanding of the components of motility that will enhance but not impede absorption may help in the design of rational antimotility therapy.

Summary and Conclusions

Diarrhea is the major health problem in travelers to developing countries. Travel to high-risk areas in Latin America, Africa, the Middle East, and Asia is associated with diarrhea rates of 20 to 50 percent. The syndrome is caused by an infection acquired by ingesting fecally contaminated food or beverages. *Escherichia coli*, a common species of enteric bacteria, is the leading pathogen, although a host of other bacteria, viruses, and protozoa have been implicated in some cases. Prudent dietary and hygienic practices should be followed, and they will prevent some, but not all, diarrhea. Antimicrobial agents are not recommended for prevention of TD. Such widespread usage in millions of travelers would cause many side effects, including some severe ones, while preventing a disease that has had no reported mortality. Instead of universal antimicrobial prophylaxis, a more sensible approach is rapid institution of effective treatment that can shorten the disease to 30 hours or less in most people. For mild diarrhea, an antimotility drug such as diphenoxylate or loperamide could be taken. Alternatively, bismuth subsalicylate, which works somewhat slower, con be used. For more severe diarrhea, an antimicrobial drug may be used for treatment, and trimethoprim/sulfamethoxazole, trimethoprim alone, and doxycycline are among the choices. These drugs could be carried by the traveler for use in the event of illness. Oral rehydration should be instituted when necessary.

The millions of Americans who travel annually to developing countries and their physicians must be warned of the potential risks of prophylactic antimicrobial drugs, with the attendant side effects in otherwise healthy individuals, and should be informed of the alternative method of prompt, effective treatment for diarrhea.

Members of the Consensus Development Panel Were:

Sherwood L. Gorbach, M.D.
(Chairman)
Professor of Medicine and Microbiology
Tuffs University School of Medicine
Chief, Infectious Diseases Division
New England Medical Center
Boston, Massachusetts

Charles C.J. Carpenter, M.D.
Professor and Chairman
Department of Medicine
Case Western Reserve University
University Hospitals of Cleveland
Cleveland, Ohio

Robert Grayson, M.D.
Clinical Professor of Pediatrics
University of Miami School of Medicine
Miami, Florida

Joyce D. Gryboski, M.D.
Professor of Pediatrics
Chief, Pediatric Gastroenterology
Yale University School of Medicine
New Haven, Connecticut

Richard L. Guerrant, M.D.
Professor of Medicine
Head, Division of Geographic Medicine
University of Virginia School of Medicine
Charlottesville, Virginia

Thomas R. Hendrix, M.D.
Paulson Professor of Gastroenterology
Department of Medicine
Johns Hopkins University School of Medicine
Baltimore, Maryland

Richard B. Hornick, M.D.
Chairman
Department of Medicine
University of Rochester School of Medicine and Dentistry
Rochester, New York

John S. Marr, M.D., M.P.H.
Assistant Medical Director
Exxon Corporation
New York, New York

Jerry Morris
Travel Editor
The Boston Globe
Boston, Massachusetts

B. Frank Polk, M.D.
Associate Professor of Epidemiology and Medicine
Department of Epidemiology
Johns Hopkins School of Hygiene and Public Health
Baltimore, Maryland

Somerset R. Waters
President
Child & Waters, Inc.
New York, New York

George W. Williams, Ph.D.
Chairman
Department of Biostatistics and Epidemiology
Cleveland Clinic Foundation
Cleveland, Ohio

Martin S. Wolfe, M.D.
Director Travelers' Medical Service of Washington
Washington, D.C.

Members of the Planning Committee Were:

Robert Edelman, M.D, F.A.C.P.
(Chairman)
Chief, Clinical and Epidemiological Studies Branch
Deputy Director, Microbiology and Infectious Diseases Program
National Institute of Allergy and Infectious Diseases
National Institutes of Health
Bethesda, Maryland

Herbert L. DuPont, M.D.
Professor and Director
Program in Infectious Diseases and Clinical Microbiology
University of Texas Medical School
Houston, Texas

Jerry M. Elliott
OMAR Coordinator
Program Analyst
Office of Medical Applications of Research
Office of the Director
National Institutes of Health
Bethesda, Maryland

Sherwood L. Gorbach, M.D.
Professor of Medicine and Microbiology
Tufts University School of Medicine
Chief, Infectious Diseases Division
New England Medical Center
Boston, Massachusetts

Richard Horton, M.D., M.P.H.
Medical Officer
Clinical and Epidemiological Studies Branch
Microbiology and Infectious Diseases Program
National Institute of Allergy and Infectious Diseases
National Institutes of Health
Bethesda, Maryland

Myron M. Levine, M.D., M.P.H.
Professor and Director
Center for Vaccine Development
Division of Geographic Medicine
University of Maryland School of Medicine
Baltimore, Maryland

John Nutter, Ph.D.
Chief, Office of Program Planning and Evaluation
National Institute of Allergy and Infectious Diseases
National Institutes of Health
Bethesda, Maryland

Myron G. Schultz, D.V.M., M.D.
Medical Epidemiologist
Centers for Disease Control
Atlanta, Georgia

Michael J. Bernstein
Director of Communications
Office of Medical Applications of Research
Office of the Director
National Institutes of Health
Bethesda, Maryland

Judy L. Murphy
Public Affairs Specialist
Office of Research Reporting and Public Response
National Institute of Allergy and Infectious Diseases
National Institutes of Health
Bethesda, Maryland

The Conference Was Sponsored by:

Office of Medical Applications of Research
Itzhak Jacoby, Ph.D.
Acting Director

National Institute of Allergy and Infectious Diseases
Anthony S. Fauci, M.D.
Director

Chapter 17

Some Diseases Encountered by Foreign Travelers

Chapter Contents

Section 17.1

Cholera

(Source: CDC Document No. 310101, November 19, 1992.)

Cholera is an acute intestinal infection. Cholera occurs in many of the developing countries of Africa, and Asia, where sanitary conditions are less than optimal. Most recently, cholera outbreaks have occurred in parts of Latin America.

Most infected persons have no symptoms or only mild diarrhea. However, persons with severe disease can die within a few hours after onset due to loss of fluid and salts through profuse diarrhea and, to a lesser extent, through vomiting.

Only a few cases of cholera have occurred in the United States since 1973. Even with foreign travel, the risk of infection to the U. S. traveler is very low, especially for those who follow the usual tourist itineraries and stay in standard accommodations. Worldwide cholera activity is characterized by occasional epidemics in developing countries.

The organism that causes the illness is named *Vibrio cholerae* type 0:1. During epidemics, it is spread by ingestion of food or water contaminated directly or indirectly by feces or vomitus from infected persons. Diagnosis is made by culturing the bacteria from the stool of a patient and confirming that the organism produces toxin.

The best protection is to avoid consuming food or water that may be contaminated with feces or vomitus from infected persons. The organism can grow well in some foods, such as rice, but it will not grow or survive in very acidic foods, including carbonated beverages, and is killed by heat.

A cholera vaccine is available, but normally is not recommended. Only 50% of those who take the vaccine develop immunity to cholera, and this immunity lasts only a few months.

Treatment for cholera involves rehydration with oral rehydration solution or, in the most severe cases, with intravenous solutions until the patient is able to ingest fluids. Treatment with antibiotics (usually tetracycline or doxycycline) will decrease the duration of illness and the excretion of live cholera bacteria, and will decrease the volume of fluid lost but is not necessary for successful treatment.

Cholera Vaccine Information

A cholera vaccine is available, but normally is not recommended. Only 50% of those who take the vaccine develop immunity to cholera, and this immunity lasts only a few months. No country currently requires the cholera vaccine for entry if arriving from cholera-infected countries. Consult the International Travelers Hotline for specific recommendations.

The complete vaccination schedule includes 2 doses of vaccine spaced 1 to 4 or more weeks apart. Dosages are age specific.

For infants 0-6 months of age; the vaccine is not recommended.

Data indicate that simultaneous administration of cholera and yellow fever vaccines produces less-than-normal antibody responses to both vaccines. A three week minimum interval between cholera and yellow fever vaccines is recommended. In cases where both vaccines are required and time constraints exist, then administer simultaneously or as far apart as possible.

Reactions to the vaccine are 1-2 days of pain, erythema, and induration at the site of injection; fever, malaise, and headache. Serious reactions are rare, but if experienced, re-vaccination is not advisable.

No specific information on the safety of cholera vaccine in pregnancy is available, therefore vaccination should be avoided.

Section 17.2

Malaria

(Source: Taken from "Preventing 'Turista' and Other Travelers' Ailments," *FDA Consumer*, March 1991.)

Once thought to be under control and perhaps even close to eradication, malaria has made a remarkable comeback in the past decade or two, says [Hans Lobel, M.D., chief of CDC's malaria surveillance program].

Malaria is caused by a single-cell blood parasite called plasmodium. The parasite is usually transmitted to people by the bite of an infected *Anopheles* mosquito. Symptoms start with a listless feeling, loss of appetite, muscle aches, and a low fever. After a few days, the classic symptoms appear: a fever that can reach 105 degrees Fahrenheit and teeth-rattling chills that can last 20 to 60 minutes. The fever may break and then return again on a 48-to-72-hour cycle, and it may be accompanied by nausea, diarrhea and vomiting.

Worldwide, some 200 million people are estimated to have malaria, Lobel says. Those numbers are guesses, he admits, since reliable figures are hard to come by. In Africa, he says, "most everybody has been infected." In this country, about 1,000 malaria cases a year are reported to CDC, a figure Lobel thinks represents only a third of the true numbers. According to Bruce Burlington, M.D., deputy director of FDA's Office of Drug Evaluation II, people living in Africa come "more or less into equilibrium" with malaria and don't get as sick as travelers who are newly infected.

Malaria is prevalent throughout the tropics, but the traveler's risk of contracting the disease is greatest in Africa and the island of Papua New Guinea in the Pacific near Australia. It is common but less of a risk in India and southeastern Asia, central and northeastern South America, and in Haiti. It is less prevalent in China and the Middle East. Even in high-risk regions, Lobel adds, the chances of getting malaria are much greater in rural areas than in cities.

The reasons for malaria's comeback are a familiar refrain nowadays. The mosquitoes that transmit the disease now resist what had been the most effective pesticides, and many of the parasites themselves now resist what had been the most effective drug used to prevent and treat the disease.

Actually, malaria is four diseases caused by four different species of the plasmodium organism. In particular, the form known as falciparum now widely resists chloroquine (Aralen), the drug developed in the 1940s to prevent and treat malaria. Often called "malignant malaria" or "black-water fever," falciparum is the most serious form of the disease and the one most likely to kill its victims. Resistance began to appear in the 1960s and is widespread in most places falciparum malaria is found today.

Fortunately, malaria can still be prevented and cured in most cases if diagnosed properly, Lobel says. While chloroquine remains an effective anti-malarial drug in nonresistant areas and for the non-falciparum forms, mefloquine (Lariam), approved by FDA in 1989, is now also recommended.

Travelers going to chloroquine-resistant areas who cannot take mefloquine—people taking beta blocker drugs for heart conditions or who are subject to seizures, FDA's Maxwell says—can use pyrimethamine/sulfadoxine (Fansidar) or doxycycline. Doxycycline is as effective as mefloquine, Lobel says, but cannot be used for as long a time because of its potential side effects. Doxycycline must also be taken daily rather than weekly as with chloroquine and mefloquine. Fansidar can cause an uncommon but potentially fatal rash as a side effect, so it is generally used only when other drugs aren't appropriate.

Several other drugs are sometimes prescribed for malaria by physicians in other countries. One, proguanil (Paludrine), is widely used in Great Britain and Kenya. Others include pyrimethamine (Daraprim) and pyrimethamine-dapsone (Maloprim). None are as broadly effective as mefloquine or chloroquine, some need to be used with other anti-malarial drugs, and a few have serious side effects. Nor have any been approved by FDA for malaria.

As with travelers' diarrhea, the best treatment for malaria is prevention. Americans are advised to avoid the mosquitoes that transmit the disease. Stay inside at dusk and dawn, wear long pants or long-sleeved shirts when in mosquito-infested areas, sleep in well-screened rooms or under mosquito nets, and use an insect repellant such as DEET (N, N-diethyl-m-tolumide) on exposed skin.

Section 17.3

New Drug for Malaria

(*Source: FDA Consumer*, September 1989.)

FDA recently approved a new drug to treat and prevent certain malaria infections. A major cause of illness in tropical and subtropical regions, malaria has been treated with quinine for many decades. Strains of the parasite *Plasmodium falciparum*, which cause the most serious and potentially fatal form of the disease, however, have become resistant to quinine.

The new drug, mefloquine, was approved in May for treatment and prevention of infection of malaria caused by *P. falciparum* and *P. vivax*. In clinical trials carried out in South America and South Asia involving more than 1,000 patients, the drug was shown to be highly effective in killing those parasites in individuals with mild to moderate illness. Patients with severe malaria require initial treatment with an intravenous anti-malaria drug. To complete the treatment of vivax malaria, mefloquine must be used in combination with a second malaria drug—primaquine—to clear infection in the liver and prevent relapses.

Mefloquine was also found effective in preventing malaria and is recommended for travelers to malarious areas, particularly where *P. falciparum* is resistant to other anti-malaria drugs.

The drug must be used carefully by patients taking beta blockers (heart drugs), seizure medications, or quinine because of possible interactions that may affect the heart rhythm. Also, its effects on the human fetus are not known, and women of child-bearing age who take the drug should be warned against becoming pregnant.

The Walter Reed Army Institute of Research, the World Health Organization, and Hoffmann-La Roche of Nutley, N.J., collaborated in developing mefloquine. Both the U.S. Army and Hoffmann-La Roche will distribute the drug, which Roche will market under the brand name Lariam.

Section 17.4

Continuing Quest for a Malaria Vaccine

(Source: *Research Resources Reporter*, March/April 1993.)

By producing experimental vaccines that contain fragments of malaria parasites, scientists hope one day to quell the spread of malaria, a disease that kills about 1.5 million people worldwide each year and infects an additional 300 million. To date, however, the disease-causing *Plasmodium* organisms have evaded the best efforts of vaccine developers, who are attempting to block several different stages in the parasite's complex life cycle. Studies in nonhuman primates, the only animals that can be infected with human malaria, are helping researchers to identify new molecular targets and to understand why earlier vaccines have failed.

"The monkeys offer a marvelous opportunity for understanding the human malarias," says Dr. William E. Collins, a research biologist in the malaria branch of the U.S. Centers for Disease Control (CDC) in Atlanta, Georgia. He and his colleagues at CDC design and conduct vaccine trials in monkeys to test malaria vaccines that have been developed by researchers from around the world. "To see what kind of protection a vaccine offers, we immunize monkeys and then challenge them with infective parasites to see if the antibodies that are produced are protective," Dr. Collins says. He collaborates with scientists at the Yerkes Regional Primate Research Center in Atlanta to collect large numbers of parasites from the blood of chimpanzees infected with non-fatal human malaria.

Most malaria researchers agree that there is no substitute for evaluating potential malaria vaccines in human trials. Already more than a dozen vaccine candidates have been tested in humans, but so far with limited success. "Mounting dozens of different human vaccine trials is very difficult," says Dr. Stephen L. Hoffman, director of the malaria program at the Naval Medical Research Institute in Bethesda, Maryland. "Although monkeys are not a natural host for the human malarias, they give us an idea of how humans may respond to various vaccines."

There are several drawbacks, however, to testing human malaria vaccines in monkeys, notes Dr. Ruth S. Nussenzweig, head of the department of medical and molecular parasitology at New York University (NYU) School of Medicine in New York City. "Because these animals are not very sensitive to inoculation with sporozoites [a pre-erythrocyte form of the parasite that usually enters the bloodstream through a mosquito's bite], hundreds of times more sporozoites are needed to infect monkeys than to infect humans," she says. In addition, monkeys infected with human malaria do not develop the common human symptoms—fever, chills, and drenching sweats. "The course of infection in these animals is quite different from its progression in man," she says, and the results of monkey vaccine trials cannot be directly extrapolated to predict human response. Another problem is that the monkeys' spleens must be removed before the animals can develop a persistent infection with the human sporozoite-stage parasites, creating a very artificial situation. Dr. Nussenzweig argues that monkey vaccine trials are best conducted using the species of *Plasmodium* that naturally infect monkeys, such as *Plasmodium cynomolgi* or *Plasmodium knowlesi*.

Despite these many drawbacks, nonhuman primates remain the only animal model for testing potential vaccines against the human malarias. "The monkey model has its limitations," says Dr. Hoffman, "but it could certainly hasten the development of human vaccines."

Malaria vaccines can be designed to attack several different stages of the *Plasmodium* life cycle. As the parasite travels through its mammalian and mosquito hosts, it undergoes a dramatic metamorphosis that presents several different antigenic, or immunoreactive, targets to candidate vaccines.

In recent years some malaria vaccine researchers have sought to prevent parasite fertilization in the mosquito or to block development of blood-stage organisms. But by far the most thoroughly explored potential malaria vaccines are designed to halt the pre-erythrocyte stages of malaria, the sporozoite and the liver cell parasites. Ideally, Dr. Nussenzweig says, these different approaches will be combined in the future to produce a single vaccine that blocks several stages of the *Plasmodium* life cycle.

The groundwork for sporozoite vaccine research was laid more than two decades ago in animal studies conducted by Dr. Nussenzweig and her colleagues at NYU. Studying a species of *Plasmodium* that naturally infects mice, the researchers found that mice inoculated with irradiated, killed sporozoites were protected on challenge with live sporozoites. "Afterward it was shown that monkeys and humans also can be fully protected by immunization with irradiated sporozoites," Dr. Nussenzweig says. As a commercial vaccine, however, irradiated sporozoites are entirely impractical, in part because they are difficult to produce in bulk.

Researchers have now turned to subunit vaccines that contain key immunogenic portions of sporozoite proteins. Four experimental subunit vaccines against the human parasite *Plasmodium vivax* were evaluated in squirrel monkey trials conducted by Dr. Collins in collaboration with Drs. Nussenzweig and Hoffman and their associates, along with scientists at the Walter Reed Army Institute of Research in Washington, D. C., the University of Maryland School of Medicine in Baltimore, and two pharmaceutical companies. *P. vivax* is the most common cause of human malaria worldwide. These were the first studies to test *P. vivax* sporozoite vaccines in monkeys with subsequent challenge, Dr. Collins says.

Although none of the experimental vaccines conferred a significant degree of protection compared to non-vaccinated control monkeys, all of the vaccines induced significant antibody production against the sporozoites.

The four experimental vaccines contained key fragments of the circumsporozoite (CS) protein, the predominant protein on the sporozoite's surface and a primary target for vaccine developers. "This major surface antigen has been found on all *Plasmodium* species that we have studied—rodent, monkey, and human parasites," says Dr. Elizabeth H. Nardin, assistant professor of medical and molecular parasitology at the NYU School of Medicine. All CS proteins are similar in size and structure, but their amino acid compositions are species specific, Dr. Nardin says. "The unique thing about the CS protein is its central repeat region, which is immunodominant in terms of antibody response."

The repeat region consists of a stretch of amino acids that appears many times along the CS protein chain. The repeat region of *P. vivax* parasites comprises nine amino acids that appear as a group several times along the CS protein backbone. "The antibody response against the repeat region is protective in that monoclonal antibodies specific to the repeats can protect mice from infection," adds Dr. Nardin. "One aim of vaccines based on the CS protein has always been to generate high levels of antibody against the repeat region to get a protective immune response."

In the squirrel monkey studies, however, "some of the monkeys were protected, but there was no direct correlation between high titers of antibodies and protection," Dr. Nardin says. The antibody response was polymorphic, directed against several different portions of the CS protein, but apparently the proper sections of the protein's repeat region were not targeted.

In a recent followup study, Dr. Collins and others found that two of the vaccines had induced antibody production against nonrepeat regions of the CS protein, and these antibodies could inhibit development of liver-stage parasites in vitro.

In another study Dr. Hoffman and his colleagues identified a monoclonal antibody that protects squirrel monkeys from *P. vivax* infection. To produce this monoclonal antibody, the scientists immunized mice with irradiated *P. vivax* sporozoites. The antibody specifically reacted with four amino acids—alanine, glycine, aspartic acid, and arginine (abbreviated AGDR)—along the nine-amino acid repeat region of the CS protein.

When the mouse monoclonal antibody against AGDR was administered to six monkeys at CDC, four were completely protected against challenge with *P. vivax* sporozoites, and the onset of infection was significantly delayed in the remaining two animals, says Dr. Yupin Charoenvit, a research scientist in the malaria program of the Naval Medical Research Institute.

However, when the researchers tested blood from the earlier vaccine trials, they found that none of the vaccinated squirrel monkeys had produced antibodies against AGDR. "Even though the four experimental vaccines contained the sequence AGDR, vaccinated monkeys did not produce antibodies against AGDR. Somehow AGDR was masked in those vaccines," Dr. Charoenvit says.

Drs. Hoffman and Charoenvit, together with Dr. Trevor Jones of the Naval Medical Research Institute and their colleagues at Walter Reed, are now working to develop vaccine candidates in which AGDR is unmasked and can induce production of protective antibodies. "We are trying many different carrier proteins and many different configurations. We are considering different forms of AGDR in straight chains or branched chains," says Dr. Charoenvit.

"As soon as we get these new AGDR vaccines formulated and show that they are good antibody-producers in mice, we will do a study in squirrel monkeys with Dr. Collins at CDC," adds Dr. Hoffman.

Human monoclonal antibodies directed against AGDR are another possibility for short-term human protection against *P. vivax*, Dr. Hoffman says. "These antibodies would not necessarily be useful to a villager living in Africa, but they could be very useful to a traveler going only for a few weeks or a few months to a malarious area." This type of protection, in which antibodies are transferred to and not produced by the body, is known as passive immunization. "Just as travelers are now given shots of gamma-globulin, which is essentially a mixture of antibodies, for temporary protection against hepatitis, we hope to develop a malaria antibody preparation that can circulate in the blood for several months."

Antibodies are only one component of the immune system, and many vaccine developers are now attempting to activate a second branch known as cell-mediated immunity, says Dr. Nardin. "Once the sporozoite invades the liver cells of the host it is susceptible to cell-mediated immune responses. These responses can be cytokine mediated—for example, gamma-interferon is a potent inhibitor of parasites in the cell—or involve direct cytotoxicity. With the latter response cytotoxic T-cells destroy the infected liver cells and thereby prevent development of blood-stage parasites," she says. The NYU scientists are now working to produce synthetic peptide vaccines intended to elicit both cell-mediated immune responses and antibody production.

Meanwhile investigators at the Navy are focusing on a second surface antigen known as SSP2, which was previously identified on mouse malaria sporozoites. Vaccines that expressed both the CS protein and SSP2 protected mice from malaria. The strength of this vaccine was that it mobilized both antibodies and cytotoxic T-cells against the parasite, Dr. Hoffman says. He and his colleagues say they have recently identified the SSP2 antigen on the sporozoite of the deadly human parasite *P. falciparum*. "We are now working on vaccine formulations that will induce immune responses in humans similar to what we saw in mice, particularly with the cytotoxic T-cells," Dr. Hoffman says. "We are very excited to have found the *P. falciparum* analogue for SSP2."

Despite many breakthroughs, a practical malaria vaccine for humans remains a distant prospect and will probably not be seen for a decade or more, the scientists say. Dr. Nussenzweig points out that another significant obstacle yet to be overcome is the development of effective human adjuvants, or immunity-boosting compounds, that can be delivered along with the vaccines. Adjuvants are needed because subunit vaccines are much less immunogenic than whole microbial organisms, she says.

"We are under a lot of pressure," Dr. Collins says. "Malaria is a terrifically important problem, and people want a vaccine that works. Everyone thinks that we should be able to do it overnight, but this is a long-haul project."

Plasmodium Life Cycle

Each stage of the *Plasmodium* life cycle presents different immunoreactive targets to vaccine developers. Human infection begins when a mosquito's bite injects sporozoites into the bloodstream. Parasites invade and multiply within liver cells, ultimately bursting forth as merozoites, which infect and reproduce within red blood cells (RBC). When the parasite-packed cells burst, they release more merozoites. By an incompletely understood mechanism, this bursting of blood cells causes the fever and chills that are characteristic of malaria. Some merozoites infect more red blood cells, while others are transformed to male and female gametocytes. After a mosquito draws gametocyte-laden blood, fertilization occurs in the insect's gut and the parasite again becomes a sporozoite, which travels to the insect's salivary gland awaiting the next human host.

—by Victoria L. Contie

Additional reading:

1. Millet, P., Chizzolini, C., Wirtz, R. A., et al., Inhibitory activity against sporozoites induced by antibodies directed against nonrepetitive regions of the circumsporozoite protein of *Plasmodium vinax*. *European Journal of Immunology* 22:519-524, 1992.

2. Khusmith, S., Charoenvit, Y., Kumar, S., et al., Protection against malaria by vaccination with sporozoite surface protein 2 plus CS protein. *Science* 252:715-718, 1991.

3. Charoenvit, Y., Collins, W. E., Jones, T. R., et al., Inability of malaria vaccine to induce antibodies to a protective epitope within its sequence. *Science* 251:668-671, 1991.

4. Collins, W. E., Nussenzweig, R. S., Ruebush, T. K., II, et al., Further studies on the immunization of *Saimiri sciureus boliviensis* with recombinant vaccines based on the circumsporozoite protein of *Plasmodium vivax*. *American Journal of Tropical Medicine and Hygiene* 43:576-583, 1991.

5. Collins, W. E., Nussenzweig, R. S., Ballou, W. R., et al., Immunization of *Saimiri sciureus boliviensis* with recombinant vaccines based on the circumsporozoite protein of *Plasmodium vivax*. *American Journal of Tropical Medicine and Hygiene* 40:455-464, 1989.

The research described in this article was supported by the Comparative Medicine Program of the National Center for Research Resources; the U.S. Agency for International Development; the National Institute of Allergy and Infectious Diseases; the MacArthur Foundation; the Naval Medical Research and Development Command; the U.S. Centers for Disease Control; and the U.S. Army Medical Research and Development Command.

Section 17.5

Schistosomiasis

(Source: "Snail-Borne Disease Slowed by New Drug,"
FDA Consumer, May 1983.)

Late last December [1982], the Food and Drug Administration approved a new drug, praziquantel, for the treatment of schistosomiasis, one of the world's major tropical diseases. The drug represents an important therapeutic breakthrough, for praziquantel is the first anti-parasitic drug that is effective against all types of schistosomiasis. Further, it takes only one to three doses to do its job, and it causes few side effects, making hospitalization unnecessary. All of which could be good news for the 200 to 250 million people in some 70 countries afflicted with this debilitating disease.

Schistosomiasis results from infection by one of several species of flukes, or trematode worms, called schistosomes. Three major species infect humans: *Schistosoma mansoni*, found in the Caribbean area, South America, Africa and the Middle East; *S. haematobium*, distributed throughout Africa, the Near East, Mauritius, Madagascar and Iraq; and *S. japonicum*, which, as the name suggests, is indigenous to Japan, as well as to China, the Philippines and the Celebes.

Survival and spread of any of these species depend on the availability of a human or animal host, a suitable snail to act as an intermediary host, and the right environment for the snail, which means still or slowly moving fresh water, usually (but not always) with vegetation, a water temperature of 22 to 23 degrees Celsius, and the right amount of alkalinity. Schistosomiasis does not occur naturally in the United States because we don't have the right type of snails to serve as the intermediate host.

Small dams and ponds are prime schistosome breeding areas. Humans use them for bathing, washing clothes, and as sources of water for drinking and cooking. The spread of snails is assured thanks to ducks that ferry snail eggs from one pond to another on their feet. Irrigation ditches are another factor in the spread of schistosomiasis.

The life cycle of the schistosome starts when the human host carrying the parasite contaminates the water with urine or excrement containing schistosome eggs. Within a few minutes after reaching the fresh water the eggs hatch, releasing a larva, called the miracidium. This highly mobile creature can survive about 24 hours while moving about the water looking for a snail to serve as host for the next stage of development. Miracidia are not fussy; they'll enter any snail, even though it's not the right one.

Once inside the soft tissues of a suitable snail host, the miracidia multiply and form thousands of baby worms called cercariae.

The snail is somewhat the worse for wear after this stage of schistosome development, usually living only one or two months more. At peak production 500 to 3,000 baby worms may be shed into the water daily for 200 days, although the production figures for the Far East variety are much lower (15 to 160) since its snail host is much smaller than the others.

Free of their snail hosts, the cercariae tend to swim up to the surface of the water, sinking to the bottom from time to time. They do not feed and will die within 48 hours unless a hapless human happens to enter the water. Within a few minutes a cercaria can penetrate a person's unbroken skin, although the worms may enter through the mouth. The baby worms stay in the skin about two days, then migrate via the lymphatic system to the heart and lungs. They end up in the liver where they mature and mate.

Worms of the *S. mansoni* and *S. japonicum* species then find their way to the tiny veins in the intestinal walls, a trip that takes about a month. Eggs laid there are deposited in the tissues or are swept back to the liver. Some also get into the gastrointestinal tract.

S. haematobium worms take two to three months to migrate to the bladder and ureter where their eggs are laid. Early symptoms of this infection, such as blood in the urine, are often disregarded in areas where the disease is always present. Indeed, in some African communities bloody urine is accepted as a normal occurrence of puberty.

In the early stages of schistosomiasis, the patient may have fever, cough, diarrhea, joint pains and loss of appetite. Symptoms may get worse when the worms begin laying their eggs. In fact, inflammation caused by the eggs is responsible for many of the symptoms.

The acute stage of the disease is seen most often in tourists and other visitors who are exposed for the first time. In endemic areas, infected people often aren't even aware that anything is wrong. However, in some cases the infection progresses, without symptoms, until its effects are irreversible.

Only a small number of patients get seriously ill, but heavy infection over time can lead to inflammation, obstruction and fibrosis, particularly of the liver and lower urinary tract. Chronic schistosomiasis also can cause bloody diarrhea, cor pulmonale (a form of heart disease), kidney problems and involvement of the central nervous system.

Treatment of schistosomiasis is reserved for patients who have active infections—that is, when they are shedding eggs. Modern drug therapy dates from 1918 when antimony compounds were first used in Khartoum, Sudan. Unfortunately, the side effects of these compounds—nausea, vomiting, stiff joints and muscles, a sense of constriction of the chest, dizziness and collapse—made the treatment seem worse than the disease. Miracil compounds, which were introduced shortly after World War II, were almost as bad. Later hycanthone and niridazole compounds were used. But mutagenic effects as well as undesirable side effects are associated with the two.

The newest drug on the scene, praziquantel, is effective against all three species of schistosomes. Almost immediately after administration the drug causes the worm's muscles to go into spasm. Within minutes, its skin blisters and the worm is made harmless. Existing eggs are not destroyed, but the body's immune system takes care of them by surrounding them with a fibrous sac. No major toxic reactions have been reported.

Infections from *S. mansoni* and *S. haematobium* have been cured with a single dose. A larger dose, administered in three parts on the same day, will knock out *S. japonicum*. The same dose is proving effective against *S. mekongi*, a rare new species turning up in Laotian refugees.

Also in use today are oxamniquine and metrifonate. Oxamniquine in a single oral dose is effective against *S. mansoni*. Side effects are mild and can be reduced by taking the drug after a meal and late in the day. This drug has been widely used in Africa and in Brazil. FDA has approved only the oral single dose for schistosomiasis contracted in the western hemisphere.

Metrifonate, effective only against *S. haematobium*, acts by paralyzing the infecting worm. The drug is well tolerated and the side effects—nausea, vomiting and bronchospasm—are rare. The prime disadvantage of metrifonate is that it must be given over a period of several weeks.

The three drugs—oxamniquine, metrifonate and praziquantel—may well play an important role in the community control of schistosomiasis, according to Dr. Joseph A. Cook of the Edna McConnell Clark Foundation, a New York based organization devoted

379

in part to finding ways of curing and controlling schistosomiasis. Quoted in the *Annals of Internal Medicine* (97:740-54, 1982), Dr. Cook noted that control efforts have relied heavily on killing the snail intermediate host, an "increasingly expensive, labor-intensive, never-ending" means of control. "With oral drugs it is now possible to target treatment on those who most need treatment (patients excreting the largest numbers of eggs and therefore most responsible for continuing transmission of infection)," Dr. Cook said.

Sanitary engineering and killing snails will still be needed in community control programs, Dr. Cook pointed out. "However, control of clinical disease may be achieved or the incidence greatly reduced by careful use of the currently available drugs."

—by Annabel Hecht

Annabel Hecht is a member of FDA's publications staff.

Section 17.6

Typhoid

(Source: CDC Document No. 310102, November 19, 1992.)

Typhoid fever is an acute bacterial disease caused by *Salmonella typhi*. The onset of typhoid fever is normally gradual, with fever, malaise, chills, headache, and generalized aches in the muscles and joints. The spleen is usually enlarged, there is generally a decrease in the number of white blood cells, and small, discrete, rose-colored spots may appear on the trunk. Diarrhea is infrequent, and vomiting, which may occur toward the end of the first week, is not usually severe. Abdominal distention and tenderness are common.

Salmonella typhi is transmitted by contaminated food and water and is prevalent in many developing countries of Latin America, Africa, and Asia. It became rare in the United States and other industrialized countries with the development of protected water supplies, pasteurization of milk, and improved sewage systems.

Diagnosis comes from isolation of *Salmonella typhi* from the blood or stool of an infected person. The best protection is to avoid consuming food or water that may be contaminated. For foreign travelers drinking only boiled water or carbonated beverages and eating only cooked food, lowers risk of infection. In addition vaccines are available that afford significant protection.

Chloramphenicol is the most effective drug for treatment of the acute illness if the organism is not resistant. Trimethoprim-sulfamethoxazole, ampicillin and amoxicillin are effective alternatives. The frequency of relapse does not appear to have been changed dramatically by antimicrobial therapy.

Eliminating the bacteria from carriers is difficult. A six-week course of ampicillin with probenecid has been successful for treating chronic carriers with normal gallbladders and without evidence of gallstones. A prolonged course of amoxicillin has been reported to be effective even in patients with gallstones or non-functioning gallbladders. Other effective treatments include trimethoprim-sulfamethoxazole and fluoroquinolones.

Removal of the gallbladder is also useful in eradicating the carrier state and may be necessary for patients whose illnesses relapse after therapy or who cannot tolerate antimicrobial therapy.

The incidence of typhoid fever in the United States fell from one case per 100,000 population in 1955 to 0.2 cases per 100,000 in 1966 and has since remained fairly stable. Between 1975 and 1984 62% of cases in the United States were imported, in contrast to 33% between 1967 and 1972. The major sources of imported cases between 1975 and 1984 were people coming from India and Mexico. The case-fatality rate during this time was 1.3%.

Typhoid Vaccine

Currently available vaccines have been shown to protect 70% - 90% of the recipients. Therefore, even vaccinated travelers should be cautious in selecting their food and water.

The oral vaccine consists of 4 capsules containing live attenuated bacteria. They are taken every other day for seven days. The entire 4 doses should be repeated every 5 years if the person is at continued risk. Reactions are rare and include nausea, vomiting, abdominal cramps, and skin rash.

The injectable vaccine consists of a primary series of two shots, spaced at least 4 weeks apart. A booster dose given every 3 years provides continued protection for repeated exposure. If there is insufficient time for two doses a month apart, an accelerated schedule of three shots a week apart may be administered. The accelerated schedule may be less effective. A primary series need never be repeated. Reactions to the vaccine include discomfort at the site of injection for 1-2 days, fever, malaise and headache.

Either of these vaccines may be given simultaneously with other vaccines.

Section 17.7

Typhoid Immunization: Recommendations of the Advisory Committee on Immunization Practices (ACIP)

(Source: *MMWR*, December 9, 1994.)

Summary

These revised recommendations of the Advisory Committee on Immunization Practices update previous recommendations (*MMWR* 1990;39[RR-10]:1-5). They include information on the Vi capsular polysaccharide (ViCPS) vaccine, which was not available when the previous recommendations were published.

Introduction

The incidence of typhoid fever declined steadily in the United States from 1900 to 1960 and has since remained low. From 1975 through 1984, the average number of cases reported annually was 464. During that period, 57% of reported cases occurred among persons ≥20 years of age; 62% of reported cases occurred among persons who had traveled to other countries. From 1967 through 1976, only 33% of reported cases occurred among travelers to other countries (1).

Typhoid Vaccines

Three typhoid vaccines are currently available for use in the United States: a) an oral live-attenuated vaccine (Vivotif Berna™ vaccine, manufactured from the Ty21a strain of *Salmonella typhi* (2) by the Swiss Serum and Vaccine Institute); b) a parenteral heat-phenol-inactivated vaccine that has been widely used for many years (Typhoid Vaccine, manufactured by Wyeth-Ayerst); and c) a newly licensed capsular polysaccharide vaccine for parenteral use (Typhim Vi, manufactured by Pasteur Mérieux). A fourth vaccine, an acetone-inactivated parenteral vaccine, is currently available only to the armed forces.

Although no prospective, randomized trials comparing any of the three U.S. licensed typhoid vaccines have been conducted, several field trials have demonstrated the efficacy of each vaccine. In controlled field trials conducted among schoolchildren in Chile, three doses of the Ty21a vaccine in enteric-coated capsules administered on alternate days reduced laboratory-confirmed infection by 66% over a period of 5 years (95% confidence interval [CI]=50%-77%) (3,4). In a subsequent trial in Chile, efficacy appeared to be lower: three doses resulted in only 33% (95% CI=0%-57%) fewer cases of laboratory-confirmed infection over a period of 3 years. When the data were stratified by age in this trial, children ≥10 years of age had a 53% reduction in incidence of culture-confirmed typhoid fever (95% CI=7%-77%), whereas children 5-9 years of age had only a 17% reduction (95% CI=0%-53%). This difference in age-related efficacy, however, is not statistically significant (5). In another trial in Chile, a significant decrease in the incidence of clinical typhoid fever occurred among persons receiving four doses of vaccine compared with persons receiving two (p<0.001) or three (p=0.002) doses. Because no placebo group was included in this trial, absolute vaccine efficacy could not be calculated (6).

Weekly and triweekly dosing regimens have been less effective than alternate-day dosing (3). A liquid formulation of Ty21a is more effective than enteric-coated capsules (5,7,8), but only enteric-coated capsules are available in the United States. The efficacy of vaccination with Ty21a has not been studied among persons from areas without endemic disease who travel to disease-endemic regions. The mechanism by which Ty21a vaccine confers protection is unknown; however, the vaccine does elicit both serum (2,9) and intestinal (10) antibodies and cell-mediated immune responses (11). Vaccine organisms can be shed transiently in the stool of vaccine recipients (*2,9*). However, secondary transmission of vaccine organisms has not been documented.

In field trials involving a primary series of two doses of heat-phenol-inactivated typhoid vaccine (which is similar to the currently available parenteral inactivated vaccine), vaccine efficacy over the 2½- to 3-year follow-up periods ranged from 51% to 77% (*12-14*). Efficacy for the acetone-inactivated parenteral vaccine, available only to the armed forces, ranges from 75% to 94% (*12,14,15*).

The newly licensed parenteral vaccine (Vi capsular polysaccharide [ViCPS]) is composed of purified Vi ("virulence") antigen, the capsular polysaccharide elaborated by *S. typhi* isolated from blood cultures (*16*). In recent studies, one 25µg injection of purified ViCPS produced seroconversion (i.e., at least a fourfold rise in antibody titers) in 93% of healthy U.S. adults (*17*); similar results were observed in Europe (*18*). Two field trials in disease-endemic areas have demonstrated the efficacy of ViCPS in preventing typhoid fever. In a trial in Nepal, in which vaccine recipients were observed for 20 months, one dose of ViCPS among persons 5-44 years of age resulted in 74% (95% Cl=49%-87%) fewer cases of typhoid fever confirmed by blood culture than occurred with controls (*19*). In a trial involving schoolchildren in South Africa who were 5-15 years of age, one dose of ViCPS resulted in 55% (95% Cl=30%-71%) fewer cases of blood-culture-confirmed typhoid fever over a period of 3 years than occurred with controls. The reduction in the number of cases in years 1, 2, and 3, was 61%, 52%, and 50%, respectively (*20,21*). The efficacy of vaccination with ViCPS has not been studied among persons from areas without endemic disease who travel to disease-endemic regions or among children <5 years of age. ViCPS has not been tested among children <1 year of age.

Vaccine Usage

Routine typhoid vaccination is not recommended in the United States. However, vaccination is indicated for the following groups:

- Travelers to areas in which there is a recognized risk of exposure to *S. typhi*. Risk is greatest for travelers to developing countries (e.g., countries in Latin America, Asia, and Africa) who have prolonged exposure to potentially contaminated food and drink (*22*). Multidrug-resistant strains of *S. typhi* have become common in some areas of the world (e.g., the Indian subcontinent [23] and the Arabian peninsula [24,25]), and cases of typhoid fever that are treated with ineffective drugs can be fatal. Travelers should be cautioned that typhoid vaccination is not a substitute for careful selection of food and drink. Typhoid vaccines are not 100% effective, and the vaccine's protection can be overwhelmed by large inocula of *S. typhi*.

- Persons with intimate exposure (e.g., household contact) to a documented *S. typhi* carrier.

- Microbiology laboratorians who work frequently with *S. typhi* (26).

Routine vaccination of sewage sanitation workers is not warranted in the United States and is indicated only for persons living in typhoid-endemic areas. Also, typhoid vaccine is not indicated for persons attending rural summer camps or living in areas in which natural disasters (e.g., floods) have occurred (27). No evidence has indicated that typhoid vaccine is useful in controlling common-source outbreaks.

Choice of Vaccine

The parenteral inactivated vaccine causes substantially more adverse reactions but is no more effective than Ty21a or ViCPS. Thus, when not contraindicated, either oral Ty21a or parenteral ViCPS is preferable.

Each of the three vaccines approved by the Food and Drug Administration has a different lower age limit for use among children (Figure 17.1). In addition, the time required for primary vaccination differs for each vaccine. Primary vaccination with ViCPS can be accomplished with a single injection, whereas 1 week is required for Ty21a, and 4 weeks are required to complete a primary series for parenteral inactivated vaccine (Figure 17.1). Finally, the live-attenuated Ty21a vaccine should not be used for immunocompromised persons or persons taking antibiotics at the time of vaccination (see Precautions and Contraindications).

Vaccination	Age	Dosage			
		Dose/mode of administration	Number of doses	Interval between doses	Boosting interval
Oral live-attenuated Ty21a vaccine					
Primary series	≥6 yrs	1 capsule*	4	2 days	—
Booster	≥6 yrs	1 capsule*	4	2 days	every 5 yrs
Vi capsular poly-saccharide vaccine					
Primary series	≥2 yrs	0.50 mL†	1	—	—
Booster	≥2 yrs	0.50 mL†	1	—	every 2 yrs
Heat-phenol-inactivated parenteral vaccine					
Primary series	6 mos–10 yrs	0.25 mL§	2	≥4 wks	—
	≥10 yrs	0.50 mL§	2	≥4 wks	—
Booster	6 mos–10 yrs	0.25 mL§	1	—	every 3 yrs
	≥10 yrs	0.50 mL§	1	—	every 3 yrs
	≥6 mos	0.10 mL¶	1	—	every 3 yrs

*Each orally administered capsule contains contains 2–6 x 10^9 viable *S. typhi* Ty21a and 5–50 x 10^9 nonviable *S. typhi* Ty21a.
†Intramuscularly.
§Subcutaneously.
¶Intradermally.
— Not applicable.

Figure 17.1. Dosage and schedules for typhoid fever vaccination

Vaccine Administration

Ty21a

Primary vaccination with live-attenuated Ty21a vaccine consists of one enteric-coated capsule taken on alternate days for a total of four capsules. The capsules must be kept refrigerated (not frozen), and all four doses must be taken to achieve maximum efficacy (6). Each capsule should be taken with cool liquid no warmer than 37 C (98.6 F), approximately 1 hour before a meal. Although adverse reactions to Ty21a are uncommon among children 1-5 years of age (28,29), data are unavailable regarding efficacy for this age group. This vaccine has not been studied among children <1 year of age. The vaccine manufacturer recommends that Ty21a not be administered to children <6 years of age.

ViCPS

Primary vaccination with ViCPS consists of one 0.5-mL (25-μg) dose administered intramuscularly. This vaccine has not been studied among children <1 year of age. The vaccine manufacturer does not recommend the vaccine for children <2 years of age.

Parenteral Inactivated Vaccine

Primary vaccination with parenteral inactivated vaccine consists of two 0.5-mL subcutaneous injections, each containing approximately 5 x 10^8 killed bacteria, separated by $\geq$4 weeks. The vaccine manufacturer does not recommend the vaccine for use among children <6 months of age. If the two doses of parenteral inactivated vaccine cannot be separated by $\geq$4 weeks because of time constraints, common practice has been to administer three doses of the vaccine at weekly intervals in the volumes listed above. Vaccines administered according to this schedule may be less effective, however.

Booster Doses

If continued or repeated exposure to *S. typhi* is expected, booster doses of vaccine are required to maintain immunity after vaccination with parenteral typhoid vaccines (Figure 17.1). The ViCPS manufacturer recommends a booster dose every 2 years after the primary dose if continued or renewed exposure is expected. In a study in which efficacy was not examined, revaccination of U.S. adults at either 27 or 34 months after the primary vaccination increased mean antibody titers to the approximate levels achieved with the primary dose (*17*). The optimal booster schedule for persons administered Ty21a for primary vaccination has not been determined; however, the longest reported follow-up study of vaccine trial subjects indicated that efficacy continued for 5 years after vaccination (*4*). The manufacturer of Ty21a recommends revaccination with the entire four-dose series every 5 years if continued or renewed exposure to *S. typhi* is expected. This recommendation may change as more data become available about the period of protection produced by the Ty21a vaccine. If the parenteral inactivated vaccine is used initially, booster doses should be administered every 3 years if continued or renewed exposure is expected. A single booster dose of parenteral inactivated vaccine is sufficient, even if >3 years have elapsed since the prior vaccination. When the heat-phenol-inactivated vaccine is used for booster vaccination, the intradermal route causes less reaction than the subcutaneous route (*30*). The acetone-inactivated vaccine should not be administered intradermally or by jet-injector gun because of the potential for severe local reactions (*31*).

No information has been reported concerning the use of one vaccine as a booster after primary vaccination with a different vaccine. However, using either the series of four doses of Ty21a or one dose of ViCPS for persons previously vaccinated with parenteral vaccine is a reasonable alternative to administration of a booster dose of parenteral inactivated vaccine.

Adverse Reactions

Ty21a produces fewer adverse reactions than either ViCPS or the parenteral inactivated vaccine. During volunteer studies and field trials with oral live-attenuated Ty21a vaccine, side effects were rare and consisted of abdominal discomfort, nausea, vomiting, fever, headache, and rash or urticaria (*2,7,32*) (Figure 17.2). In placebo-controlled trials, monitored adverse reactions occurred with equal frequency among groups receiving vaccine and placebo.

In several trials, ViCPS produced fever (occurring in 0%-1% of vaccinees), headache (1.5%-3% of vaccinees), and erythema or induration ≥1 cm (7% of vaccinees) (*17,20,33*) (Figure 17.2). In the study conducted in Nepal, the ViCPS vaccine produced fewer local and systemic reactions than did the control (the 23-valent pneumococcal vaccine) (*19*). Among schoolchildren in South Africa, ViCPS produced less erythema and induration than did the control bivalent meningococcal vaccine (*20*). In a direct comparison, ViCPS produced reactions less than half as frequently as parenteral inactivated vaccine, probably because ViCPS contains negligible amounts of bacterial lipopolysaccharide (*33*).

Parenteral inactivated vaccines produce several systemic and local adverse reactions, including fever (occurring in 6.7%-24% of vaccinees), headache (9%-10% of vaccinees), and severe local pain and/or swelling (3%-35% of vaccinees) (Figure 17.2) 21%-23% of vaccinees missed work or school because of adverse reactions (*12,13,34*). More severe reactions, including hypotension, chest pain, and shock, have been reported sporadically.

Vaccine	Reactions		
	Fever	Headache	Local reactions
Ty21a*	0%– 5%	0%– 5%	Not applicable
ViCPS	0%– 1%	1.5%– 3%	Erythema or induration ≥1 cm: 7%
Parenteral inactivated	6.7%–24%	9%–10%	Severe local pain or swelling: 3%–35%

*The side effects of Ty21a are rare and mainly consist of abdominal discomfort, nausea, vomiting, and rash or urticaria.

Figure 17.2. Common adverse reactions of typhoid fever vaccines

Precautions and Contraindications

The theoretical possibility for decreased immunogenicity when Ty21a, a live bacterial vaccine, is administered concurrently with immunoglobulin, antimalarials, or viral vaccines has caused concern (*35*). However, because Ty21a is immunogenic even in persons with preexisting antibody titers (*29*), its immunogenicity should not be affected by simultaneous administration of immunoglobulin. Mefloquine can inhibit the growth of the live Ty21a strain in vitro; if this antimalarial is administered, vaccination with Ty21a should be delayed for 24 hours. The minimum inhibitory concentration of chloroquine for Ty21a is >256 µg/mL; this antimalarial should not affect the immunogenicity of Ty21a (*36,37*). The vaccine manufacturer advises that Ty21a should not be administered to persons receiving sulfonamides or other antimicrobial agents; Ty21a should be administered ≥24 hours after an antimicrobial dose. No data exist on the immunogenicity of Ty21a when administered concurrently or within 30 days of viral vaccines (e.g., oral polio, measles/mumps/rubella, or yellow fever vaccines). In the absence of such data, if typhoid vaccination is warranted, it should not be delayed because of the administration of viral vaccines.

No data have been reported on the use of any of the three typhoid vaccines among pregnant women. Live-attenuated Ty21a should not be used among immunocompromised persons, including those persons known to be infected with human immunodeficiency virus. The two available parenteral vaccines present theoretically safer alternatives for this group. The only contraindication to vaccination with either

ViCPS or with parenteral inactivated vaccine is a history of severe local or systemic reactions following a previous dose.

References

1. Ryan CA, Hargrett-Bean NT, Blake PA. *Salmonella typhi* infections in the United States, 1975-1984: increasing role of foreign travel. Rev Infect Dis 1989;11:1-8.

2. Gilman RH, Hornick RB, Woodward WE, et al. Evaluation of a UDP-glucose-4-epimeraseless mutant of *Salmonella typhi* as a live oral vaccine. J Infect Dis 1977;136:717-23.

3. Levine MM, Ferreccio C, Black RE, Germanier R, Chilean Typhoid Committee. Large-scale field trial of Ty21a live oral typhoid vaccine in enteric-coated capsule formulation. Lancet 1987;329:1049-52.

4. Levine MM, Taylor DN, Ferreccio C. Typhoid vaccines come of age. Pediatr Infect Dis J 1989;8:374-81.

5. Levine MM, Ferreccio C, Cryz S, Ortiz E. Comparison of enteric-coated capsules and liquid formulation of Ty21a typhoid vaccine in randomised controlled field trial. Lancet 1990;336:891-4.

6. Ferreccio C, Levine MM, Rodriguez H, Contreras R, Chilean Typhoid Committee. Comparative efficacy of two, three, or four doses of TY21a live oral typhoid vaccine in enteric-coated capsules: a field trial in an endemic area. J Infect Dis 1989;159:766-9.

7. Simanjuntak CH, Paleologo FP, Punjabi NH, et al. Oral immunisation against typhoid fever in Indonesia with Ty21a vaccine. Lancet 1991;338:1055-9.

8. Wahdan MH, Série C, Cerisier Y, Sallam S, Germanier R. A controlled field trial of live *Salmonella typhi* strain Ty 21a oral vaccine against typhoid: three-year results. J Infect Dis 1982;145:292-5.

9. Hornick RB, Dupont HL, Levine MM, et al. Efficacy of a live oral typhoid vaccine in human volunteers. Dev Biol Stand 1976;33:89-92.

10. Cancellieri V, Fara GM. Demonstration of specific IgA in human feces after immunization with live Ty21a *Salmonella typhi* vaccine. J Infect Dis 1985;151:482-4.

11. Murphy JR, Baqar S, Muñoz C, et al. Characteristics of humoral and cellular immunity to *Salmonella typhi* in residents of typhoid-endemic and typhoid-free regions. J Infect Dis 1987;156:1005-9.

12. Yugoslav Typhoid Commission. A controlled field trial of the effectiveness of acetone-dried and inactivated and heat-phenol-inactivated typhoid vaccines in Yugoslavia. Bull WHO 1964;30:623-30.

13. Hejfec LB, Salmin LV, Lejtman MZ, et al. A controlled field trial and laboratory study of five typhoid vaccines in the USSR. Bull WHO 1966;34:321-9.

14. Ashcroft MT, Singh B, Nicholson CC, Ritchie JM, Sobryan E, Williams F. A seven-year field trial of two typhoid vaccines in Guyana. Lancet 1967;290:1056-9.

15. Polish Typhoid Committee. Controlled field trials and laboratory studies on the effectiveness of typhoid vaccines in Poland, 1961-64. Bull WHO 1966;34:211-22.

16. Robbins JD, Robbins JB. Reexamination of the protective role of the capsular polysaccharide (Vi antigen) of *Salmonella typhi*. J Infect Dis 1984;150:436-49.

17. Keitel WA, Bond NL, Zahradnik JM, CramtonTA, RobbinsJB. Clinical and serological responses following primary and booster immunization with *Salmonella typhi* Vi capsular polysaccharide vaccines. Vaccine 1994;12:195-9.

18. Ambrosch F, Fritzell B, Gregor J, et al. Combined vaccination against yellow fever and typhoid fever: a comparative trial. Vaccine 1994;12:625-8.

19. Acharya IL, Lowe CU, Thapa R, et al. Prevention of typhoid fever in Nepal with the Vi capsular polysaccharide of *Salmonella typhi*. N Engl J Med 1987;317:1101-4.

20. Klugman KP, Gilbertson IT, Koornhof HJ, et al. Protective activity of Vi capsular polysaccharide vaccine against typhoid fever. Lancet 1987;330:1165-9.

21. Klugman KP, Koornhof HJ, Robbins JB. Immunogenicity and protective efficacy of Vi vaccine against typhoid fever three years after immunization [Abstract]. Bangkok, Thailand: Second Asia-Pacific Symposium on Typhoid Fever and Other Salmonellosis, 1994.

22. Edelman R, Levine MM. Summary of an international workshop on typhoid fever. Rev Infect Dis 1986;8:329-49.

23. Rao PS, Rajashekar V, Varghese GK, Shivananda PG. Emergence of multidrug-resistant *Salmonella typhi* in rural southern India. Am J Trop Med Hyg 1993;48:108-11.

24. Wallace M, Yousif AA. Spread of multiresistant *Salmonella typhi* (letter). Lancet 1990;336:1065-6.

25. Elshafie SS, Rafay AM. Chloramphenicol-resistant typhoid fever—an emerging problem in Oman. Scand J Infect Dis 1992;24:819-20.

26. Blaser MJ, Hickman FW, Farmer III JJ, Brenner DJ, Balows A, Feldman RA. *Salmonella typhi*: the laboratory as a reservoir of infection. J Infect Dis 1980;142:934-8.

27. Blake PA. Communicable disease control. In: Gregg MB, ed. The public health consequences of disasters. Atlanta: US Department of Health and Human Services, Public Health Service, CDC, 1989;7-12.

28. Murphy JR, Grez L, Schlesinger L, et al. Immunogenicity of *Salmonella typhi* Ty21a vaccine for young children. Infect Immun 1991;59:4291-3.

29. Cryz SJ, Vanprapar N, Thisyakorn U, et al. Safety and immunogenicity of *Salmonella-typhi* Ty21a vaccine in young Thai children. Infect Immun 1993;61:1149-51.

30. Iwarson S, Larsson P. Intradermal versus subcutaneous immunization with typhoid vaccine. J Hyg (Lond) 1978;84:11-6.

31. Edwards EA, Johnson DP, Pierce WE, Peckinpaugh RO. Reactions and serologic responses to monovalent acetone-inactivated typhoid vaccine and heat-killed TAB when given by jet-injection. Bull WHO 1974;51:501-5.

32. Cryz SJ,Jr. Post-marketing experience with live oral Ty21a vaccine (letter). Lancet 1993;341:49-50.

33. Cumberland NS, Roberts JS, Arnold WSG, Patel RK, Bowker CH. Typhoid Vi: a less reactogenic vaccine. J Int Med Res 1992;20:247-53.

34. Ashcroft MT, Ritchie JM, Nicholson CC. Controlled field trial in British Guiana school children of heat-killed-phenolized and acetone-killed lyophilized typhoid vaccines. Amer J Hyg 1964;79:196-206.

35. Wolfe MS. Precautions with oral live typhoid (Ty 21a) vaccine (letter). Lancet 1990;336:631-2.

36. Brachman PS, Metchock B, Kozarsky PE. Effects of antimalarial chemoprophylactic agents on the viability of the Ty21a typhoid vaccine strain (letter). Clin Infect Dis 1992;15:1057-8.

37. Horowitz H, Carbonaro CA. Inhibition of the *Salmonella-typhi* oral vaccine strain, Ty21a, by mefloquine and chloroquine (letter). J Infect Dis 1992;166:1462-4.

Chapter 18

United States Public Health Service Recommendations to International Travelers

Introduction

Recommendations for individuals engaging in international travel apply primarily to vaccinations and prophylactic measures generally advisable for U.S. travelers planning to spend time in areas of the world where diseases such as measles, poliomyelitis, typhoid fever, viral hepatitis, and malaria occur either in endemic form or epidemic form and, therefore, pose a threat to their health. In addition, some countries require an International Certificate of Vaccination against yellow fever as a condition for entry. The majority of U.S. international travelers probably do not need any additional immunizations or prophylaxis, provided their routine immunization status is up-to-date according to the standards of the Public Health Service Advisory Committee on Immunization Practices (ACIP).

The extent to which advisory statements can be made specific for each country and each disease is limited by the lack of reliable data. Although data on the occurrence of many of these diseases are published regularly by WHO, these figures represent only a small percentage of the total number of cases that actually occur—in fact, many countries do not report these diseases at all. Furthermore, communicable diseases are not well reported by practicing physicians, and in

Taken from HHS Pub. No. (CDC) 94-8280, *Health Information for International Travel, 1994.*

395

some countries where the number of physicians is inadequate, many cases never come to medical attention. For these reasons, any recommendations must be interpreted with care.

In general, the risk of acquiring illness when engaging in international travel depends on the areas of the world to be visited—travelers in developing countries are at greater risk than those traveling in developed areas. In most developed countries (i.e., Canada, Australia, New Zealand, Japan, and the continent of Europe), the risk to the general health of the traveler will be no greater than that incurred throughout the United States. However, a higher risk of measles, mumps, and rubella may exist. Likewise, in many developed countries such as Germany, Ireland, Italy, Spain, Sweden, and the United Kingdom, pertussis immunization is not as widely practiced as in the United States, and the risk of acquiring pertussis is greater. In the countries in Africa, Asia, South America, Central America, Mexico, the South Pacific, Middle East, and Far East, as well as parts of Eastern Europe and the former Soviet Union, living conditions and standards of sanitation and hygiene vary considerably, and immunization coverage levels may be low. Thus the risk of acquiring disease also can vary greatly in these locations. Travelers visiting primarily tourist areas on itineraries that do not include travel or visits in rural areas have less risk of exposure to food or water that is of questionable quality. Travelers who visit smaller cities off the usual tourist routes, who spend time in small villages or rural areas for extended periods, or who expect to have extended contact with children are at greater risk of acquiring infectious diseases, because of exposure to water and food of uncertain quality and closer contact with local residents who may harbor the organisms that cause such diseases. Consequently, the added protection of booster or additional doses of certain vaccines and other prophylaxis is recommended for these persons.

More detailed comments can be found in Chapter 19 "Specific Recommendations for Vaccination and Prophylaxis."

General Recommendations on Human Immunodeficiency Virus (HIV) Infection and Acquired Immunodeficiency Syndrome (AIDS)

Acquired immunodeficiency syndrome (AIDS) is a severe, often life-threatening, illness caused by the human immunodeficiency virus (HIV). The incubation period for AIDS is very long and variable, ranging from a few months to many years. Some individuals infected with HIV have remained asymptomatic for more than a decade. Currently, there is no vaccine to protect against infection with HIV. Although there is no cure for AIDS, treatments for HIV infection and prophylaxis for several opportunistic diseases that characterize AIDS are available as a result of intense international research efforts.

HIV infection and AIDS have been reported worldwide. Comprehensive surveillance systems are lacking in many countries, so that the true number of cases is likely to be far greater than the numbers officially reported from some, particularly the non-industrialized nations. The number of persons infected with HIV is estimated by WHO to be in the range of 13-14 million worldwide. Because HIV infection and AIDS are globally distributed, the risk to international travelers is determined less by their geographic destination than by their individual behavior.

The global epidemic of HIV infection and AIDS has raised several issues regarding HIV infection and international travel. The first is the need of information for international travelers regarding HIV transmission and how HIV infection can be prevented.

HIV infection is preventable. HIV is transmitted through sexual intercourse, needlesharing, by medical use of blood or blood components, and perinatally from an infected woman. HIV is not transmitted through casual contact; air, food, or water routes; contact with inanimate objects; or through mosquitoes or other arthropod vectors. The use of any public conveyance (e.g., airplane, automobile, boat, bus, train) by persons with AIDS or HIV infection does not pose a risk of infection for the crew or other passengers.

Travelers are at risk if they:

- have sexual intercourse (heterosexual or homosexual) with an infected person;

- use or allow the use of contaminated, unsterilized syringes or needles for any injections or other skin-piercing procedures including acupuncture, use of illicit drugs, steroid injections, medical/dental procedures, ear piercing, or tattooing;

- use infected blood, blood components, or clotting factor concentrates. HIV infection by this route is a rare occurrence in those countries or cities where donated blood/plasma is screened for HIV antibody.

Travelers should avoid sexual encounters with a person who is infected with HIV or whose HIV-infection status is unknown. This includes avoiding sexual activity with intravenous drug users and persons with multiple sexual partners, such as male or female prostitutes. Condoms decrease, but do not entirely eliminate, the risk of transmission of HIV. Persons who engage in vaginal, anal, or oral-genital intercourse with anyone who is infected with HIV or whose infection status is unknown should use latex condoms. Use of spermicides with condoms may provide additional protection.

In many countries, needlesharing by IV drug users is a major source of HIV transmission and other infections such as hepatitis B and C. Do not use drugs intravenously or share needles for any purpose. In the United States, Australia, New Zealand, Canada, Japan, and western European countries, the risk of infection of transfusion-associated HIV infection has been virtually eliminated through required testing of all donated blood for antibodies to HIV.

If produced in the United States according to procedures approved by the Food and Drug Administration, immune globulin preparations (such as those used for the prevention of hepatitis A and B) and hepatitis B virus vaccine undergo processes that are known to inactivate HIV and therefore these products should be used as indicated.

In less-developed nations, there may not be a formal program for testing blood or biological products for antibody to HIV. In these countries, use of unscreened blood clotting factor concentrates or those of uncertain purity should be avoided (when medically prudent). If transfusion is necessary, the blood should be tested, if at all possible, for HIV antibodies by appropriately-trained laboratory technicians using a reliable test. For WHO blood transfusion guidelines for international travelers, see [Chapter 15].

Needles used to draw blood or administer injections should be sterile, preferably of the single-use disposable type, and prepackaged in a sealed container. Insulin-dependent diabetics, hemophiliacs or other persons who require routine or frequent injections should carry a supply of syringes, needles and disinfectant swabs (e.g., alcohol wipes) sufficient to last their entire stay abroad.

International travelers should be aware that some countries serologically screen incoming travelers (primarily those with extended visits, such as for work or study) and deny entry to persons with AIDS and those whose test results indicate infection with HIV. Persons who are intending to visit a country for a substantial period or to work or study abroad should be informed of the policies and requirements of the particular country. This information is usually available from consular officials of individual nations.

General Recommendations on Vaccination and Prophylaxis

The Advisory Committee on Immunization Practices (ACIP) meets periodically and makes recommendations to the Public Health Service. Benefits and risks are associated with the use of all immunobiologics—no vaccine is completely effective or completely safe. The recommendations represent a balancing of scientific evidence of benefits and risks in order to achieve optimal levels of protection against infectious or communicable diseases. The recommendations include information on general immunization issues and on the use of specific vaccines. When these recommendations are revised, they are published in the MMWR.

Vaccinations against diphtheria, tetanus, pertussis, measles, mumps, rubella, poliomyelitis, and *Haemophilus influenzae* type b meningitis and invasive disease are routinely administered in the United States, usually in childhood. Routine vaccination against hepatitis B virus infection also is now recommended for all infants beginning either at birth or at 2 months of age. If persons do not have a history of adequate protection against these diseases, immunizations appropriate to their age and previous immunization status should be obtained, whether or not international travel is planned. Text and [accompanying Figures] present recommendations for use, the number of doses, dose intervals, boosters, side effects, precautions and contraindications of vaccines and toxoids which may be indicated for travelers. For specific vaccines and toxoids, additional details on background, side effects, adverse reactions, precautions, and contraindications are available in the appropriate ACIP statements.

Age At Which Immunobiologics Are Administered

Factors which influence recommendations concerning the age at which a vaccine is administered include the age-specific risks of the disease and its complications, the ability of individuals of a given age to respond to the vaccine(s), and the potential interference with the immune response by passively transferred maternal antibody. Vaccines are recommended for the youngest age group at risk of develop-

399

ing the disease whose members are known to develop an adequate antibody response to vaccination.

The routine immunization recommendations and schedules for infants and children in the United States (Figures 18.1 and 18.2) do not provide specific guidelines for infants and young children who will travel internationally before the age when specific vaccines and toxoids are recommended routinely or before the primary vaccination series has been completed. The section titled "Immunization Schedule Modifications for International Travel for Infants and Inadequately Immunized Young Children <2 Years of Age" provides revised recommendations and schedules for active immunization and, when appropriate, passive immunization of such infants and children.

Spacing of Immunobiologics

Multiple Doses of Same Antigen

Some products require more than 1 dose for adequate protection. The use of multiple reduced doses that together equal a full immunizing dose, the use of smaller divided doses, or the use of doses given at less than recommended intervals may lessen the antibody response and is not endorsed or recommended; such doses should not be counted as part of the vaccination series. It is unnecessary to restart an interrupted series of a vaccine or toxoid or to add extra doses. However, some products require periodic booster doses to maintain protection.

Simultaneous Administration

Experimental evidence and extensive clinical experience have strengthened the scientific basis for giving certain vaccines at the same time. Most of the widely used antigens can safely and effectively be given simultaneously (i.e., on the same day) without impairing antibody responses or increasing rates of adverse reactions. This knowledge is particularly helpful for international travelers for whom exposure to several infectious diseases may be imminent.

In general, inactivated vaccines can be administered simultaneously at separate sites. However, when vaccines commonly associated with local or systemic reactions e.g., cholera, parenteral typhoid, and plague are given simultaneously, the reactions might be accentu-

Figure 18.1. Recommended schedule for routine active vaccination of infants and children

Vaccine	At birth (before hospital discharge)	1–2 months	2 months[†]	4 months	6 months	6–18 months	12–15 months	15 months	4–6 years (before school entry)
Diphtheria-tetanus-pertussis[§]			DTP	DTP	DTP			DTaP/DTP[¶]	DTaP/DTP
Polio, live oral			OPV	OPV	OPV**				OPV
Measles-mumps-rubella							MMR		MMR[††]
Haemophilus influenzae type b conjugate									
HbOC/PRP-T[§, §§]			Hib	Hib	Hib		Hib[¶¶]		
PRP-OMP[§§]			Hib	Hib			Hib[¶¶]		
Hepatitis B***									
Option 1	HepB	HepB[†††]				HepB[†††]			
Option 2		HepB[†††]	HepB[†††]	HepB[†††]		HepB[†††]			

*See Table 3 for the recommended immunization schedule for infants and children up to their seventh birthday who do not not begin the vaccination series at the recommended times or who are >1 month behind in the immunization schedule.

[†]Can be administered as early as 6 weeks of age.

[§]Two DTP and Hib combination vaccines are available (DTP/HbOC [TETRAMUNE™]; and PRP-T [ActHIB™, OmniHIB™] which can be reconstituted with DTP vaccine produced by Connaught).

[¶]This dose of DTP can be administered as early as 12 months of age provided that the interval since the previous dose of DTP is at least 6 months. *Diphtheria and tetanus toxoids and acellular pertussis vaccine (DTaP) is currently recommended only for use as the fourth and/or fifth doses of the DTP series among children aged 15 months through 6 years (before the seventh birthday).* Some experts prefer to administer these vaccines at 18 months of age.

**The American Academy of Pediatrics (AAP) recommends this dose of vaccine at 6–18 months of age.

[††]The AAP recommends that two doses of MMR should be administered by 12 years of age with the second dose being administered preferentially at entry to middle school or junior high school.

[§§]HbOC: [HibTITER®](Lederle Praxis). PRP-T: [ActHIB™, OmniHIB™] (Pasteur Merieux). PRP-OMP: [PedvaxHIB®] (Merck, Sharp, and Dohme). A DTP/Hib combination vaccine can be used in place of HbOC/PRP-T.

[¶¶]After the primary infant Hib conjugate vaccine series is completed, any of the licensed Hib conjugate vaccines may be used as a booster dose at age 12–15 months.

***For use among infants born to HBsAg-negative mothers. The first dose should be administered during the newborn period, preferably before hospital discharge, but no later than age 2 months. Premature infants of HBsAg-negative mothers should receive the first dose of the hepatitis B vaccine series at the time of hospital discharge or when the other routine childhood vaccines are initiated. (All infants born to HBsAg-positive mothers should receive immunoprophylaxis for hepatitis B as soon as possible after birth.)

[†††]Hepatitis B vaccine can be administered simultaneously at the same visit with DTP (or DTaP), OPV, Hib, and /or MMR.

Figure 18.2. *Recommended Accelerated Immunization Schedule for Infants and Children <7 Years of Age Who Start the Series Late* or Who Are >1 Month Behind in the Immunization Schedule+ (i.e., Children for Whom Compliance With Scheduled Return Visits Cannot be Assured)*

Timing	Vaccine(s)	Comments
First visit (≥4 months of age)	DTP[§], OPV, Hib[¶,§], Hepatitis B, MMR (should be given as soon as child is age 12–15 months)	All vaccines should be administered simultaneously at the appropriate visit
Second visit (1 month after first visit)	DTP[§], Hib[¶,§], Hepatitis B	
Third visit (1 month after second visit)	DTP[§], OPV, Hib[¶,§]	
Fourth visit (6 weeks after third visit)	OPV	
Fifth visit (≥6 months after third visit)	DTaP[§] or DTP, Hib[¶,§], Hepatitis B	
Additional visits (Age 4–6 yrs)	DTaP[§] or DTP, OPV, MMR	Preferably at or before school entry.
(Age 14–16 yrs)	Td	Repeat every 10 yrs through-out life.

DTP	Diphtheria-tetanus-pertussis
DTaP	Diphtheria-tetanus-acellular pertussis
Hib	Haemophilus influenzae type b conjugate
MMR	Measles-mumps-rubella
OPV	Poliovirus vaccine, live oral, trivalent
Td	Tetanus and diphtheria toxoids (for use among persons ≥7 years of age

*If initiated in the first year of life, administer DTP doses 1, 2, and 3, and OPV doses 1, 2, and 3 according to this schedule; administer MMR when the child reaches 12–15 months of age.

[†]See individual ACIP recommendations for detailed information on specific vaccines.

[§]Two DTP and Hib combination vaccines are available (DTP/HbOC [TETRAMUNE™]; and PRP-T [ActHIB™, OmniHIB™] which can be reconstituted with DTP vaccine produced by Connaught). DTaP preparations are currently recommended only for use as the fourth and/or fifth doses of the DTP series among children 15 months through 6 years of age (before the seventh birthday). DTP and DTaP should not be used on or after the seventh birthday.

[¶]The recommended schedule varies by vaccine manufacturer. For information specific to the vaccine being used, consult the package insert and ACIP recommendations. Children beginning the Hib vaccine series at age 2–6 months should receive a primary series of three doses of HbOC [HibTITER®] (Lederle-Praxis), PRP-T [ActHIB™, OmniHIB™] (Pasteur Merieux; SmithKline Beecham; Connaught), or a licensed DTP-Hib combination vaccine; or two doses of PRP-OMP [PedvaxHIB®] (Merck, Sharp, and Dohme). An additional booster dose of any licensed Hib conjugate vaccine should be administered at 12–15 months of age and at least 2 months after the previous dose. Children beginning the Hib vaccine series at 7–11 months of age should receive a primary series of two doses of an HbOC, PRP-T, or PRP-OMP-containing vaccine. An additional booster dose of any licensed Hib conjugate vaccine should be administered at 12–18 months of age and at least 2 months after the previous dose. Children beginning the Hib vaccine series at ages 12–14 months should receive a primary series of one dose of an HbOC, PRP-T, or PRP-OMP-containing vaccine. An additional booster dose of any licensed Hib conjugate vaccine should be administered 2 months after the previous dose. Children beginning the Hib vaccine series at ages 15-59 months should receive one dose of any licensed Hib vaccine. Hib vaccine should not be administered after the fifth birthday except for special circumstances as noted in the specific ACIP recommendations for the use of Hib vaccine.

Figure 18.4. Recommended Immunization Schedule for Persons ≥ 7 Years of Age Not Vaccinated at the Recommended Time in Early Infancy

Timing	Vaccine(s)	Comments
First visit	Td[†], OPV[§], MMR[¶], and Hepatitis B**	Primary poliovirus vaccination is not routinely recommended for persons ≥18 years of age.
Second visit (6–8 weeks after first visit)	Td, OPV, MMR[††,¶], Hepatitis B**	
Third visit (6 months after second visit)	Td, OPV, Hepatitis B**	
Additional visits	Td	Repeat every 10 years throughout life.

MMR	Measles-mumps-rubella
OPV	Poliovirus vaccine, live oral, trivalent
Td	Tetanus and diphtheria toxoids (for use among persons ≥7 years of age)

*See individual ACIP recommendations for details.

[†]The DTP and DTaP doses administered to children <7 years of age who remain incompletely vaccinated at age ≥7 years should be counted as prior exposure to tetanus and diphtheria toxoids (e.g., a child who previously received two doses of DTP needs only one dose of Td to complete a primary series for tetanus and diphtheria).

[§]When polio vaccine is administered to previously unvaccinated persons ≥18 years of age, inactivated poliovirus vaccine (IPV) is preferred. For the immunization schedule for IPV, see specific ACIP statement on the use of polio vaccine.

[¶]Persons born before 1957 can generally be considered immune to measles and mumps and need not be vaccinated. Rubella (or MMR) vaccine can be administered to persons of any age, particularly to nonpregnant women of child-bearing age.

**Hepatitis B vaccine, recombinant. Selected high-risk groups for whom vaccination is recommended include persons with occupational risk, such as health-care and public-safety workers who have occupational exposure to blood, clients and staff of institutions for the developmentally disabled, hemodialysis patients, recipients of certain blood products (e.g., clotting factor concentrates), household contacts and sex partners of hepatitis B virus carriers, injecting drug users, sexually active homosexual and bisexual men, certain sexually active heterosexual men and women, inmates of long-term correctional facilities, certain international travelers, and families of HBsAg-positive adoptees from countries where HBV infection in endemic. Because risk factors are often not identified directly among adolescents, universal hepatitis B vaccination of teenagers should be implemented in communities where injecting drug use, pregnancy among teenagers, and/or sexually transmitted diseases are common.

[††]The ACIP recommends a second dose of measles-containing vaccine (preferable MMR to assure immunity to mumps and rubella) for certain groups. Children with no documentation of live measles vaccination after the first birthday should receive two doses of live measles-containing vaccine not less than 1 month apart. In addition, the following persons born in 1957 or later should have documentation of measles immunity (i.e., two doses of measles-containing vaccine [at least one of which being MMR], physician-diagnosed measles, or laboratory evidence of measles immunity): a) those entering post-high school educational settings; b) those beginning employment in health-care settings who will have direct patient contact; and c) travelers to areas with endemic measles.

ated. Whenever feasible, it is preferable to administer these vaccines on separate occasions.

When administered at the same time and at separate sites, DTP, OPV, and MMR have produced seroconversion rates and rates of side effects similar to those observed when the vaccines are administered separately. Simultaneous vaccination of infants with DTP, OPV (or IPV), and either Hib vaccine or hepatitis B vaccine has resulted in acceptable response to all antigens. Routine simultaneous administration of DTP (or DTaP), OPV (or IPV), Hib vaccine, MMR, and hepatitis B vaccine is encouraged for children who are the recommended age to receive these vaccines and for whom no specific contraindications exist at the time of the visit. Administration of MMR and Hib vaccine at 12 to 15 months of age, followed by DTP (or DTaP, if indicated) at 15-18 months, remains an acceptable alternative for children with caregivers known to be compliant with other health-care recommendations and who are likely to return for future visits; hepatitis B vaccine can be administered at either of these two visits. DTaP may be used instead of DTP only for the fourth and fifth dose in children 15 months of age through 6 years (i.e., before the seventh birthday).

Hepatitis B vaccine administered with yellow fever vaccine is as safe and efficacious as when these vaccines are administered separately. Measles and yellow fever vaccines have been administered together safely and with full efficacy of each of the components.

The antibody response of yellow fever and cholera vaccines is decreased if administered simultaneously or within a short time of each other. If possible, yellow fever and cholera vaccinations should be separated by at least 3 weeks. If there are time constraints and both vaccines are necessary, the injections can be administered simultaneously or within a 3-week period with the understanding that antibody response may not be optimal.

Decisions on the need for yellow fever and/or cholera immunizations should take into account the amount of protection afforded by the vaccine, the importance of vaccination versus environmental or hygienic practices in avoiding disease exposure, and whether there is an actual vaccination requirement for entry into a country. Certain countries require yellow fever vaccination with documentation in an International Certificate of Vaccination. Yellow fever vaccine is highly effective in protecting against a disease with substantial mortality for which no therapy exists. The currently used cholera vaccine provides only limited protection of brief duration; few indications exist for its use.

Limited data suggest that the immunogenicity and safety of Japanese encephalitis (JE) vaccine is not compromised by simultaneous administration with DTP vaccine. No data exist on the effect of concurrent administration of other vaccines, drugs (e.g. chloroquine, mefloquine), or biologicals on the safety and immunogenicity of JE Vaccine.

Non-Simultaneous Administration

Inactivated vaccines generally do not interfere with the immune response to other inactivated vaccines or to live vaccines. In general, an inactivated vaccine can be given either simultaneously or at any time before or after a different inactivated vaccine or a live vaccine. An exception, as noted above, is the recommendation that yellow fever and cholera vaccines should be separated by at least 3 weeks, if possible.

Theoretically, the immune response to one live-virus vaccine might be impaired if administered within 30 days of another live- virus vaccine; however no evidence exists for currently available vaccines to support this concern, whenever possible, live virus vaccines administered on different days should be administered at least 30 days apart. However, OPV and MMR vaccine can be administered at any time before, with, or after each other, if indicated.

Live virus vaccines can interfere with an individual's response to tuberculin testing. Tuberculin testing, if otherwise indicated, can be done on the day that live viral vaccines are administered or 4-6 weeks later.

Immune Globulin (IG Preparations—Formerly Called Immune Serum Globulin and Immunoglobulin.)

When certain live attenuated vaccines are given with immune globulin preparations, vaccine viruses might not successfully replicate and antibody response can be diminished. IG preparations do not interfere with the immune response to either OPV or yellow fever vaccine. However, immune globulin can inhibit the immune response to other parenterally-administered live-attenuated vaccine viruses (measles, mumps, rubella); the duration of inhibition is related to the dose of immune globulin. Administration of MMR and its component vaccines should be delayed for a) at least 3 months after administration of pooled or specific immune globulin given in doses to prevent hepatitis A, hepatitis B, or tetanus prophylaxis, b) at least 4 months after rabies prophylaxis, c) at least 5 months after measles or varicella prophylaxis, and d) at least 6 months after receipt of whole blood or packed red blood cells or measles prophylaxis [in] an immuno-compromised person. Receipt of higher doses of immune globulins in immunocompromised persons or receipt of intravenous immune globulin or certain other blood products may interfere with the immune response to MMR vaccine for longer periods. The General Recommendations on Immunization (MMWR:1994;43(RR-I) should be consulted for specific guidance on MMR vaccination following use of these products.

Because of imminent exposure to disease, immune globulin administration may become necessary after MMR or its individual component vaccines have been given, and interference can occur. Vaccine virus replication and stimulation of immunity usually will occur within 1-2 weeks after vaccination. If the interval between administration of these vaccines and the subsequent administration of an immune globulin preparation is 14 days or longer, vaccine need not be readministered. If the interval is less than 14 days, the vaccine should be readministered a) at least 3 months after hepatitis A, hepatitis B, or tetanus prophylaxis, b) at least 4 months after rabies prophylaxis, and c) at least 5 months after measles or varicella prophylaxis, unless serologic testing indicates that antibodies have been produced. If administration of immune globulin becomes necessary because of imminent exposure to disease, MMR or its component vaccines can be administered simultaneously with immune globulin, with the recognition that vaccine-induced immunity may be compromised. The vaccine should be administered in a site remote from that chosen for the immune globulin inoculation. Vaccination should be repeated after the interval noted above unless serologic testing indicates antibodies have been produced.

Immune globulin preparations interact minimally with inactivated vaccines and toxoids. Therefore, inactivated vaccines can be given simultaneously or at any time interval after or before an immune globulin product is used. However, vaccines should be administered at sites different than the immune globulin.

Hypersensitivity to Vaccine Components

Vaccine components can cause allergic reactions in some recipients. These reactions can be local or systemic, and can include mild to severe anaphylaxis or anaphylactic-like responses. The vaccine components responsible can include: (1) vaccine antigen, (2) animal proteins, (3) antibiotics, (4) preservatives, and (5) stabilizers. The most common animal protein allergen is egg protein in vaccines prepared using embryonated chicken eggs (e.g., influenza fever, yellow fever) or chicken embryo cell cultures (e.g., mumps and measles). Generally, persons who are able to eat eggs or egg products safely may receive these vaccines, while persons with histories of anaphylactic allergy (e.g., hives, swelling of the mouth and throat, difficulty breathing, hypotension, or shock) to eggs or egg proteins ordinarily should not.

Screening persons by asking whether they can eat eggs without adverse effects is a reasonable way to identify those who might be at risk from receiving measles, mumps, MMR, yellow fever and influenza vaccines. Protocols requiring caution have been developed for testing and vaccinating with measles and mumps vaccines those persons with anaphylactic reactions to egg ingestion. (1991 Redbook—Report of the Committee on Infectious Diseases. (Peter G., LePow ML., McCracken, GH Jr., Phillips CF, editors, American Academy of Pediatrics; 1991, Greenberg MA, et al. Safe administration of mumps-measles-rubella vaccine in egg-allergic children. J. Pediatr 1988; 113:504-506. Lavi S., et al. Administration of measles, mumps, and rubella virus vaccine (live) to egg-allergic children. JAMA 1990;263:269-271. Kemp A, et al. Measles immunization in children with clinical reactions to egg protein. AJDC 1990;144:33-35). A regimen for administering influenza vaccine to children with egg hypersensitivity and severe asthma has also been published. (Murphy and Strunk. J. Pediatr 1985;106:931-3).

Some vaccines contain preservatives (e.g., thimerosal, a mercurial compound) or trace amounts of antibiotics (e.g., neomycin) to which patients may be hypersensitive. Persons administering vaccines should carefully review the information provided in the package insert before deciding if the rare patient with such hypersensitivity should receive the vaccine(s). No currently recommended vaccine contains penicillin or penicillin derivatives. Some vaccines (e.g., MMR and its individual component vaccines) contain trace amounts of neomycin. This amount is less than would usually be used for the skin test to determine hypersensitivity. However, persons who have experienced anaphylactic reactions to neomycin should not receive these vaccines. Most often, neomycin allergy is a contact dermatitis—a manifestation of a delayed-type (cell-mediated) immune response—rather than anaphylaxis. A history of delayed-type reactions to neomycin is not a contraindication to receiving these vaccines.

Certain bacterial vaccines, such as cholera, DTP, plague, and parenteral typhoid, are frequently associated with local or systemic adverse effects. These reactions appear to be of a toxic rather than a hypersensitivity nature and are difficult to link with a specific sensitivity to vaccine components. On rare occasions, urticarial or anaphylactic reactions have been reported in DTP, DT, Td, or tetanus toxoid recipients. Appropriate skin testing can be performed to determine sensitivity to tetanus toxoid before discontinuing its use. (Jacobs RL, et al. Adverse reactions to tetanus toxoid. JAMA 1982;247:40-42). Alternatively, the need for a booster dose of tetanus toxoid can be evaluated by serologic testing.

Altered Immunocompetence

Killed or inactivated vaccines do not represent a damper to immunocompromised persons and generally should be administered as recommended for healthy persons. Frequently, however, the immune response to these vaccines is suboptimal.

Virus replication after administration of live, attenuated-virus vaccines can be enhanced in persons with immunodeficiency diseases, and in those with suppressed capacity for immune response, as occurs with leukemia, lymphoma, generalized malignancy, or therapy with corticosteroids, alkylating agents, antimetabolites, or radiation. Severe complications have been reported following vaccination with live attenuated virus vaccines and with live bacterial vaccines (e.g., BCG) in patients with leukemia, lymphoma and other persons with suppressed capacity for immune response. In general, patients with such conditions should not be given live vaccines. Vaccine recommendations specific for persons infected with Human Immunodeficiency Virus (HIV) are found under the individual diseases in [Chapter 19] "Specific Recommendations for Vaccinations and Prophylaxis."

OPV should not be given to any immunocompromised patient, their household members, or their close contacts. If polio immunization is indicated for these persons, IPV is recommended. Because of the possibility of immunodeficiency in other children born to a family in which there has been a case of congenital immunodeficiency, family members should not receive OPV until the immune status of the recipient and other children in the family is known.

Patients with leukemia in remission whose chemotherapy has been terminated for at least 3 months may receive live virus vaccines.

Most experts agree that steroid therapy usually does not contraindicate administration of live virus vaccine when it is short-term; low to moderate dose; (<2 weeks); long-term, alternate-day treatment with short-acting steroids; maintenance physiologic doses (replacement therapy); or administered topically (i.e., skin or eyes) by aerosol; or by intra-articular, bursal or tendon injection.

Children infected with HIV should receive on schedule all of the routinely recommended inactivated childhood vaccines (i.e., DTP, Hib, and hepatitis B vaccine) whether or not they are symptomatic. IPV is the polio vaccine of choice for HIV-infected asymptomatic and symptomatic persons and their household members and other close contacts. Limited studies of MMR immunization of asymptomatic and symptomatic HIV-infected persons have not documented unusual or severe adverse events. Because disease can be severe in such persons, MMR vaccine is recommended for all asymptomatic HIV-infected persons and should also be considered strongly for all those who are symptomatic. Pneumococcal vaccine is recommended for any person >2 years of age with HIV infection. Because influenza may result in serious illness and complications, vaccination against influenza is a prudent precaution in HIV-infected persons.

Vaccination of Persons with Acute Illnesses

The decision to administer or delay vaccination because of a current or recent acute illness depends largely on the severity of the symptoms and their etiology. Although a moderate or severe febrile illness is sufficient reason to postpone vaccination, minor illnesses, such as diarrhea, mild upper-respiratory infection with or without low-grade fever, or other low-grade febrile illness are not contraindications to vaccination. Likewise, antimicrobial therapy is not a contraindication to vaccination. In persons whose compliance with medical care cannot be assured, it is particularly important to take every opportunity to provide appropriate vaccinations. Persons with moderate or severe illness with or without fever should be vaccinated as soon as they have recovered from the acute phase of the illness. This precaution is to avoid superimposing adverse effects from the vaccine on the underlying illness or mistakenly attributing a manifestation of the underlying illness to the vaccine.

Routine physical examinations or temperature measurements are not prerequisites for vaccinating infants and other persons who appear to be in good health. Asking if the person is ill, postponing vaccination for those with moderate or severe acute illnesses, and vaccinating those without contraindications are appropriate procedures in immunization programs.

Vaccination During Pregnancy

Risk from vaccination during pregnancy is largely theoretical. The benefit of vaccination among pregnant women usually outweighs the potential risk when a) the risk for disease exposure is high, b) infection would pose a special risk to the mother or fetus, and c) the vaccine is unlikely to cause harm.

OPV can be administered to pregnant women who are at substantial risk of imminent exposure to natural infection. Although OPV is preferred, IPV may be considered if full immunization can be completed before the anticipated exposure. Pregnant women travelling to areas where the risk of yellow fever is high should receive a yellow fever vaccine. Under these circumstances, the small theoretical risk from vaccination is far outweighed by the risk of yellow fever infection. Known pregnancy is a contraindication for rubella, measles, and mumps vaccines. Although of theoretical concern, no case of congenital rubella syndrome or abnormalities attributable to a rubella vaccine virus infection have been observed in infants born to susceptible mothers who received rubella vaccine during pregnancy.

Persons who receive measles, mumps, or rubella vaccines can shed these viruses but generally do not transmit them. These vaccines can be administered safely to the children of pregnant women. Although live polio virus is shed by persons recently vaccinated with OPV (particularly after the first dose), this vaccine can also be administered to the children of pregnant women because experience has not revealed any risk of polio vaccine virus to the fetus.

Japanese encephalitis vaccine poses an unknown but theoretical risk to the developing fetus, and the vaccine should not be administered routinely during pregnancy. Pregnant women who must travel to an area where risk of JE is high should be vaccinated when the theoretical risks of immunization are outweighed by the risk of infection to the mother and developing fetus.

No evidence exists to indicate that tetanus and diphtheria toxoids administered during pregnancy are teratogenic. Pregnant women who are unvaccinated, especially those whose child may be

Figure 18.4. *Vaccination During Pregnancy*

	Vaccine	Indications for vaccination during pregnancy
Live virus vaccine		
Measles	Live-attenuated	Contraindicated.
Mumps		
Rubella		
Yellow fever	Live-attenuated	Contraindicated except if exposure to yellow fever virus is unavoidable.
Poliomyelitis	Trivalent live-attenuated (OPV)	Persons at substantial risk of exposure to polio.
Inactivated virus vaccines		
Hepatitis B	Recombinant produced, purified hepatitis B surface antigen	Pregnancy is not a contraindication.
Influenza	Inactivated type A and type B virus vaccines	Usually recommended only for patients with serious underlying disease. Consult health authorities for current recommendations.
Japanese Encephalitis	Killed virus	Should reflect actual risks of disease and probable benefits of vaccine.
Poliomyelitis	Killed virus (IPV)	OPV preferred when immediate protection of pregnant females is needed; however, IPV is alternative if complete vaccination series can be administered before exposure.
Rabies	Killed virus Rabies IG	Substantial risk of exposure.
Live bacterial vaccines		
Typhoid (Ty21a)	Live bacterial	Should reflect actual risks of disease and probable benefits of vaccine.
Inactivated bacterial vaccines		
Cholera	Killed bacterial	Should reflect actual risks of disease and probable benefits of vaccine.
Typhoid		
Plague	Killed bacterial	Selective vaccination of exposed persons.
Meningococcal	Polysaccharide	Only in unusual outbreak situations.
Pneumococcal	Polysaccharide	Only for high-risk persons.
Haemophilus b conjugate	Polysaccharide-protein	Only for high-risk persons.
Toxoids		
Tetanus-diphtheria (Td)	Combined tetanus-diphtheria toxoids, adult formulation	Lack of primary series, or no booster within past 10 years.
Immune globulins, pooled or hyperimmune	Immune globulin or specific globulin preparations	Exposure or anticipated unavoidable exposure to measles, hepatitis A, hepatitis B, rabies, or tetanus.

born under unhygienic conditions (i.e., without sterile technique), should receive two doses of Td 4-8 weeks apart before delivery. Pregnant women in similar circumstances who are only partially vaccinated against tetanus should complete the 3-dose primary series. Depending on when the woman seeks prenatal care and the required interval between doses, one or two doses of Td can be administered before delivery. Previously immunized pregnant women who have not received a Td vaccination within the last 10 years should receive a booster dose.

There is no convincing evidence of risk from vaccinating pregnant women with other inactivated virus or bacteria vaccines or toxoids. In addition, there is no known risk to the fetus from passive immunization of pregnant women with immune globulin.

Immunization Schedule Modifications for International Travel for Infants and Inadequately Immunized Young Children <2 years of Age

Routine Childhood Vaccine Preventable Diseases (Measles, Mumps, Rubella, Polio, Diphtheria, Tetanus, Pertussis, Haemophilus influenzae *type b, and Hepatitis B)*

Diphtheria and tetanus toxoid and pertussis vaccine. Diphtheria is an endemic disease in many developing countries. Tetanus is ubiquitous worldwide. Pertussis is common in developing countries and in other countries where routine immunization against pertussis is not practiced widely. Because the risk of contracting pertussis in other countries and of diphtheria in developing countries is higher than in the United States, children who will be leaving the United States should be as well immunized as is possible before departing. Optimum protection against diphtheria, tetanus, and pertussis in the first year of life is achieved with 3 doses of DTP, the first administered at 6-8 weeks of age and the next two at 4-8 week intervals, as is generally the practice in the United States. A fourth dose of DTP 6-12 months after the third dose or diphtheria and tetanus toxoids and acellular pertussis vaccine (DTaP), at 15 months, maintains protection. Infants traveling to areas where diphtheria and/ or pertussis are endemic or epidemic preferably should have received 3 doses; the first dose may be given to infants as young as 4 weeks of age and the next 2 doses at intervals of no less than 4 weeks. Two doses of DTP received at intervals of at least 4 weeks may provide some protection particularly against diphtheria and tetanus, while a single dose is of little protective benefit. Parents who are traveling with young infants should be informed that infants who have not received 3 doses of DTP are at greater risk of contracting pertussis than children who have been adequately vaccinated. Infants and other children less than 7 years of age who at the time of travel have received less than 3 doses of DTP and who will remain for extended periods in areas of increased risk of exposure to pertussis and/or diphtheria should complete their remaining doses at 4-week intervals.

For infants and children traveling internationally or remaining in areas of increased risk of exposure, reducing the interval between the third and fourth doses of the primary series to 6 months may be considered.

Measles vaccine. Measles is an endemic disease in many developing countries and in other countries where measles immunization is not routinely practiced. Because the risk of contracting measles in many countries is far greater than in the United States, children should be as well protected as possible before departing from the United States. Measles vaccine, preferably in combination with rubella and mumps vaccines, i.e., MMR vaccine, should be administered to all children 12-15 months of age and older. A second dose is currently recommended for all children, and is usually given at school entry (Figure 18.1).

The age at vaccination should be lowered for infants traveling to areas where measles is endemic or epidemic. Infants 6-11 months of age who will be traveling to areas where measles is endemic or epidemic should receive a dose of single measles antigen vaccine before departure, although MMR may be used if single antigen measles vaccine is not available. Children vaccinated prior to their first birthday must be revaccinated with two doses of MMR vaccine on or after their first birthday and at least 1 month apart. The optimal age for the first revaccination is 12-15 months. The second revaccination dose should normally be given at school entry. Since virtually all infants less than 6 months of age will be protected by maternally derived antibodies, no additional means to provide protection against measles is generally necessary in this age group.

Mumps and rubella vaccine(s). Because the risk of serious disease from infection with either mumps or rubella in infants is so

413

small, mumps or rubella vaccine generally should not be administered to children below the age of 12 months, unless measles vaccine is indicated and single antigen measles vaccine is not available. However, parents of children less than 12 months of age should be immune to mumps and rubella so they will not become infected if their infants develop illness.

Polio vaccine. Trivalent oral polio vaccine (OPV) is the vaccine of choice for all infants and children if there are no contraindications to vaccination (see Chapter 19). Inactivated polio vaccine (IPV) also is available.

When time permits, children traveling to polio-endemic areas should receive at least 3 doses of OPV at intervals of at least 6 weeks. Children who have received 3 prior doses of OPV should receive a fourth dose if at least 6-8 weeks have elapsed since the third dose. In the United States, the Advisory Committee on Immunization Practices (ACIP) recommends that a primary series of 3 doses of oral poliovirus vaccine (OPV) be given at 2, 4, and 6 months of age. The OPV series may start as early as 6 weeks of age and at intervals of at least 6 weeks. However, in polio endemic areas, the "Expanded Programme on Immunization" of the World Health Organization recommends that a dose of OPV be given in the newborn period, e.g., at birth or before 6 weeks of age, with 3 additional doses (the primary series) given subsequently at 6, 10, and 14 weeks of age. While ideally the ACIP recommendations on age and intervals between doses of OPV should be followed, if travel to an endemic country will occur before a child is 6 weeks of age, a dose of OPV should be given prior to travel. A dose of vaccine administered before 6 weeks of age should not be counted as part of the standard 3-dose primary series. If the child remains in an endemic country, the child should receive the first dose of the standard 3-dose primary series no sooner than 4 weeks after the newborn period dose and the remaining 2 doses of the primary series at 4-week intervals. If the child has left the endemic area, the first dose of the primary series should be given 6-8 weeks after the newborn period dose, the second dose 6-8 weeks after the first dose and the third dose of the primary series 6-8 weeks after the second as is now recommended by the ACIP.

Children traveling to an endemic country who have received a first or second dose of the primary series of OPV but lack sufficient time to complete the primary series schedule as generally practiced in the United States should receive their second and/or third doses of

OPV 4 weeks after their prior dose(s). Children with less than a primary series at the time of departure to an endemic area and who remain in an endemic area should complete the 3-dose primary series within the endemic area with doses at 4-week intervals.

No data or recommendations are available for the use of IPV prior to 6 weeks of age. Otherwise, if IPV is indicated, a primary series of IPV consists of 3 doses which can be given at 2, 4, and 15-18 months of age. The interval between doses 1 and 2 should be 6-8 weeks and between doses 2 and 3 at least 6 months.

Haemophilus influenzae type b Conjugate Vaccine.

Haemophilus influenzae type b is an endemic disease worldwide. Risk of acquiring disease may be higher in developing countries than in the United States. In the United States, three types of *Haemophilus influenzae* type b conjugate vaccines (HbCV) are recommended for use in infants beginning at 6 weeks of age, and a fourth is recommended for use as a primary vaccination only in children age 15 months and older. Two of the Hib conjugates vaccines for infants are also available as combined DTP-Hib vaccines. Routine vaccination is recommended beginning at 2 months of age for all U.S. children. The number and timing of remaining doses depend on the type of conjugate vaccine used (see *Haemophilus influenzae* type b section, Chapter 19, for additional details). If vaccination is started at >7 months of age, fewer doses may be required. The same conjugate vaccine should preferably be used for all doses in the primary series. If, however, different vaccines are administered, a total of three doses of Hib conjugate vaccine is adequate. After completion of the primary infant vaccination series, any of the licensed Hib conjugate vaccines may be used for the booster dose at 12-15 months.

Infants and children should have optimal protection prior to travel. If previously unvaccinated, children less than 15 months of age should ideally receive at least 2 vaccine doses prior to travel. An interval as short as 1 month is acceptable.

Children between 15 months and 2 years of age require a single dose of vaccine.

Hepatitis B Vaccine. Since November, 1991, hepatitis B vaccine has been recommended for all infants beginning either at birth or by 2 months of age. Infants and young children who have not previously been vaccinated and who are traveling to areas with highly endemic hepatitis B virus (HBV) infection may be at risk if they are

415

directly exposed to blood from the local population. Circumstances in which HBV transmission could occur include receipt of blood transfusions not screened for HBsAg, exposure to unsterilized needles (or other medical/dental equipment) in local health facilities, or continuous close contact with local children who have open skin lesions (impetigo, scabies, scratched insect bites). Such exposures are most likely to occur if the child is living for long periods in smaller cities or rural areas and in close contact with the local population. Children who will live in an HBV endemic area for six or more months and who are expected to have the above exposures should receive the 3 doses of hepatitis B vaccine. The interval between doses 1 and 2 should be 1-2 months. Between doses 2 and 3 the interval should be a minimum of 2 months however, 4-12 months is preferred. [See Figure 18.1] for the suggested schedule, and [Chapter 19] for vaccine specific doses.

Other Vaccines and Immune Globulin

Cholera vaccine. The risk of cholera to U.S. travelers of any age is so low that it is questionable whether vaccination is of benefit. No data are available concerning the efficacy or side effects of cholera vaccine in children less than 6 months of age. Cholera vaccine is not recommended for children less than 6 months of age. Breast-feeding is protective against cholera; careful preparation of formula and food from safe water and foodstuffs should protect nonbreast-fed infants. If a child less than 6 months of age is to travel to areas requiring cholera immunization, a medical waiver should be obtained before travel. For older infants and children traveling to countries that require vaccination, a single dose of vaccine is sufficient to satisfy country requirements.

Typhoid vaccine. Typhoid vaccination is not required for international travel. No data are available concerning the efficacy of typhoid vaccine in infants. Breast-feeding is likely to be protective against typhoid; careful preparation of formula and food from safe water and foodstuffs should protect nonbreast-fed infants. Typhoid vaccine is recommended for older children traveling to areas where there is a recognized risk of exposure to *Salmonella typhi*.

Yellow fever vaccine. Because immunization of infants against yellow fever is associated with an increased risk of encephalitis, the recommendation for vaccination should be considered on an individual basis. Although the risk has not been clearly defined, 14 of 18 reported cases of post-vaccination encephalitis were in infants under 4 months of age. The ACIP and the World Health Organization recommend that yellow fever vaccine should be administered to children ≥9 months of age if they are traveling to or living in areas of South America and Africa where yellow fever infection is officially reported (see "Summary of Health Information for International Travel", also known as Blue Sheet) or to countries that require yellow fever immunization. Children 9 months of age or older also should be immunized if they travel outside urban areas within the yellow fever endemic zone. Infants 6-9 months of age should be vaccinated only if they travel to areas of ongoing epidemic yellow fever, and a high level of protection against mosquito bites is not possible. Immunization of children 4-6 months of age should be considered only under unusual circumstances (consult CDC), and in no instance should infants under 4 months of age receive yellow fever vaccine. Information on yellow fever risk is also available from the CDC travel hotline, telephone (404) 332-4559.

Immune globulin for Hepatitis A. Infants and children traveling to developing countries are at increased risk of acquiring hepatitis A virus infection, especially if their travel is outside usual tourist routes, if they will be eating food or drinking water in settings of questionable sanitation, or if they will be in contact with local young children in settings of poor sanitation. Although hepatitis A is rarely severe in children under age 5 years, infected children efficiently transmit infection to older children and adults. Immune globulin (IG) should be given to infants and children as prophylaxis in the same schedule as recommended for adults.

Other diseases. See [Chapter 19] for discussion of malaria and diarrhea in infants.

Breast-Feeding

Neither killed nor live vaccines affect the safety of breast-feeding for mothers or infants. Breast-feeding does not adversely affect immunization and is not a contraindication for any vaccine. Breast-fed infants should be vaccinated according to routine recommended schedules.

Inactivated or killed vaccines do not multiply within the body. Therefore they should pose no special risk for mothers who are breast-

417

feeding or for their infants. Although live vaccines do multiply within the mother's body, most have not been demonstrated to be excreted in breast milk. Although rubella vaccine virus may be transmitted in breast milk, the virus usually does not infect the infant, and if it does, the infection is well tolerated. There is no contraindication for vaccinating breast-feeding mothers with yellow fever vaccine. Breast-feeding mothers can receive OPV without any interruption in the feeding schedule.

Adverse Events Following Immunization: Reporting

Modern vaccines are extremely safe and effective. However, adverse events following immunization have been reported with all vaccines. These range from frequent, minor, local reactions to extremely rare, severe, systemic illness such as paralysis associated with OPV. Information on side effects and adverse events following specific vaccines and toxoids are discussed in detail in each ACIP statement. Health care providers are required by law to report selected adverse events occurring after vaccination with DTP, DT, Td, MMR, MR, measles, OPV, and IPV. Events reportable are listed in MMWR 1988;37:197-200 and, in general, are events usually requiring the recipient to seek medical attention. These events, and all temporally associated events following receipt of all other vaccines severe enough to require the recipient to seek medical attention, should be reported to the Vaccine Adverse Event Reporting System (VAERS) (telephone: 1-800-822-7967) maintained by the Centers for Disease Control and Prevention and the Food and Drug Administration.

Communicable Diseases in Disasters

Natural disasters can contribute to the transmission of some diseases; however, unless the causative agent is in the environment, transmission cannot take place. Studies of flood and earthquake disasters have shown that communicable disease outbreaks rarely result. Natural disasters often disrupt water supplies and sewage systems. Epidemic typhoid has been conspicuously absent following natural disasters in developing countries where typhoid is endemic. It takes several weeks for typhoid antibodies to develop and even then immunization provides only moderate protection. Floods pose no additional risk of typhoid.

Of greatest importance in preventing enteric disease transmission when water and sewage systems have been disrupted is to assure that water and food supplies are safe to consume. When contamination is suspected, water should be boiled or appropriately disinfected.

Chapter 19

U.S. Public Health Service Specific Recommendations for Vaccination and Prophylaxis

Acquired Immunodeficiency Syndrome (AIDS)

There is no vaccine available to prevent infection with human immunodeficiency virus (HIV), the virus that causes AIDS. For general information on HIV and AIDS and how to prevent HIV infection, please refer to [the section on AIDS in Chapter 18]; or call (800) 342-AIDS, toll free from the U.S. or its territories. (For Spanish speaking callers, (800) 344-SIDA, or for hearing-impaired callers with teletype equipment (800) AIDS-TTY).

Scientists have reviewed the safety and efficacy of vaccines (such as for measles, yellow fever, influenza, pneumococcal, and other infections) in persons with HIV infection or AIDS. No increased incidence of adverse reactions to inactivated vaccines has been noted in these persons. However, administration of live organism vaccines may carry increased risks of adverse reactions (see especially the sections on polio and yellow fever). The likelihood of successful immune response is reduced in some HIV-infected persons (depending on the degree of immunodeficiency), but the risk of serious adverse effects remains low. On the other hand, because of their immunodeficiency, many HIV-infected persons are at increased risk for complications of vaccine-preventable diseases. Thus, the risk benefit balance usually tips in favor of administration of vaccine to HIV-infected persons. Nonetheless, ad-

---

Taken from HHS Pub. No. (CDC) 94-8280, *Health Information for International Travel, 1994.*

ministration should be backed up by behaviors to prevent infections (e.g., avoid mosquito bites in yellow fever areas; avoid exposure to measles or chickenpox patients).

Please refer to the sections that follow regarding specific information for persons with HIV infection or AIDS. Particular attention should be paid to the section on tuberculosis (TB) because persons with HIV infection are more likely to develop clinical TB if they are exposed and infected with tubercle bacilli. All HIV-infected persons should have a tuberculin skin test as part of their routine medical care and especially prior to and upon return from travel to an area where TB is endemic.

African Sleeping Sickness (African Trypanosomiasis)

African trypanosomiasis is confined to tropical Africa between 15° North and 20° South latitude. It is transmitted by the bite of the tsetse fly, a large gray-brown insect approximately the size of a honeybee, which bites during the day. Chronic trypanosomiasis (caused by the parasite *Trypanosoma brucei gambiense*) may not cause symptoms until months to years following travel to an endemic area, but the incubation period of acute trypanosomiasis (caused by the parasite *Trypanosoma brucei rhodesiense*) ranges from 6 to 28 days, and travelers frequently become ill during their trips or shortly after returning home. Fever, rash or skin lesions, lethargy, and confusion are usually the predominate signs and symptoms.

Although the risk to international travelers is relatively low, persons traveling to game parks and sparsely inhabited areas should take precautions. Tsetse flies appear to be attracted to moving vehicles and dark, contrasting colors. The flies are capable of biting through lighter weight clothing. Areas of heavy infestation tend to be sporadically distributed and are usually well known to local inhabitants. Avoidance of such areas is the best means of prevention. Travelers at risk should use "deet" containing insect repellents liberally and wear clothing of wrist and ankle length that blends with the background environment and is constructed of heavy, e.g., canvas weight, fabric (see "Protection Against Mosquitoes and Other Arthropod Vectors, in Chapter 15).

422

Amebiasis

Amebiasis, which is caused by the protozoan parasite *Entamoeba histolytica*, occurs worldwide, especially in regions with poor sanitation. Infection is acquired by the fecal-oral route either by person-to-person contact or indirectly by eating or drinking fecally contaminated food or water. Travelers to developing countries are advised to follow the precautions included under "Risks From Food and Drink" [in Chapter 15].

The clinical spectrum of intestinal amebiasis ranges from asymptomatic infection to fulminant colitis. Most infected persons do not have symptoms. In infected persons who are symptomatic, the most common symptom is diarrhea. The diarrhea may evolve to painful, bloody bowel movements, with or without fever (amebic dysentery). Occasionally, amebiasis causes disease outside the intestines, most notably in the liver. Most patients with amebic liver abscesses develop fever and abdominal pain within 25 months of becoming infected with the parasite. For recommendations about treating amebiasis, refer to The Medical Letter (Drugs for Parasitic Infections. 1992;34:17-26).

American Trypanosomiasis (Chagas' Disease)

Chagas' disease occurs throughout much of the Western hemisphere from Mexico to Argentina. The disease is caused by the protozoan parasite, *T. cruzi*. Acute infection may be asymptomatic or accompanied by a febrile illness with meningoencephalitis and/or myocarditis. Manifestations of chronic infection include cardiomyopathy and intestinal "mega" syndromes, e.g., megaesophagus and megacolon. Chagas' disease is usually transmitted by contact with feces of an infected reduviid ("cone nose" or "kissing") bug; transmission may also occur through blood transfusion or via transplacental infection. Reduviid bugs typically infest buildings constructed of mud, adobe brick, or palm thatch, particularly those with cracks or crevices in the walls and roof. Avoidance of overnight stays in dwellings infested by the reduviid bug vector reduces the risk of acquiring the infection. Alternate preventive measures include insecticide spraying of infested houses and the use of bed netting. The latter is recommended if camping or sleeping out-of-doors in highly endemic areas. In some regions, travelers should be aware that blood for transfusion may not be routinely tested or treated for trypanosomiasis. While anti-trypanosomal treatment exists for acute disease, currently there is no accepted anti-parasitic treatment for chronic infection. Persons with chronic cardiac or mega-syndromes may, however, benefit from symptomatic therapy.

Cholera

Cholera is an acute intestinal infection caused by *Vibrio cholerae* O-group 1 or O-group 139. The infection is often mild and self-limited or subclinical. Persons with severe cases respond dramatically to simple fluid- and electrolyte-replacement therapy. Infection is acquired primarily by ingesting contaminated water or food; person-to-person transmission is rare.

Currently no country or territory requires vaccination as a condition for entry. Local authorities, however, may continue to require documentation of vaccination against cholera; in such cases, a single dose of vaccine is sufficient to satisfy local requirements. The risk of cholera to U. S. travelers is so low that it is questionable whether vaccination is of benefit. Persons following the usual tourist itinerary who use standard accommodations in countries reporting cholera are at virtually no risk of infection. Travelers to cholera-infected areas are advised to avoid eating uncooked food, especially fish and shellfish, and to peel fruits themselves. Carbonated bottled water and carbonated soft drinks are usually safe.

Currently available vaccines have been shown to provide only about 50 percent effectiveness in reducing clinical illness from *Vibrio cholerae* O1 infection for 3-6 months after vaccination, with the greatest protection for the first 2 months. Illness caused by the recently discovered *Vibrio cholerae* O-group 139 is probably unaffected by currently available vaccines.

For persons vaccinated in the United States for travel to countries where local authorities may still request documentation of cholera vaccination, a single dose of vaccine is sufficient to satisfy local requirements. The complete primary series is suggested only for special high-risk groups that work and live in highly endemic areas under less than adequate sanitary conditions. The primary series need never be repeated for the booster doses to be effective. Figure 19.1 summarizes the recommended doses for primary and booster vaccinations. Cholera vaccine is not recommended for infants under 6 months of age. [A discussion of cholera immunization for infants who will be

424

traveling is included in Chapter 18. For information about the timing of the administration of Yellow Fever and Cholera vaccines, see the Yellow Fever section later in this chapter.]

| Doses | Intradermal route* | Subcutaneous or intramuscular route | | | Comments |
	5 years of age and over	6 months-4 years of age	5-10 years of age	>10 years of age	
Primary series: 1 & 2	0.2 ml	0.2 ml	0.3 ml	0.5 ml	Give 1 week to 1 month or more apart
Booster	0.2 ml	0.2 ml	0.3 ml	0.5 ml	1 dose every 6 months

*Higher levels of protection (antibody) may be achieved in children less than 5 years of age by the subcutaneous or intramuscular routes.

Figure 19.1. Cholera Vaccine

Precautions and Contraindications

Reactions. Vaccination often results in 1-2 days of pain, erythema, and induration at the site of injection. The local reaction may be accompanied by fever, malaise, and headache. Serious reactions to vaccination are extremely rare. If a person has experienced a serious reaction to the vaccine, revaccination is not advisable.

Pregnancy. Specific information is not available on the safety of cholera vaccine during pregnancy. Therefore, it is prudent on theoretical grounds to avoid vaccinating pregnant women.

Dengue Fever

Dengue fever/dengue hemorrhagic fever is a viral disease transmitted by urban *Aedes* mosquitoes, usually *Aedes aegypti*. There are four dengue viruses which are immunologically related, but which do not provide cross-protective immunity.

Dengue fever is characterized by sudden onset, high fever, severe frontal headache, joint and muscle pain. Many patients have nausea, vomiting, and rash. The rash appears 3 to 5 days after onset of fever and may spread from torso to arms, legs, and face. The disease is usually benign and self-limited, although convalescence may be prolonged. Many cases of subclinical or nonspecific infection occur, but dengue may also present as a severe and fatal hemorrhagic disease called dengue hemorrhagic fever (DHF). There is no specific treatment for dengue infection and no vaccines are available.

Dengue fever is a rapidly expanding disease in most tropical areas of the world. In the past 20 years, it has become the most important arbovirus disease of humans. There are now over 2 billion persons at risk of infection and millions of cases occur each year. Epidemics caused by all four virus serotypes have become progressively more frequent and larger. Since 1982, major epidemics have occurred for the first time in over 30 years in Brazil, Costa Rica, Venezuela, Bolivia, Paraguay, Peru, and Ecuador in the Americas; Kenya, Somalia, Djibouti, Mozambique, Angola, and Burkina Faso in Africa; and China and Taiwan in Asia. In 1994, dengue viruses are endemic in most tropical countries of the South Pacific, Asia, the Caribbean Basin, Mexico, Central and South America, and Africa (see map). It is not possible to accurately predict future dengue incidence, but it is anticipated that there will be increased dengue transmission in all tropical areas of the world during the next several years.

The incidence of the severe disease, DHF, has increased dramatically in Southeast Asia in the past 20 years, with major epidemics occurring in most countries every 3 to 4 years. Dengue hemorrhagic fever first occurred in the Americas in 1981, with a major epidemic in Cuba. A second major epidemic of DHF occurred in Venezuela in 1989-90. DHF has also been confirmed as sporadic cases in many countries of the region including Mexico, El Salvador, Honduras, Nicaragua, Colombia, Brazil, Suriname, French Guiana, Curacao, Aruba, St. Lucia, Puerto Rico, and the Dominican Republic. Although not completely understood, current data suggest that virus strain, together with age, immune status, and genetic background of the human host are the most important risk factors for developing DHF. In Asia, children under the age of 15 years who are experiencing a second dengue infection appear to have the highest risk. Although adults can also develop DHF, this suggests that most international travelers from nonendemic areas such as the United States are at low risk for severe dengue infection.

The principal vector mosquito, *Aedes aegypti*, prefers to feed on humans during the daytime and most frequently is found in or near human habitations. There are two peaks of biting activity, in the

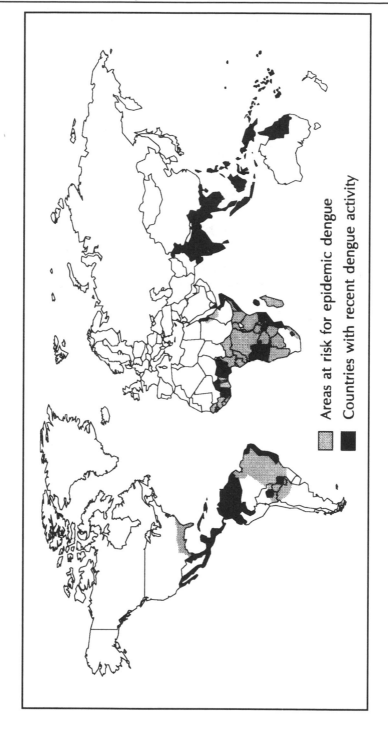

Figure 19.2. World Distribution of Dengue—1994

Areas at risk for epidemic dengue

Countries with recent dengue activity

morning for several hours after daybreak and in the late afternoon for several hours before dark. The mosquito may feed at any time during the day, however, especially indoors, in shady areas, or when it is overcast. Larval habitats include artificial water containers such as discarded tires, barrels, buckets, flower vases/pots, cans, and cisterns.

The risk of dengue infection for the international traveler appears to be small, unless an epidemic is in progress. However, cases of dengue are confirmed every year in travelers returning to the U.S. from visits to endemic areas. Travelers to endemic and epidemic areas, therefore, should take precautions to avoid mosquito bites. Travelers can reduce their risk of acquiring dengue by remaining in well-screened areas when possible, by wearing clothing that adequately covers the arms and legs, and by applying mosquito repellent. The most effective repellents are those containing N,N diethylmethylbenzamide (DEET) at a concentration equal to or greater than 20 percent. High concentration (>30% DEET) products for the skin, particularly in children, should be avoided.

Travelers should advise their physician of any acute febrile illness occurring within 3 weeks after returning from an endemic area. Physicians should notify the state health department of any suspected or confirmed case of dengue.

Diphtheria, Tetanus, and Pertussis

Diphtheria remains a serious disease throughout much of the world. Most cases occur in unimmunized or inadequately immunized persons.

Tetanus is a global health problem. The disease occurs almost exclusively in persons who are unimmunized or inadequately immunized or whose history is unknown. In developing countries most reported illness occurs in infants and young children.

Pertussis primarily occurs in children and is common in countries where immunization is not generally provided. It is highly communicable, often associated with complications, and has a relatively high case-fatality ratio in infants.

Immunizations for Persons Less Than 7 Years of Age

Simultaneous immunization against diphtheria, tetanus, and pertussis during infancy is recommended. Because the incidence and severity of pertussis decreases with age and because the vaccine may cause side effects and adverse reactions, pertussis vaccination is not recommended for children after their seventh birthday or for adults.

Primary immunization for children up to the seventh birthday consists of four doses of DTP vaccine (Official name: Diphtheria and Tetanus Toxoids and Pertussis Vaccine Adsorbed), the first three doses given at 4-to 8-week intervals and the fourth dose given 6 to 12 months after the third dose, (generally at 15 months of age) to maintain adequate immunity during the preschool years. Ideally, immunization should begin at 6 weeks-two months of age. Once the primary series is started, interrupting the recommended schedule or delaying subsequent doses does not require restarting a series. A booster dose is recommended between 4 and 6 years of age. The booster dose is not necessary if the fourth dose in the primary series was given after the fourth birthday. Children inadequately immunized for their age should be brought up-to-date prior to travel. For children less than 7 years of age with a contraindication to the pertussis component of DTP, DT should be used. [See Chapter 18 for a discussion of the DTP immunization schedule modifications for infants who will be traveling.]

In December 1991, the Food and Drug Administration approved a new vaccine for use, diphtheria and tetanus toxoids and acellular pertussis vaccine (DTaP). This vaccine is licensed *only* for use as the fourth and fifth doses for children who have previously been vaccinated against diphtheria, tetanus, and pertussis with three doses of whole-cell diphtheria and tetanus toxoids and pertussis vaccine (DTP) and is not licensed for the initial three-dose series in infants and children; whole-cell DTP should continue to be used for these initial doses. Because it causes less fever and fewer local reactions and other common systemic symptoms, DTaP is preferred for the fourth and fifth vaccine doses; however, whole-cell DTP continues to be an acceptable alternative for these doses. DTaP is not licensed for use in children <15 months of age or after the seventh birthday. The fourth dose should be given at least 6 months after the third dose of whole-cell DTP and is usually administered to children 15-18 months of age. A dose of DTaP may be given as the fifth dose in the series for children aged 4-6 years who have received either all four prior doses as whole-cell vaccine or three doses of whole-cell DTP plus one dose of DTaP; this fifth dose should be given before the child enters kindergarten or elementary school. The fifth dose in the vaccination series is not necessary if the fourth dose was given on or after the fourth birthday.

Immunizations for Persons 7 Years of Age and Older

For primary immunization, persons 7 years of age or older should receive three doses of the formulation of tetanus-diphtheria toxoid for adult use (Td) (Official name: Tetanus and Diphtheria Toxoids Adsorbed for Adult Use). The first two doses are given 4 to 8 weeks apart and the third dose 6 to 12 months after the second. Once the primary series is started, interrupting the regular schedule or delaying subsequent doses does not require restarting a series. Two doses of Td received at intervals of at least 4 weeks may provide some protection, while a single dose is of little benefit.

A Td booster should be given whenever 10 or more years have elapsed since completion of a primary series or the last booster dose. ACIP recommendations [MMWR 1991;40 (No.RR-10)] on tetanus and diphtheria prevention should be consulted for further details.

Adverse Reactions

Local reactions (generally erythema and induration with or without tenderness) are common after the administration of vaccines containing diphtheria, tetanus, and pertussis antigens. Mild systemic reactions such as fever, drowsiness, fretfulness, and anorexia occur frequently. Moderate-to-severe systemic events, including high fever (i.e., temperature of 40.5°C [105°F] or higher); persistent, or inconsolable crying lasting 3 or more hours; collapse (hypotonic-hyporesponsive episode); or short-lived convulsions (usually febrile) occur infrequently. These events appear to be without sequelae. Rarely, severe neurologic events, such as a prolonged convulsion or encephalopathy, have occurred after receiving DTP. However, a causal relation between receipt of DTP vaccine and permanent brain damage has not been demonstrated. The receipt of DTP is not causally related to sudden infant death syndrome (SIDS).

Rarely, anaphylactic reactions have been reported after receiving a preparation containing diphtheria, tetanus and/or pertussis. Arthus-type hypersensitivity reactions, characterized by severe local reactions, may follow receipt of tetanus toxoid, particularly in adults who have received frequent (e.g., annual) boosters of tetanus toxoid.

The rates of local reactions, fever, and other common systemic symptoms following receipt of DTaP are lower than those following whole-cell DTP vaccination.

Precautions and Contraindications

Neurologic conditions characterized by changing developmental findings are considered contraindications to receipt of pertussis vaccine. Such disorders include uncontrolled epilepsy, infantile spasms, and progressive encephalopathy. Children who because of perinatal complications or other phenomena are felt to be at an increased risk of latent onset of central nervous system disorders should have immunization with DTP or DT [Official name: Diphtheria and Tetanus Toxoids Adsorbed (for pediatric use)] (but not OPV) delayed until further observation and study have clarified the child's neurologic status. The decision whether to commence immunization with DTP or with DT should be made no later than the child's first birthday. Infants and children with stable neurologic conditions such as cerebral palsy and developmental delay or even well-controlled seizures may be vaccinated. The occurrence of a single seizure (not temporally associated with DTP) does not contraindicate DTP vaccination, particularly if the seizures can be satisfactorily explained. Parents of infants and children with personal or family histories of convulsion should be informed of the increased risk of simple febrile seizures following immunization. Acetaminophen, 15 mg/kg, every 4 hours for 24 hours, should be given to children with such histories to reduce the possibility of postvaccination fever. Infants and children who have received one or more doses of DTP and who experience a neurologic disorder (e.g., a seizure) not temporally associated with the vaccination, but before the next scheduled dose, should have their neurologic status evaluated and clarified before a subsequent dose of DTP is given, or the decision made to use DT instead.

When an infant or child returns for the next dose of DTP, the parent should always be questioned about any adverse events that might have occurred following the previous dose. Further vaccination with DTP is contraindicated if an anaphylactic reaction immediately followed a DTP dose, or if an encephalopathy not due to another identifiable cause occurred within 7 days of receipt of DTP. If any of the following events occur in temporal relation to receipt of DTP, the decision to give subsequent doses of vaccine containing the pertussis component should be carefully considered. Although these events were considered absolute contraindications in previous ACIP recommendations, there may be circumstances, such as a high incidence of pertussis, in which the potential benefits outweigh possible risks, particularly because these events are not associated with permanent sequelae. The following events were previously considered contraindications and are now considered precautions:

1. Temperature of 40.5°C (105°F) or greater within 48 hours not due to another identifiable cause.

2. Collapse or shock-like state (hypotonic-hyporesponsive episode) within 48 hours.

3. Persistent, inconsolable crying lasting 3 or more hours, occurring within 48 hours.

4. Convulsions with or without fever occurring within 3 days.

If the decision is to discontinue further vaccination with DTP, DT should be substituted for any remaining scheduled doses of DTP.

The only contraindication to tetanus and diphtheria toxoids is a history of a neurologic or severe hypersensitivity reaction following a previous dose. There is no evidence that tetanus and diphtheria toxoids are teratogenic.

Encephalitis, Japanese

Japanese encephalitis (JE) is a mosquito-borne viral encephalitis that occurs chiefly in the summer and autumn in the temperate regions and the northern tropical zones of Bangladesh, China, India, Japan, Kampuchea, Korea, Laos, Myanmar, Nepal, Thailand, Viet Nam, and eastern areas of Russia. In other endemic, chiefly tropical, areas seasonal patterns of disease activity are associated principally with the rainy season. These areas include the tropical zones of south India, Indonesia, Malaysia, Philippines, Singapore, Sri Lanka, Taiwan, and south Thailand.

Most infections are asymptomatic, but among patients who develop a clinical illness, the case-fatality rate may be as high as 30%. Serious sequelae of central nervous system infection are reported in 30% of survivors. In endemic areas, children are at greatest risk of infection, however, multiple factors such as occupation, recreational exposure, gender (possibly reflecting exposure), previous vaccination, and naturally acquired immunity, alter the potential for infection and illness. A higher case-fatality rate is reported in the elderly, but serious sequelae are more frequent in the very young, possibly because they are more likely to survive a severe infection.

JE virus is transmitted chiefly by the bites of mosquitoes in the *Culex vishnui* complex: the individual vector species in specific geographic areas differ. In China and many endemic areas in Asia, *Culex tritaeniorhyncus* is the principal vector. This species feeds outdoors beginning at dusk and during evening hours, and has a wide host range including domestic animals, birds, and man. Larvae are found in flooded rice fields, marshes, and small stable collections of water around cultivated fields. The vectors are present in greatest numbers from June through September throughout their distribution and are inactive in temperate zones during winter months. Swine and certain species of wild birds function as viremic reservoir hosts in the transmission cycle. Habitats supporting the transmission cycle of JE virus are principally in rural, agricultural regions. In many areas of Asia, however, the appropriate ecological conditions for virus transmission occur near or occasionally within urban centers.

The risk to short-term travelers and persons who confine their travel to urban centers is low. Persons at greatest risk are those living for prolonged periods of time in rural areas where JE is endemic or epidemic. In temperate areas such as China, the risk of transmission during the winter months is negligible. In subtropical and tropical areas, transmission may occur at a low level throughout the year but risk is greatest during the rainy season and early dry season when mosquito populations are highest. Travel in rural areas where rice culture and pig farming are common increases the risk of contracting JE. In these areas, travelers are advised to stay in screened or air-conditioned rooms, to use insecticidal space sprays as necessary, and mosquito repellents and protective clothing to avoid mosquito bites.

Vaccination

JE vaccine licensed in the United States is manufactured by Biken, Osaka, Japan and distributed by Connaught Laboratories, Inc. (use of names is for identification only and does not imply endorsement by the Public Health Service or the U.S. Department of Health and Human Services). Other JE vaccines are made by several companies in Asia, but are not licensed in the U.S. Vaccination should only be considered for persons who plan to live in areas where JE is endemic or epidemic and for travelers whose activities include trips into rural, farming areas. Short-term travelers (less than 30 days), especially those whose visits are restricted to major urban areas are at a lower risk for acquiring JE and, generally, should not receive the vaccine. Individual consideration of travelers' risk should include an evaluation of their itinerary and activities and information on the current level of JE activity in the country.

The recommended primary immunization series is three doses of 1.0 ml each, administered subcutaneously on days 0, 7, and 30. An abbreviated schedule of days 0, 7, and 14 can be used when the longer schedule is impractical because of time constraints. Two doses given a week apart may be used in unusual circumstance, but will confer short-term immunity in only 80% of vaccinees. The last dose should be administered at least 10 days before the commencement of travel to ensure an adequate immune response and access to medical care in the event of delayed adverse reactions. Immunization route and schedules for children 1 to 3 years of age is identical except that doses of 0.5 ml should be administered. No data are available on vaccine efficacy and safety in children less than 1 year of age. The full duration of protection is unknown, however, preliminary data indicate that neutralizing antibodies persist for at least 3 years after primary immunization. In children whose primary immunization series included 0.5 ml dosing, a booster dose of 1.0 ml may be administered 2 years after the primary series.

Adverse Reactions

JE vaccine is associated with local reactions and mild systemic side effects (fever, headache, myalgias, malaise) in about 20% of vaccinees. More serious allergic reactions including generalized urticaria, angioedema, respiratory distress, and anaphylaxis have occurred within minutes to as long as two weeks after immunization. Reactions have been responsive to therapy with epinephrine, antihistamines and/or steroids. Vaccinees should be observed for 30 minutes after immunization and warned about the possibility of delayed allergic reactions. The full course of immunization should be completed 10 or more days before departure and vaccinees should be advised to remain in areas with access to medical care. Persons with a past history of urticaria appear to have a greater risk for developing more serious allergic reactions and this must be considered when weighing the risks and benefits of the vaccine. A history of allergy to JE or other mouse-derived vaccines is a contraindication to further immunization.

Contraindications

Persons with known hypersensitivity to the vaccine should not be vaccinated. Persons with multiple allergies, especially a history of allergic urticaria or angioedema, are at higher risk for allergic complications from JE vaccinations.

Vaccination during pregnancy should be avoided unless the risk of Japanese encephalitis outweighs the theoretical risk of vaccination.

Encephalitis, Tickborne

Tickborne encephalitis (TBE) is a viral infection of the central nervous system. It occurs in Russia and other countries that comprised the former Soviet Union and Europe chiefly from April through August when *Ixodes ricinus*, the principal tick vector is active. The incidence of TBE is highest in Austria, the Czech Republic, Slovakia, Germany, Hungary, Poland, Switzerland, Russia, Ukraine, Belarus, and northern Yugoslavia. The disease occurs at a lower frequency in Bulgaria, Romania, Denmark, France, the Aland Islands and neighboring Finnish coastline, and along the coastline of southern Sweden, from Uppsala to Karlshamn. Serologic evidence for TBE infection or sporadic cases have been reported in Albania, Greece, Italy, Norway, and Turkey. A closely related disease, Russian spring-summer encephalitis, transmitted by *Ix. persulcatus* ticks, occurs in China, Korea and eastern areas of Russia. The severity of disease, incidence of sequelae, and case-fatality rates are higher in the far east and eastern regions of Russia and lower in western and central Europe.

Human infections follow bites of infected *Ix. ricinus* ticks, usually in persons who visit or work in forested areas. Infection also may be acquired by consuming unpasteurized dairy products from infected cows, goats, or sheep. The risk to travelers who do not visit forested areas or consume unpasteurized dairy products is low. Travelers should be advised to avoid tick infested endemic areas and to protect themselves from tick bites by dressing appropriately and using repellents. The repellent N,N diethylmethylbenzamide (deet) can be applied either to clothing or directly on the skin. Compounds containing permethrin have an acaricidal and repellent effect and are used chiefly to treat clothing. Consumption of unpasteurized dairy products should be avoided. Effective killed vaccines are commercially available in Europe from Immuno, Vienna, Austria, and Behring, Germany. Vaccination has been temporally-associated with Guillain Barré syndrome in several cases. The vaccine is recommended only for travelers with a high risk of exposure.

Giardiasis

Giardiasis occurs worldwide. Transmission occurs after ingestion of fecally contaminated water or food, from exposure to fecally contaminated environmental surfaces, and from person-to-person by the fecal-oral route. Symptoms include diarrhea, abdominal cramps, fatigue, weight loss, flatulence, anorexia, or nausea, in various combinations, and usually lasting for more than 5 days. Fever and vomiting are uncommon. There is no known chemoprophylaxis. To prevent infection, travelers to disease-endemic areas should follow the precautions included [in Chapter 15].

Haemophilus Influenzae Type b Meningitis and Invasive Disease

Haemophilus influenzae causes meningitis and other severe bacterial illnesses (e.g., pneumonia, septic arthritis, epiglottitis and sepsis), primarily among children less than 5 years of age. Severe disease is most common in children 6 months to 1 year of age, but approximately 20-35 percent of severe disease occurs in children 18 months of age or older. It was the most common cause of bacterial meningitis in the United States before use of Haemophilus b conjugate vaccines (HbCV) dramatically reduced incidence of this disease. The risk of exposure to persons with the organism and the disease while traveling outside the United States is at least as high as that within the United States.

Three different HbCV are licensed for use in children—Haemophilus b conjugate vaccine (Diphtheria CRM_{197} Protein Conjugate) (HbOC), Haemophilus b conjugate vaccine (Meningococcal Protein Conjugate) (PRP-OMP), and Haemophilus b conjugate vaccine (Diphtheria Toxoid Conjugate) (PRP-D). Two of these vaccines, HbOC and PRP-OMP, were licensed for infant use in 1990. All children should be immunized beginning at 2 months of age with one of these two vaccines as outlined in Figure 19.3. Since no data exist regarding the interchangeability of different vaccines, the same conjugate vaccine should be used throughout the entire vaccination series. PRP-D is recommended only for children 15 months of age and older. Children who have had invasive *H. influenzae* type b disease when they were less than 24 months of age should still receive HbCV following the above recommendations, since most fail to mount an immune response to the clinical disease. In contrast, children 24 months of age or older who have reliably diagnosed invasive disease do not need vaccination.

Vaccine	2 months	4 months	6 months	12–15 months
HbOC/PRP-T**	dose 1	dose 2	dose 3	booster
PRP-OMP	dose 1	dose 2		booster
PRP-D*	—	—	—	—

*PRP-D is recommended only for children ≥15 months of age.
**Two combination DTP-Hib vaccines are currently available.

Figure 19.3. *Recommended* Haemophilus influenzae *type b (Hib) routine vaccination schedule*

Side Effects and Adverse Reactions

HbCV is considered relatively free of side effects. Redness and/or swelling following receipt of the current HbCV occurs in less than 2 percent of recipients. About 1 out of every 100 recipients will have a fever of 101.3° F or higher. These reactions begin within 24 hours and generally subside rapidly. Severe hypersensitivity reactions have been rare.

Precautions and Contraindications

Recurrent upper respiratory diseases, including otitis media and sinusitis, are not considered indications for vaccination. HbOC or PRP-D vaccines should not be considered as an immunizing agent against diphtheria. PRP-OMP should not be considered as an immunizing agent against meningococcal disease.

Hepatitis, Viral, Type A

Hepatitis A is an enterically transmitted viral disease which is highly endemic throughout the developing world but of low endemicity in developed countries such as the United States. In developing countries, hepatitis A virus (HAV) is usually acquired during childhood, most frequently as an asymptomatic or mild infection. Transmission may occur by direct person-to-person contact; or from contaminated water, ice or shellfish harvested from sewage-contaminated water; or from fruits, vegetables or other foods which are eaten uncooked, but which may become contaminated during handling. HAV is inactivated by boiling or cooking to 85°C (1 minute); cooked foods cannot serve as vehicles for disease unless contaminated after cooking. Adequate chlorination of water as recommended in the United States will inactivate HAV.

The risk of acquiring HAV infection for U.S. citizens traveling abroad varies with living conditions, length of stay, and incidence of hepatitis A in the area visited. Travelers to North America except Mexico and developed countries in Europe, Japan, Australia, and New Zealand are at no greater risk of infection than in the United States. For travelers to developing countries, risk of infection increases with duration of travel, and will be highest in those who live in or visit rural areas, trek in back country areas, or frequently eat or drink in settings of poor sanitation. Nevertheless, a recent study has shown that many cases of travel-related hepatitis A occur in travelers with "standard" tourist itineraries, accommodations and food consumption behaviors.

In developing countries, travelers should minimize their risk of hepatitis A and other enteric diseases by avoiding potentially contaminated water or food. Drinking water (and beverages with ice) of unknown purity, uncooked shellfish, and uncooked fruits or vegetables which are not peeled or prepared by the traveler should be avoided.

Immune globulin (IG) (formerly called immune serum globulin and gamma globulin) prophylaxis is recommended for travelers to developing countries, especially those who will be living in or visiting rural areas, eating or drinking in settings of poor or uncertain sanitation, or who will have close contact with local persons, particularly young children, in settings with poor sanitation. Persons who plan to reside in developing countries should receive IG regularly.

For travelers, a single dose of IG of 0.02 ml/kg is recommended if travel is for less than 3 months. For prolonged travel or residence in developing countries, 0.06 ml/kg should be given every 5 months (for approximate dosages see Figure 19.4). For persons who require repeated IG prophylaxis, screening for total antibodies to HAV (antiHAV) before travel may be useful to define susceptibility and eliminate unnecessary doses of IG in those who are immune. [See

Chapter 18 for a discussion of the IG immunization schedule for infants who will be traveling.]

Inactivated hepatitis A virus vaccines have been developed and shown to be effective in preventing hepatitis A. Detailed recommendations regarding use of the hepatitis A vaccine will follow its licensure, and it is likely that such recommendations will include persons at risk of infection due to travel.

Length of stay	Body weight		Dose volume*	Comments
	lb	kg**		
Short-term travel (<3 mos)	<50	<23	0.5 ml	Dose volume depends on body weight and length of stay
	50-100	23-45	1.0 ml	
	>100	>45	2.0 ml	
Long-term travel (>3 mos)	<22	<10	0.5 ml	
	<50	<23	1.0 ml	
	50-100	23-45	2.5 ml	
	>100	>45	5.0 ml	

*For intramuscular injection.
**kg = approximately 2.2 lbs.

Figure 19.4. Immune Globulin for Protection Against Viral Hepatitis A

Safety

Immune globulin prepared in the United States has few side effects (primarily soreness at the injection site) and has never been shown to transmit infectious agents (hepatitis B virus [HBV], hepatitis C virus [HCV] or human immunodeficiency virus [HIV]). Recent specific laboratory studies have additionally shown that immune globulins prepared by the Cohn-Oncley procedure (the standard procedure used in U.S.-manufactured preparations) carry no risk of transmission of HIV. Pregnancy is not a contraindication to using immune globulin.

Hepatitis, Viral, Type B

The risk of hepatitis B virus (HBV) infection for international travelers is generally low, except for certain travelers in countries with high HBV endemicity. Factors to consider when assessing risk include: 1) the prevalence of HBV carriers in the local population, 2) the extent of direct contact with blood, or secretions, or of intimate sexual contact with potentially infected persons, and 3) the duration of travel.

The prevalence of HBV carriers is high (8% or more) in all socio-economic groups in certain areas (see map): all of Africa, Southeast Asia including China, Korea, Indonesia, and the Philippines; the Middle East except Israel; South and Western Pacific Islands, interior Amazon Basin, and certain parts of the Caribbean, i.e., Haiti and the Dominican Republic. It is moderate (2%-7%) in South Central and Southwest Asia, Israel, Japan, Eastern and Southern Europe and Russia, and most of Middle and South America. In Northern and Western Europe, North America, Australia and New Zealand, HBV carrier prevalence is low (1% or less) in the general population.

HBV is primarily transmitted through activities which result in exchange of blood or blood-derived fluids; and through sexual activity, either heterosexual or homosexual, between an infected and a susceptible person. Principle activities which may result in blood exposure include work in health care fields, i.e., medical, dental, laboratory which entail direct exposure to human blood; receipt of blood transfusions which have not been screened for HBV; and having dental, medical, or other exposure to needles (e.g., acupuncture, tattooing, or injecting drug use) which have not been appropriately sterilized. In addition, in less developed areas, open skin lesions in children or adults due to factors such as impetigo, scabies, and scratched insect bites, may play a role in disease transmission if direct exposure to wound exudates occurs.

Hepatitis B vaccination is currently recommended for all persons who work in health care fields (medical, dental, laboratory or other) which entail exposure to human blood. Previously unvaccinated persons who will work in health care fields for any duration in high or moderate HBV endemicity areas are strongly advised to receive hepatitis B vaccine prior to such travel. Hepatitis B vaccination should also be considered for persons who plan to reside for 6 months or more in areas with moderate to high levels of endemic HBV transmission and who will have any of the previously discussed types of contact with the local population. In particular, persons who anticipate sexual contact with the local population, who will live in rural areas and/or have daily physical contact with local populations; and persons who are likely to seek medical, dental or other treatment in local facilities during their stay should receive the vaccine. Vaccination should be considered for short-term travelers (<6 months) who will have direct contact with blood, or sexual contact with residents of areas with moderate to high levels of endemic HBV transmission.

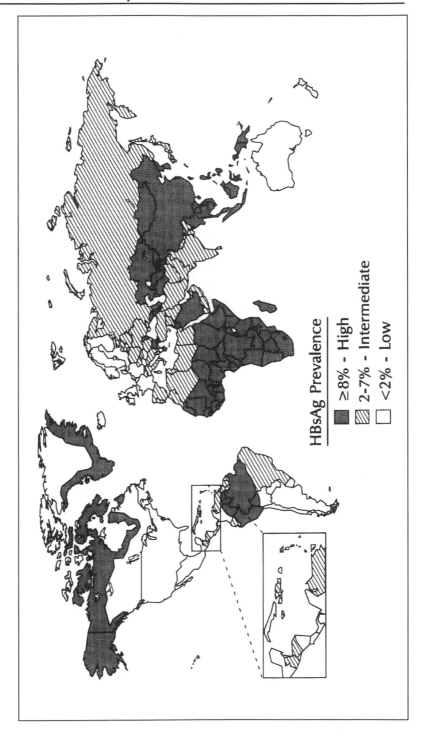

Figure 19.5. Geographic Distribution of Hepatitis B Prevalence

Two types of hepatitis B vaccines have been licensed in the United States. One, which was manufactured from plasma of HBV carriers is no longer produced in the United States. The currently available vaccines are produced through recombinant DNA technology by common bakers yeast into which the gene for hepatitis B surface antigen (HBsAg) has been inserted.

Primary vaccination consists of three intramuscular doses of vaccine. The recommended dose varies by product and the recipient's age (Figure 19.6). When the vaccine is administered as a 3-dose series, the second dose should be given 1 month after the first dose, and the third dose 6 months after the first dose. Alternatively, the vaccine produced by one manufacturer is licensed to be administered as a 4-dose schedule at 0, 1, 2, and 12 months. Vaccination should ideally begin at least 6 months before travel in order to complete the full vaccine series prior to departure. Since some protection is provided by one or two doses, the vaccine series should be initiated, if indicated, even if it cannot be completed prior to departure. However, optimal protection is not conferred until after the final (3rd or 4th) vaccine dose. There is no evidence of interference between hepatitis B vaccine and other simultaneously administered vaccine(s) or with immunoglobulin.

Group	Recombivax HB[*]		Engerix-B[*]	
	Dose (µg)	(mL)	Dose (µg)	(mL)
Infants of HBsAg-negative mothers and children <11 years	2.5	(0.5)[†]	10	(0.5)
Infants of HBsAg-positive mothers; prevention of perinatal infection	5	(0.5)[§]	10	(0.5)
Children and adolescents 11-19 years	5	(0.5)[§]	20	(1.0)
Adults ≥20 years	10	(1.0)[§]	20	(1.0)
Dialysis patients and other immuno-compromised persons	40	(1.0)[¶]	40	(2.0)**

[*]Both vaccines are routinely administered in a three-dose series. Engerix-B also has been licensed for a four-dose series administered at 0, 1, 2, and 12 months.
[†]New pediatric formulation.
[§]Previously licensed formulation; may be used to deliver the appropriate age-specific dosage to infants of HBsAg-negative mothers and children <11 years.
[¶]Special formulation.
**Two 1.0-mL doses given at one site, in a four-dose schedule at 0, 1, 2, 6 months.

Figure 19.6. Recommended doses of currently licensed hepatitis B vaccines

The optimum site of injection in adults is the deltoid muscle; vaccination in the buttocks results in poorer antibody response. Long term studies of healthy adults and children indicate that immunologic memory remains intact for at least 10 years and confers protection against chronic HBV infection, even though hepatitis B surface antibody (anti-HBs) levels may become low or decline below detectable levels. For children and adults whose immune status is normal, booster doses of vaccine are not recommended, nor is serologic testing to assess antibody levels necessary. [See Chapter 18 for a discussion of the hepatitis B immunization schedule for infants who will be traveling.]

Safety

Hepatitis B vaccines have been shown to be safe when administered to both adults and children. Over 4 million adults have been vaccinated in the United States, and at least that many children have received hepatitis B vaccine worldwide. The major side-effects observed with hepatitis B vaccines have been soreness and redness at the site of injection. In the United States, surveillance of adverse reactions has shown a possible association between Guillain Barré syndrome (GBS) and receipt of the first dose of plasma-derived hepatitis B vaccine. Available data from reporting systems for adverse events do not indicate an association between receipt of recombinant vaccine and GBS.

Pregnancy

On the basis of limited experience, there is no apparent risk of adverse events to developing fetuses when hepatitis B vaccine is administered to pregnant women. The vaccine contains only non-infectious HBsAg particles, and should cause no risk to the fetus. In contrast, HBV infection in a pregnant woman may result in serious disease for the mother and chronic infection for the newborn. Therefore, neither pregnancy or lactation should be considered a contraindication to the use of this vaccine for persons at risk.

Hepatitis E (Enterically Transmitted Non-A, Non-B Hepatitis, Epidemic Non-A, Non-B; Fecal-Oral Non-A, Non-B)

In recent years, epidemic and endemic transmission of hepatitis E virus (HEV) spread by water or close personal contact has been reported from several areas of Asia (Afghanistan, Bangladesh, China, Central Asian Republics of the former Soviet Union, Indonesia, Malaysia, Mongolia, Myanmar, Pakistan, and India), North Africa, and from rural areas of central Mexico. Such epidemics generally affect adults and cause an unusually high mortality in pregnant women. HEV has been transmitted to experimental animals and the virus has been cloned and sequenced. Several experimental assays to detect antibody to HEV (anti-HEV) have been developed; however, none are yet available for commercial use. Several imported cases of hepatitis E have been identified in American travelers, but hepatitis E has not been recognized as an endemic disease in the United States or Western Europe and it is not known whether HEV is present in these areas.

Travelers to areas where hepatitis E occurs (see above) may be at some risk of acquiring this disease by close contact with cases or through contaminated food or water. Immune globulin (IG) prepared from plasma collected in non-HEV endemic areas has not been effective in preventing clinical disease during hepatitis E outbreaks. The efficacy of IG prepared from plasma collected in HEV endemic areas is unclear. Travelers to these areas should receive IG for protection against hepatitis A, but they should not assume that they are protected against hepatitis E. The best prevention of infection is to avoid potentially contaminated food and water, as with hepatitis A and other enteric infections.

Lassa Fever

Lassa fever is a severe, often fatal, hemorrhagic fever that occurs in rural areas of West Africa, and is caused by a virus transmitted from asymptomatically infected rodents to man. The risk of infection in international travelers is considered small. Treatment with the antiviral drug ribavirin may be life-saving. The Special Pathogens Branch, DVRD, NCID, CDC is the only national laboratory responsible for research and diagnosis on highly lethal hemorrhagic fever viruses, such as Lassa virus. These viruses do not exist naturally in the United States and there are no vaccines currently available.

Leishmaniasis

Leishmaniasis is a parasitic disease acquired in tropical and subtropical areas of the world. Persons become infected through the bite of some species of sand flies. In the Western Hemisphere, the infection usually is acquired in rural areas; but in the Eastern Hemisphere, infection may be acquired in some urban areas as well. The disease most commonly manifests either in a cutaneous (skin) form or in a visceral (internal organ) form. Cutaneous leishmaniasis is characterized by one or more skin sores (either open or closed) that develop weeks to months after a person is bitten by infected sand flies. The manifestations of visceral leishmaniasis, such as fever, enlargement of the spleen and liver, and anemia, typically develop months, but sometimes years after a person becomes infected.

Vaccines and drugs for preventing infection are not currently available. Preventive measures for the individual traveler are aimed at reducing contact with sand flies. Outdoor activities should be avoided when sand flies are most active (dusk to dawn). Although sand flies are primarily night-time biters, infection may be acquired during the daytime if resting sand flies are disturbed. Sand fly activity in an area may easily be underestimated because sand flies are noiseless fliers, and rare bites may go unnoticed.

Protective clothing and insect repellent should be used for supplementary protection. Clothing should cover as much of the body as possible and tolerable in the climate. Repellent with DEET (N,N-diethylmethylbenzamide) (DEET) should be applied to exposed skin and under the edges of clothing, such as under the ends of sleeves and pant legs. It should be applied according to the manufacturer's instructions; repeated applications may be necessary under conditions of excessive perspiration, wiping, and washing. Although impregnation of clothing with permethrin may provide additional protection, it does not eliminate the need for repellent on exposed skin and should be repeated after every five washings.

Contact with sand flies can be reduced by mechanical means, such as bed nets and screening of doors and windows. Fine-mesh netting (at least 18 holes to the linear inch; some sources say even finer) is required for an effective barrier against sand flies, which are about one-third the size of mosquitoes. However, such closely woven bed nets may be difficult to tolerate in hot climates. Impregnating bed nets and window screens with permethrin aerosol may provide some protection, as may spraying dwelling with insecticides.

445

Malaria

Malaria in humans is caused by one of four protozoan species of the genus *Plasmodium*: *P. falciparum, P. vivax, P. ovale,* and *P. malariae.* All are transmitted by the bite of an infected female *Anopheles* mosquito. Occasionally transmission occurs by blood transfusion or congenitally from mother to fetus. The disease is characterized by fever and flu-like symptoms, including chills, headache, myalgias, and malaise; these symptoms may occur at intervals. Malaria may be associated with anemia and jaundice, and *P. falciparum* infections may cause kidney failure, coma, and death. Deaths due to malaria are preventable.

Information on malaria risk in specific countries is derived from various sources, including the World Health Organization. While this is the most accurate information available at the time of publication, factors that may vary from year to year, such as local weather conditions, mosquito vector density, and prevalence of infection, can have a marked effect on local malaria transmission patterns.

Checklist for Travelers to Malarious Areas

The following is a checklist of key issues to be considered in advising travelers.

Risk of malaria. Travelers should be informed about the risk of malaria infection and the presence of drug-resistant *P. falciparum* malaria in their areas of destination.

Anti-mosquito measures. Travelers should know how to protect themselves against mosquito bites.

Chemoprophylaxis. Travelers should be:

- Advised to start prophylaxis before travel, and to use prophylaxis continuously while in malaria-endemic areas, and for four weeks after leaving such areas.

- Questioned about drug allergies and other contraindications for use of drugs to prevent malaria.

- Advised which drug to use for prophylaxis, and, if chloroquine is used, whether Fansidar® should be carried for presumptive self-treatment. (Use of names for identification only and does not imply endorsement by the Public Health Service or the U.S. Department of Health and Human Services.)

- Informed that antimalarial drugs can cause side effects; if these side effects are serious, medical help should be sought promptly and use of the drug discontinued.

- Warned that they may acquire malaria even if they use malaria chemoprophylaxis.

In case of illness. Travelers should be:

- Informed that symptoms of malaria may be mild, and that they should suspect malaria if they experience unexplained fever or other symptoms such as persistent headaches, muscular aching and weakness, vomiting, or diarrhea.

- Informed that malaria may be fatal if treatment is delayed. Medical help should be sought promptly if malaria is suspected, and a blood sample should be taken and examined for malaria parasites on one or more occasions.

- Reminded that self-treatment should be taken only if prompt medical care is not available and that medical advice should still be sought as soon as possible after self-treatment.

Special categories. Pregnant women and young children require special attention because they cannot use some drugs (mefloquine and doxycycline).

(Adapted from International Travel and Health, World Health Organization, Geneva, 1991)

Risk of Acquiring Malaria

Malaria transmission occurs in large areas of Central and South America, Hispaniola, sub-Saharan Africa, the Indian subcontinent, Southeast Asia, the Middle East, and Oceania. The estimated risk of a traveler acquiring malaria varies markedly from area to area. This variability is a function of the intensity of transmission within the various regions and of the itinerary and time and type of travel. From 1980-1992, 2,548 cases of *P. falciparum* among U.S. civilians were reported to the CDC. Of these, 2,096 (82%) were acquired in sub-Saharan Africa; 191 (8%) were acquired in Asia; 129 (5%) were acquired in the Caribbean and South America; and 132 (5%) were acquired in other parts of the world. During this time period there were 45 fatal malaria infections among U.S. civilians; 44 (98%) were caused by *P. falciparum,*—of which 36 (82%) were acquired in sub-Saharan Africa.

Thus, most imported *P. falciparum* malaria among American travelers was acquired in Africa south of the Sahara, even though only 130,000 arrivals from the United States were reported by countries in that region in 1991. In contrast, 20 million arrivals from the United States were reported that year in other countries with malaria (including 15 million travelers to Mexico, (World Tourism Organization). This disparity in the risk of acquiring malaria reflects the fact that travelers to Africa tend to spend considerable time, including evening and nighttime hours, in rural areas where malaria risk is highest. Travelers to Asia and South America, however, spend most of their time in urban or resort areas where there is limited, if any, risk of exposure and travel to rural areas mainly during daytime hours when the risk of infection is limited.

Estimating the risk of infection for different categories of travelers is difficult and may be significantly different even for persons who travel or reside temporarily in the same general areas within a country. For example, tourists staying in air conditioned hotels may be at lower risk than backpackers or adventure travelers. Similarly, longer-term residents living in screened and air-conditioned housing are less likely to be exposed than are missionaries or Peace Corps volunteers.

Drug Resistance

Resistance of *P. falciparum* to chloroquine has been confirmed or is probable in all countries with *P. falciparum* malaria except the Dominican Republic, Haiti, Central America west of the Panama Canal, Egypt, and most countries in the Middle East. In addition, resistance to both chloroquine and Fansidar® is widespread in Thailand, Myanmar (formerly Burma), Cambodia, and the Amazon basin area of South America, and resistance has also been reported in sub-Saharan

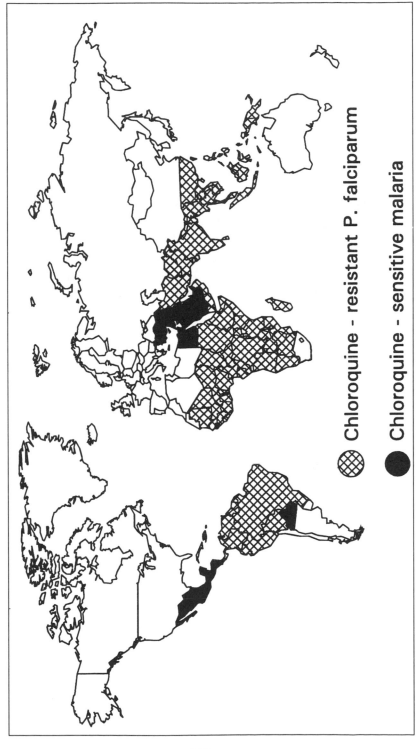

Figure 19.7. Distribution of Malaria and Chloroquine-resistant Plasmodium falciparum, *1994*

Chloroquine - resistant P. falciparum

Chloroquine - sensitive malaria

Africa. Resistance to mefloquine has been confirmed in those areas of Thailand with malaria transmission.

General Advice for Travelers to Malaria-Endemic Areas

All travelers to malarious areas of the world are advised to use an appropriate drug regimen and personal protection measures to prevent malaria; however, travelers should be informed that regardless of methods employed, malaria still may be contracted. Malaria symptoms can develop as early as 8 days after initial exposure in a malaria-endemic area and as late as several months after departure from a malarious area, after chemoprophylaxis has been terminated. Travelers should understand that malaria can be treated effectively early in the course of the disease, but that delay of appropriate therapy can have serious or even fatal consequences. Individuals who have symptoms of malaria should seek prompt medical evaluation, including thick and thin blood smears, *as soon as possible.*

Personal Protection Measures

Because of the nocturnal feeding habits of *Anopheles* mosquitoes, malaria transmission occurs primarily between dusk and dawn. Travelers should take protective measures to reduce contact with mosquitoes especially during these hours. Such measures include remaining in well-screened areas, using mosquito nets, and wearing clothes that cover most of the body. Additionally, travelers should be advised to purchase insect repellent before travel for use on exposed skin. The most effective repellents contain N,N diethylmethyltoluamide (DEET), an ingredient in many commercially available insect repellents. The actual concentration of DEET varies among repellents and can be as high as 95%. Repellents with DEET concentrations between 30% and 35% are quite effective and the effect should last for about 4 hours. Rarely, children exposed to DEET have had toxic encephalopathy. The possibility of adverse reactions to DEET will be minimized if the following precautions are taken: apply repellent sparingly and only to exposed skin or clothing; avoid applying high-concentration products to the skin; do not inhale or ingest repellents or get them in the eyes; avoid applying repellents to portions of children's hands that are likely to have contact with eyes or mouth; never use repellents on wounds or irritated skin; wash repellent-treated skin after coming indoors. If a reaction to insect repellent is suspected, wash treated skin and seek medical attention.

Travelers should use a pyrethroid-containing flying-insect spray in living and sleeping areas during evening and nighttime hours. In addition, persons who will not be staying in rooms which are well-screened or air-conditioned should take additional precaution, which include sleeping under mosquito netting, i.e., bednets. Permethrin (Permanone®) may be sprayed on clothing and bednets for additional protection against mosquitoes. Bednets are more effective if they are treated with permethrin or deltamethrin insecticides. In the United States permethrin spray can be used, while overseas permethrin or deltamethrin liquid may be purchased for the treatment of bednets.

Drug	Adult dose	Pediatric dose
Mefloquine (Lariam®)	228 mg base (250 mg salt) orally, once/week	15-19 kg: 1/4 tab/wk 20-30 kg: 1/2 tab/wk 31-45 kg: 3/4 tab/wk >45 kg: 1 tab/wk
Doxycycline	100 mg orally, once/day	>8 years of age: 2 mg/kg of body weight orally/day up to adult dose of 100 mg/day
Chloroquine phosphate (Aralen®)	300 mg base (500 mg salt) orally, once/week	5 mg/kg base (8.3 mg/kg salt) orally, once/week, up to maximum adult dose of 300 mg base
Hydroxychloroquine sulfate (Plaquenil®)	310 mg base (400 mg salt) orally, once/week	5 mg/kg base (6.5 mg/kg salt) orally, once/week, up to maximum adult dose
Proguanil	200 mg orally, once/day in combination with weekly chloroquine	<2 years: 50 mg/day 2-6 years: 100 mg/day 7-10 years: 150 mg/day >10 years: 200 mg/day
Primaquine	15 mg base (26.3 mg salt) orally, once/day for 14 days	0.3 mg/kg base (0.5 mg/kg salt) orally once/day for 14 days

Figure 19.8. Drugs Used in the Prophylaxis of Malaria

Drug	Adult dose	Pediatric dose weight (kg): tablet(s)
Pyrimethamine-sulfadoxine (Fansidar®)	3 tablets (75 mg pyrimethamine and 1,500 mg sulfadoxine), orally as a single dose	5-10: 1/2 11-20: 1 21-30: 1 1/2 31-45: 2 >45: 3

Figure 19.9. Drug Used in the Presumptive Treatment of Malaria

Chemoprophylaxis

In choosing an appropriate chemoprophylactic regimen before travel, persons should consider several factors. The travel itinerary should be reviewed in detail and compared with the information on areas of risk within a given country to determine whether the traveler will actually be at risk of acquiring malaria. Whether the traveler will be at risk of acquiring drug-resistant *P. falciparum* malaria should also be determined. In addition, it should be established whether the traveler has previously experienced an allergic or other reaction to the antimalarial drug of choice and whether medical care will be readily accessible during travel.

Malaria chemoprophylaxis should preferably begin 1-2 weeks before travel to malarious areas (except for doxycycline, which can begin 1-2 days before). This allows any potential side effects to be evaluated and treated by the traveler's physician before departure. Chemoprophylaxis should continue during travel in the malarious areas and for 4 weeks after leaving the malarious areas.

Chemoprophylactic Regimens [to be used in conjunction with up-to-date, country-specific information available from the U.S. Department of Public of Health and Human Services, Public Health Service].

- *Regimen A:* For travel to areas of risk where chloroquine-resistant *P. falciparum* has NOT been reported, once-weekly use of chloroquine *alone* is recommended. Chloroquine is usually well tolerated. The few people who experience uncomfortable side effects may tolerate the drug better by taking it with meals, or in divided, twice-weekly doses. As an alternative, the related compound hydroxychloroquine may be better tolerated. Chloroquine prophylaxis should begin 1-2 weeks before travel to malarious areas. It should be continued weekly during travel in malarious areas and for 4 weeks after a person leaves such areas. (See Figure 19.8 for recommended dosages.)

- *Regimen B:* For travel to areas of risk where chloroquine-resistant *P. falciparum* exists, use of mefloquine *alone* is recommended. Mefloquine is usually well tolerated but precautions should be observed as described in the section on adverse reactions. Mefloquine prophylaxis should begin 1-2 weeks before travel to malarious areas. It should be continued weekly during travel in malarious areas and for 4 weeks after a person leaves such areas. Mefloquine can be used for long-term prophylaxis. (See Figure 19.8 for recommended dosages.) Note: In some foreign countries a fixed combination of mefloquine and Fansidar® is marketed under the name Fansimef®. Fansimef® should not be confused with mefloquine, and it is not recommended for prophylaxis of malaria because of the severe adverse reactions associated with prophylactic use of Fansidar®.

Alternatives to Mefloquine. Persons who travel to areas where drug-resistant *P. falciparum* is endemic and for whom mefloquine is not recommended may elect to use an alternative regimen, as follows:

- Doxycycline *alone* taken daily is an alternative regimen for travelers who cannot tolerate mefloquine or for whom the drug is not recommended. Doxycycline is as effective as mefloquine for travel to most malarious areas. However, it is also the only available effective prophylactic drug for prophylaxis for travelers to malaria endemic areas of Thailand. Travelers who use doxycycline should be cautioned about the possible side effects as described in the section on adverse reactions. Doxycycline prophylaxis should begin 1-2 days before travel to malarious areas. It should be continued daily during travel in malarious areas and for 4 weeks after the traveler leaves such areas. (See Figure 19.8 for recommended dosages.)

- Chloroquine *alone* taken weekly is only recommended for those travelers to areas with drug-resistant *P. falciparum* who cannot use mefloquine or doxycycline, for example pregnant women and children less than 15 kg. Limited data suggest that the combination of chloroquine with daily proguanil (Paludrine®) is more effective than chloroquine alone in Africa, but not in Thailand and Papua New Guinea. Therefore, travelers to Africa who use chloroquine for prophylaxis should, if possible, also take 200 mg daily (adult) of proguanil. Proguanil is not available commercially in the United States but can be obtained in Canada, Europe and many African countries.

453

Self-treatment. Travelers who elect to use chloroquine either alone or with daily proguanil (except those with histories of sulfonamide intolerance) should be given a treatment dose of Fansidar® to be carried during travel. These travelers should take the Fansidar® promptly if they have a febrile illness during their travel *and if professional medical care is not readily available within 24 hours*; however, they should be aware that this self-treatment of a possible malarial infection is only a temporary measure and that prompt medical evaluation is imperative. They should continue their weekly chloroquine prophylaxis after presumptive treatment with Fansidar®. (See Figure 19.8 for recommended dosages for prophylaxis and Figure 19.9 for presumptive treatment with Fansidar.)

Mefloquine should not be used for self-treatment because of the frequency of serious side effects (e.g., hallucinations, convulsions) that have been associated with the high dosages of mefloquine used for treatment of malaria.

Halofantrine (Halfan) is an antimalarial drug which is licensed in the United States but is not commercially available, although the drug is available in many other countries. Halofantrine is not recommended for self-treatment of malaria because of potentially serious electrocardiogram changes which have been documented following treatment doses of halofantrine; these changes may be accentuated in the presence of other antimalarial drugs that can decrease myocardial conduction (for example mefloquine).

Primaquine: Prevention of Relapses of *P. vivax* and *P. ovale*. *P. vivax* and *P. ovale* parasites can persist in the liver and cause relapses for as long as 4 years after routine chemoprophylaxis is discontinued. Travelers to malarious areas should be alerted to this risk and if they develop malaria symptoms after leaving a malarious area, they should report their travel history and the possibility of malaria to a physician as soon as possible. Primaquine decreases the risk of relapses by acting against the liver stages of *P. vivax* and *P. ovale*. Primaquine is administered after the traveler has left a malaria-endemic area, usually during the last 2 weeks of prophylaxis.

Since most malarious areas of the world (except Haiti) have at least one species of relapsing malaria, travelers to these areas have some risk of acquiring either *P. vivax* or *P. ovale*. Prophylaxis with primaquine is generally indicated only for persons who have had prolonged exposure in malaria-endemic areas, e.g., missionaries and

Peace Corps Volunteers. Although the actual risk to travelers with less intense exposure is difficult to define, most people can tolerate the standard regimen of primaquine, with the exception of individuals deficient in glucose-6-phosphate dehydrogenase (G6PD) (see discussion of adverse reactions). (See Figure 19.8 for recommended dosages.)

Adverse Reactions and Contraindications to Antimalarials. The frequent or serious side effects of recommended antimalarials are discussed below. In addition, physicians should review the prescribing information in standard pharmaceutical reference texts and in the manufacturers' package inserts.

Chloroquine and **hydroxychloroquine** rarely cause serious adverse reactions when taken at prophylactic doses for malaria. Minor side effects that may occur include gastrointestinal disturbance, headache, dizziness, blurred vision, and pruritus, but generally these effects do not require that the drug be discontinued. High doses of chloroquine, such as those used to treat rheumatoid arthritis, have been associated with retinopathy, but this serious side effect has not been associated with routine weekly malaria prophylaxis. Chloroquine and related compounds have been reported to exacerbate psoriasis. Chloroquine may interfere with the antibody response to human diploid cell rabies vaccine when the vaccine is administered intradermally.

Mefloquine has rarely been associated with serious adverse reactions (e.g., psychoses, convulsions) at prophylactic dosage, but these reactions are more frequent with the higher dosages used in treatment. Minor side effects observed with prophylactic doses, such as gastrointestinal disturbance, insomnia, and dizziness, tend to be transient and self-limited.

Mefloquine is *contraindicated* for use by travelers with a known hypersensitivity to mefloquine and is not recommended for use by, children <15 kg. (30 lbs.), pregnant women, and travelers with a history of epilepsy or psychiatric disorder. A review of the data suggest that mefloquine may be used in persons concurrently on beta blockers, if they have no underlying arrhythmia. However, mefloquine is not recommended for persons with cardiac conduction abnormalities until additional data is available. It has not been established that mefloquine is contraindicated for travelers involved in tasks requiring fine coordination and spatial discrimination, such as airline pilots.

All studies to date confirm that mefloquine is well tolerated when used for prophylaxis; however, monitoring the occurrence of severe adverse reactions is important because such reactions are possible. Users of mefloquine prophylaxis who experience serious adverse reactions should consult their physician, and the reactions should be reported to the Malaria Section, CDC, telephone (404) 488-7760.

Doxycycline may cause photosensitivity, usually manifested as an exaggerated sunburn reaction. The risk of such a reaction can be minimized by avoiding prolonged, direct exposure to the sun; using sunscreens that absorb long-wave ultraviolet (UVA) radiation; and taking the drug in the evening. In addition, doxycycline use is associated with an increased frequency of monilial vaginitis. Gastrointestinal side effects (nausea or vomiting) may be minimized by taking the drug with a meal. Doxycycline is contraindicated in pregnancy and in children less than 8 years of age.

Fansidar® is contraindicated in persons with a history of sulfonamide intolerance and in infants less than 2 months of age.

Proguanil rarely causes serious adverse reactions at prophylactic dosage. Reported side effects include nausea, vomiting, mouth ulcers, and hair loss.

Primaquine may cause severe hemolysis in G6PD-deficient individuals. Before primaquine is used, G6PD deficiency should be ruled out by appropriate laboratory testing.

Chemoprophylaxis for Children. Children of any age can contract malaria. Consequently, the indications for prophylaxis are identical to those described for adults. Mefloquine is not indicated for children <15 kg. (30 lbs.). Doxycycline is contraindicated in children <8 years of age. (See recommended dosages in Figure 19.8.) Children who cannot take mefloquine or doxycycline can be given chloroquine (with proguanil for travel to sub-Saharan Africa) for prophylaxis. Young children should avoid travel to areas with chloroquine-resistant *P. falciparum*, unless they can take a highly effective drug, such as mefloquine or doxycycline.

Chloroquine phosphate is manufactured in the United States in tablet form only and has a very bitter taste. Pediatric doses should be calculated carefully according to body weight. Pharmacists can pulverize tablets and prepare gelatin capsules with calculated pediatric doses. Mixing the powder in food or drink may facilitate the weekly administration of chloroquine to children. Alternatively, chloroquine in suspension is widely available overseas. Parents should calculate the dose and volume to be administered based on body weight, because the concentration of chloroquine base varies in different suspensions.

OVERDOSE OF ANTIMALARIAL DRUGS CAN BE FATAL. THE MEDICATION SHOULD BE STORED IN CHILDPROOF CONTAINERS OUT OF THE REACH OF CHILDREN.

Prophylaxis During Pregnancy. Malaria infection in pregnant women may be more severe than in nonpregnant women. In addition, malaria may increase the risk of adverse pregnancy outcomes including prematurity, abortion, and stillbirth. For these reasons, and because chloroquine has not been found to have any harmful effects on the fetus when used in the recommended doses for malaria prophylaxis, pregnancy is not a contraindication for malaria prophylaxis with chloroquine or hydroxychloroquine. However, because no chemoprophylactic regimen is completely effective in areas with drug-resistant *P. falciparum*, women who are pregnant or likely to become so should avoid travel to such areas.

Mefloquine is not recommended for use during pregnancy according to the current FDA licensure agreement. A review of mefloquine use in pregnancy, from clinical trials or reports of inadvertent use of mefloquine during pregnancy, does not suggest that its use is associated with adverse fetal outcomes. Consequently, mefloquine can be considered by health care providers for prophylaxis in women in their second or third trimester of pregnancy where exposure to chloroquine-resistant *P. falciparum* is unavoidable. Until more data is available, women of childbearing potential who are taking mefloquine for malaria prophylaxis should take reliable contraceptive precautions for the duration of prophylaxis and for 2 months after the last dose of mefloquine. Women exposed to mefloquine during the first trimester of pregnancy or their health care providers are asked to report the exposure to the Malaria Section, CDC, telephone (404) 488-7760, for inclusion in a registry to assess pregnancy outcomes.

Doxycycline is contraindicated for malaria prophylaxis during pregnancy. Adverse effects of tetracyclines on the fetus include discoloration and dysplasia of the teeth and inhibition of bone growth. During pregnancy, tetracyclines are indicated only to treat life-threatening infections due to multidrug-resistant *P. falciparum*.

Proguanil has been widely used for several decades and no adverse effects on pregnancy or fetus have been established.

Primaquine should not be used during pregnancy because the drug may be passed transplacentally to a G6PD-deficient fetus and cause hemolytic anemia *in utero*. Whenever radical cure or terminal prophylaxis with primaquine is indicated during pregnancy, chloroquine should be given once a week until delivery, at which time primaquine may be given.

Prophylaxis While Breast-feeding. Very small amounts of antimalarial drugs are secreted in the breast milk of lactating women. The amount of drug transferred is not thought to be harmful to a nursing infant. Because the quantity of antimalarials transferred in breast milk is insufficient to provide adequate protection against malaria, infants who require chemoprophylaxis should receive the recommended dosages of antimalarials listed in Figure 19.8.

Malaria Hotline

Detailed recommendations for the prevention of malaria are available 24 hours a day by phone or fax by calling the CDC Malaria Hotline at (404) 332-4555.

Measles (Rubeola)

Measles is often a severe disease frequently complicated by middle ear infection or bronchopneumonia. Since vaccine licensure in 1963, measles elimination efforts in the United States have resulted in record low numbers of reported measles cases. Although the number of reported measles cases increased in 1989- 1991, chances remain low that individuals will be exposed to natural measles; unvaccinated persons may reach older ages still susceptible to measles. The risk of exposure to measles outside the United States may be high. As many as 20 percent of all the cases reported in the United States between 1981 and 1991 were internationally imported cases or resulted from an imported case. Many of these were among returning U.S. citizens exposed abroad. Although vaccination against measles is not a requirement for entry into any country, all travelers are strongly urged to be immune to measles. In general, persons can be considered immune to measles if they have documentation of physician-diagnosed measles, laboratory evidence of measles immunity, or proof of receipt of two doses of live measles vaccine on or after the first birthday. Consideration should be given to providing one-dose of measles vaccine to persons born in or after 1957 who travel abroad who have not previously received 2 doses of measles vaccine, and who do not have other evidence of measles immunity, unless there is a contraindication. Most persons born before 1957 are likely to have been infected naturally and generally need not be considered susceptible. However, measles vaccine may be given to older persons if there is reason to believe they may be susceptible.

A single dose of live, attenuated measles vaccine (official name: Measles Virus Vaccine, Live, Attenuated) administered subcutaneously in the volume specified by the manufacturer induces antibody formation in at least 95% of susceptibles vaccinated at 15 months of age or older. A second dose is expected to induce immunity in most vaccinees who do not respond to the first dose. The use of a combined vaccine including rubella and/or mumps vaccine should be considered to insure immunity to these viruses. (See Chapter 18 for a discussion of measles immunization schedule modifications for infants who will be traveling.)

Side Effects and Adverse Reactions

Primary vaccination may be associated with mild fever and transient rash beginning 7-12 days after vaccination and usually lasting several days. About 5%-15% of vaccinees may develop fever of 103°F (39.4°C) or higher. Central nervous system conditions including encephalitis and encephalopathy (less than 1 case for every million doses administered) have been reported. However, the incidence rate of these conditions following measles vaccination is lower than the observed incidence rate of encephalitis of unknown etiology suggesting the reported neurologic disorders may be caused by other factors. These adverse events should be anticipated only in susceptible vaccinees and do not appear to be age-related. After revaccination, reactions should be expected to occur only among the small proportion of persons who failed to respond to the first dose. There is no evidence of a greater risk of reaction to live measles vaccine for those who have previously received live measles vaccine or had natural measles. Although recipients of killed vaccine (available in the United States from 1963-1967) may be more likely to experience local and systemic reactions after revaccination with live measles vaccine, these individuals should be revaccinated to avoid the severe atypical form of disease which often occurs after their exposure to natural measles.

Precautions and Contraindications

Pregnancy. Live measles vaccine when given as a component of MR or MMR should not be given to females known to be pregnant or who might become pregnant within 3 months after vaccination. Women who are given monovalent measles vaccine should not become pregnant for at least 30 days after vaccination. This precaution is based on the theoretical risk of fetal infection.

Febrile Illness. Although vaccination of persons with severe febrile illness should be postponed until recovery, minor illnesses such as upper respiratory infections with or without low grade fever do not preclude vaccination.

Allergies. Live measles vaccine is produced in chick embryo cell culture. Hypersensitivity reactions very rarely follow the administration of live measles vaccine. Most of these reactions are considered minor and consist of wheal and flare or urticaria at the injection site. However, persons with a history of anaphylactic reactions (hives, swelling of the mouth and throat, difficulty breathing, hypotension or shock) subsequent to egg ingestion should be vaccinated only with extreme caution. Protocols have been developed for vaccinating such individuals (J. Pediatr. 1983;102:196-199, J. Pediatr. 1988;113:504-6). Evidence indicates that persons are not at increased risk if they have egg allergies that are not anaphylactic in nature. Such persons should be vaccinated in the usual manner. There is no evidence to indicate that persons with allergies to chickens or feathers are at increased risk of reaction to the vaccine.

Since measles vaccine contains trace amounts of neomycin ($25\mu g$), persons who have experienced anaphylactic reactions to topically or systemically administered neomycin should not receive measles vaccine. Most often, neomycin allergy is manifested as a contact dermatitis which is a delayed-type (cell-mediated) immune response rather than anaphylaxis. In such individuals, the adverse reaction, if any, to $25\mu g$ of neomycin in the vaccine would be an erythematous, pruritic nodule or papule at 48-96 hours. A history of contact dermatitis to neomycin is not a contraindication to receiving measles vaccine.

Simultaneous Administration of Measles Vaccines. Live measles-containing vaccine may be administered simultaneously (but in a different site) with any other live or inactivated vaccine. Inactivated vaccines and oral polio virus vaccine may be administered at any time before or after live measles containing vaccine. However, if live measles vaccine and live yellow fever vaccine are not administered simultaneously they should be separated by an interval of at least 30 days.

Recent Administration of Immune Globulin (IG)* or Other Antibody-Containing Blood Products (*formerly called immune serum globulin and gamma globulin). Vaccination should be administered at least 14 days before the administration of antibody-containing blood products, such as IG. Because passively acquired antibodies might interfere with the response to the vaccine, MMR should be delayed following administration of blood products. The length of the delay varies from 3-11 months depending on the type of blood product received.

Tuberculosis. Tuberculosis may be exacerbated by natural measles infection. There is no evidence, however, that live measles virus vaccine has such an effect. Therefore, tuberculosis skin testing should not be a prerequisite for measles vaccination. If tuberculin skin testing is needed for other reasons, it can be performed the same day the measles vaccine is administered. Otherwise, the test should be postponed for 4-6 weeks because measles vaccination may temporarily suppress tuberculin reactivity.

Altered Immunity. Replication of live measles vaccine virus may be enhanced in patients with immune deficiency diseases and by the suppressed immune responses that occur with leukemia, lymphoma, generalized malignancy, and therapy with corticosteroids, alkylating drugs, antimetabolites and radiation. Patients with such conditions should not be given live measles virus vaccine. However, because of the risk of severe measles in symptomatic HIV-infected persons, and because limited studies of measles, mumps, and rubella (MMR) immunization in symptomatic patients have not documented serious or unusual adverse events, administration of measles vaccine alone or in combination with rubella and mumps vaccine should be considered for all susceptible HIV-infected travelers, regardless of the presence or absence of symptoms.

Meningococcal Disease

Vaccination against meningococcal disease is not a requirement for entry into any country, but it is required for pilgrims to Mecca, Saudi Arabia, for the annual Hajj. Vaccine is indicated for travelers to countries recognized as having epidemic meningococcal disease. In sub-Saharan Africa epidemics of meningococcal disease occur frequently during the dry season (December through June) particularly in the savannah areas extending from Mali eastward to Ethiopia known as the meningitis belt (see Figure 19.10). Recent epidemics have also occurred in Kenya, Tanzania and Burundi. Meningococcal disease in Americans traveling in such areas is rare. However, because of the lack of established surveillance and timely reporting from many of these countries, travelers to the meningitis belt during the dry season should receive meningococcal vaccine, especially if prolonged contact with the local populace is likely. In addition, travelers to Kenya, Tanzania, and Burundi should also receive the vaccine. Advisories for travelers to other countries will be issued when epidemics of meningococcal disease are recognized.

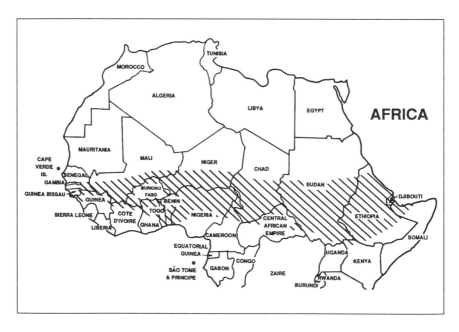

Figure 19.10. Areas with frequent epidemics of meningococcal meningitis

462

Serogroup A is the most common cause of epidemics outside the United States, but serogroup C and serogroup B, can also cause epidemic disease. One formulation of meningococcal polysaccharide vaccine is currently available in the United States—quadrivalent A/C/Y/W-135 vaccine (official name: Meningococcal Polysaccharide Vaccine—Quadrivalent groups A/C/Y/W-135). The vaccine is available, in single and multiple dose vials, and is distributed in the United States by Connaught Laboratories. Production of the bivalent vaccine has been discontinued. No vaccine is yet available to offer protection against serogroup B. Meningococcal vaccines are chemically defined antigens consisting of purified bacterial capsular polysaccharides, each inducing serogroup-specific immunity. Serogroup A vaccine has not been shown to be effective in children less than 3 months of age, and may be less than fully effective in children 3-11 months of age. Serogroup C vaccine has not been shown to be effective in children less than 2 years of age. The group Y and W-135 polysaccharides have been shown to be safe and immunogenic in adults; the response of children to these polysaccharides is unknown.

Figure 19.11 provides information on the use of meningococcal vaccine.

Type of vaccine	Dose	Dose volume[*]	Comments
Quadrivalent A/C/Y/W-135	Primary: 1	As indicated by manufacturer	Duration of immunity is unknown, but appears to be at least 3 years in those 4 years of age or older. Revaccination after 2 or 3 years should be considered for children first vaccinated at less than 4 years of age who continue to be at high risk.

[*]For subcutaneous injection.

Figure 19.11. Meningococcal Vaccine

Precautions and Contraindications

Reactions. Adverse reactions to meningococcal vaccine are infrequent and mild, consisting principally of localized erythema that lasts for 1-2 days. Up to 2% of young children develop fever transiently after vaccination.

463

Pregnancy. The safety of meningococcal vaccines in pregnant women has not been established, although the use of the vaccine in pregnant women during an epidemic in Brazil resulted in no adverse effects. On theoretical grounds, it is prudent not to use them unless there is a substantial risk of infection.

Mumps

Mumps is primarily a disease of school-age children. Vaccination against mumps is not a requirement for entry into any country. Susceptible children, adolescents, and adults should be vaccinated with a single dose of vaccine (official name: Mumps Virus Vaccine, Live) unless vaccination is contraindicated. Combination with measles and rubella vaccines (MMR) is the vaccine of choice. Mumps vaccine can be of particular value for children approaching puberty and for adolescents and adults, particularly males, who have not had mumps. Persons can be considered susceptible unless they have documentation of (1) previous vaccination on or after the first birthday, (2) physician-diagnosed mumps, or (3) laboratory evidence of immunity. Many persons in the United States will receive two doses of mumps vaccine as a result of the new two dose schedule for MMR vaccination which is now recommended in the United States. Most adults born before 1957 are likely to have been infected naturally and generally may be considered immune, even if they did not have clinically recognizable disease. Because there is no evidence that persons who have previously either received the vaccine or had mumps are at any risk of local or systemic reactions from receiving live mumps vaccine, testing for susceptibility before vaccination is unnecessary. (See Chapter 18 for a discussion of mumps immunization schedule modifications for infants who will be traveling.)

Side Effects and Adverse Reactions

Parotitis temporally related to receipt of vaccine has been reported rarely. Allergic reactions including rash, pruritis, and purpura have been associated temporally with mumps vaccination but are uncommon, usually mild and of brief duration. Very rarely, manifestations of CNS involvement, such as febrile seizures, aseptic meningitis, unilateral nerve deafness, and encephalitis within 30 days of mumps vaccination, are reported. Almost all have recovered completely.

Precautions and Contraindications

Pregnancy. Although mumps virus is capable of infecting the placenta and fetus, there is no good evidence that it causes congenital malformations in humans. However, because of a theoretical risk to the developing fetus, mumps vaccine should not be given to pregnant women, and vaccinated women should not become pregnant within 3 months of vaccination.

Febrile Illness. Although vaccination of persons with serious illnesses should be postponed until recovery, minor illnesses such as upper respiratory infections with or without low grade fever do not preclude vaccination.

Allergies. Live mumps vaccine is produced in chick-embryo cell culture. Persons with a history of anaphylactic reactions (hives, swelling of the mouth and throat, difficulty breathing, hypotension, or shock) subsequent to egg ingestion should be vaccinated only with extreme caution. Several investigators have developed special protocols for vaccinating such individuals (J. Pediatr. 1983;102:196-199, J. Pediatr. 1988;113:5046). Evidence indicates that persons are not at increased risk if they have egg allergies that are not anaphylactic in nature. Such persons may be vaccinated in the usual manner. There is no evidence to indicate that persons with allergies to chickens or feathers are at increased risk of reaction to the vaccine.

Since mumps vaccine contains trace amounts of neomycin ($25\mu g$), persons who have experienced anaphylactic reactions to topically or systemically administered neomycin should not receive mumps vaccine. A history of contact dermatitis to neomycin is not a contraindication to receiving mumps vaccine. Live mumps virus vaccine does not contain penicillin.

Simultaneous Administration of Mumps Vaccine. Mumps vaccine may be administered simultaneously (but in a different site) with any other live or inactivated vaccine. Inactivated vaccines and oral polio virus vaccines may be administered at any time before or after the mumps vaccine. However, if the mumps vaccine is not given simultaneously with the yellow fever vaccine, they should be administered at least 30 days apart.

Recent Administration of Immune Globulin (IG*) or Other Antibody-Containing Blood Products (*formerly called immune serum globulin and immunoglobulin). Vaccine should be administered at least 14 days before administration of IG or other blood products because passively acquired antibodies might interfere with the response to the vaccine. Administration of MMR should be delayed following administration of blood products. The length of the delay varies from 3-11 months depending on the type of blood product received. Mumps vaccination using products that do not contain measles vaccine should be deferred for at least 3 months after administration of blood products.

Altered Immunity. Replication of the mumps vaccine virus may be potentiated in patients with immune deficiency diseases and by the suppressed immune responses that occur with leukemia, lymphoma, generalized malignancy, or with therapy with corticosteroids, alkylating drugs, antimetabolites, or radiation. Patients with such conditions should not be given live mumps virus vaccine. However, mumps vaccination generally given as MMR can be considered for susceptible HIV-infected travelers, regardless of symptoms. There is no contraindication to using mumps vaccine, since limited studies of measles, mumps, and rubella (MMR) immunization in symptomatic HIV-infected patients have not documented serious or unusual adverse events.

Onchocerciasis (River blindness)

Onchocerciasis is endemic in over 25 nations in western and central Africa. Endemic foci are also present in the Arabian peninsula, (Yemen and Saudia Arabia) and in Latin America (Southern Mexico, Guatemala, Colombia, Venezuela, Ecuador, Brazil). The disease is caused by the pre-larval (microfilaria) and adult stages of the nematode, *Onchocerca volvulus* and results in debilitating dermatitis, subcutaneous nodules, lymphadenitis, and visual impairment, including blindness. Onchocerciasis is transmitted by the bite of female *Simulium* flies (black flies) that bite by day and are found near freely flowing rivers and streams. Short-term travelers to onchocerciasis-endemic regions, such as most tourists, appear to be at low risk for this condition. However, temporary residents and others who visit endemic regions for 3 months or more and live or work near black fly habitats are at increased risk for infection. Infections tend to occur in expatriate groups such as missionaries and their families, field scientists, and Peace Corps volunteers. Most reported cases have been acquired in Sierra Leone, Liberia, Zaire, and Cameroon. No effective chemoprophylaxis is available. Protective measures include avoidance of black fly habitats and the use of personal protection measures against biting insects such as those outlined in the section on malaria.

Plague

Plague continues to be enzootic in rural rodent populations in several continents with occasional outbreaks among commensal rodents in villages and small towns. Urban outbreaks are rare and limited. Wild rodent plague poses a real, though limited, risk to humans. When domestic or peridomestic rodents become involved in urban or populated areas, humans are at markedly increased risk of exposure. Wild rodent plague exists in the western third of the United States, in widely scattered areas of South America, in northcentral, eastern and southern Africa, Madagascar, Iranian Kurdistan, along the frontier between Yemen and Saudi Arabia, central and southeast Asia (Myanmar, China, Indonesia, Mongolia, Vietnam), and the eastern USSR. In recent years, human plague has been reported from Angola, Kenya, Lesotho, Madagascar, Mozambique, Namibia, South Africa, Botswana, Tanzania, Uganda, Zimbabwe, Zaire, Myanmar, China, Mongolia, Vietnam, United States, USSR, Brazil, Bolivia, Ecuador and Peru. Risk to travelers in any of these areas is small.

The efficacy of plague vaccine in humans has not been demonstrated in a controlled trial. Only limited indirect data are available that suggest the vaccine may offer protection against acquiring plague.

Vaccination against plague is not required by any country as a condition for entry. There are few indications to vaccinate persons other than those who are at particularly high risk of exposure because of research activities or certain field activities in epizootic areas. In most of the countries of Africa, Asia, and Americas where plague is reported, the risk of exposure exists primarily in rural mountainous or upland areas. Vaccination is infrequently indicated for most travelers to countries reporting cases, particularly if their travel is limited to urban areas with modern hotel accommodations.

Selective vaccination might be considered but is not required for persons who will have direct contact with wild or commensal rodents or other animals in plague-epizootic areas, persons who will reside or work in plague-enzootic rural areas where avoidance of rodents and fleas is difficult, and laboratory personnel or veterinarians who work regularly with *Yersinia pestis* organisms or potentially plague-infected animals in enzootic areas. Primary and booster vaccinations are summarized in Figure 19.12. Travelers who genuinely may be at risk for acquiring plague should consider antibiotic chemoprophylaxis with tetracycline 500 mg. q.i.d. during periods of exposure in an active epizootic or epidemic area. The recommendation for tetracycline chemoprophylaxis is inferred from experience with the drug in treating plague. Controlled trials that demonstrate the efficacy of tetracycline chemoprophylaxis in preventing plague have not been reported.

Dose	Dose Volume[*]				Comments
	<1 year of age	1-4 years of age	5-10 years of age	>10 years of age	
Primary series: 1 2 & 3	0.2 ml 0.04 ml	0.4 ml 0.08 ml	0.6 ml 0.12 ml	1.0 ml 0.2 ml	Give doses 1 and 2, 4 weeks apart; give dose 3, 3-6 months after dose 2.
Booster:	0.02-0.04 ml	0.04-0.08 ml	0.06-0.12 ml	0.1-0.1 ml	Give 2 booster doses 6 months apart; thereafter, 1 booster dose at 1-2 year intervals if risk of exposure persists.

[*]For intramuscular injection.

Figure 19.12. Plague Vaccine

Reactions

Mild pain, erythema, and side effects such as induration at the injection site occur frequently. With repeated doses, fever, headache, and malaise are more common and tend to be more severe. Sterile abscesses occur rarely. No fatal or disabling complications have been reported.

468

Poliomyelitis

Travelers to countries where poliomyelitis is epidemic or endemic are considered to be at increased risk of poliomyelitis and should be fully immunized. In general, travelers to developing countries should be considered to be at increased risk of exposure to wild poliovirus. A primary series consists of either three doses of trivalent oral polio vaccine (OPV) (official name: Poliovirus Vaccine, Live, Oral, Trivalent) or enhanced-potency inactivated polio vaccine (IPV) (official name: Poliovirus Vaccine, Inactivated). Unvaccinated or partially vaccinated travelers should complete a primary series with the vaccine that is appropriate to their age and previous immunization status. Persons who have previously received a primary series may need additional doses of a polio vaccine before traveling to areas with an increased risk of exposure to wild poliovirus (see Figures 19.13 and Figure 19.14).

Children and Adolescents

Trivalent oral polio vaccine (OPV) is the vaccine of choice for all infants, children, and adolescents (up to 18th birthday) if there are no contraindications to vaccination with OPV. Those who have not completed a primary series should do so (Figure 19.13). If time is a limiting factor, at least one dose of OPV should be given. Those who have completed a primary series of OPV (or a primary series and a supplementary dose administered between 4 and 6 years of age) should be given, **once**, a single additional dose of OPV. Likewise, those who have completed a primary series of any type IPV (or a primary series and a supplementary dose administered between 4 and 6 years of age) should be given a dose of IPV or OPV. The need for further supplementary doses of OPV or IPV has not been established. (See Chapter 18 for a discussion of polio immunization schedule modifications for infants who will be traveling.)

Doses	Number of Doses	Comments
Primary series	3 (OPV)	Give doses 1, 2, and 3, 6-8 weeks apart, customarily at 2, 4, and 6 months of age. (For adults see text.)
Supplementary	1 (OPV)	Give dose 4 to children 4-6 years of age.
Additional	1 (OPV)	Give a dose, **once**, to persons traveling to developing countries.

Figure 19.13. *Oral Poliovirus Vaccine (OPV)*

469

Adults

Unvaccinated or unknown immunization status. For unvaccinated adults and adults whose immunization status is unknown who are traveling to countries in which the risk of exposure to wild polio virus is increased, primary immunization with IPV is recommended whenever this is feasible (Figure 19.14). IPV is preferred because the risk of vaccine-associated paralysis following OPV is slightly higher in adults than in children.

Three doses of IPV should be given before departure according to the schedule listed in Figure 19.14. In circumstances where time does not permit this to be done, the following alternatives are recommended:

1. If less than 3 months, but more than 2 months are available before protection is needed, 3 doses of IPV should be given at least 1 month apart.

2. If less than 8, but more than 4 weeks are available before protection is needed, 2 doses of IPV should be given at least 4 weeks apart.

3. If less than 4 weeks are available before protection is needed, a single dose of OPV or IPV is recommended.

In both #2 and #3 above, the remaining doses of vaccine should be given later, at the recommended intervals, if the person remains at increased risk.

Previously received less than full primary series of any polio vaccine. Adults who are at increased risk of exposure to poliomyelitis and who have previously received less than a primary series of OPV and/or IPV should be given the remaining required doses with either OPV or IPV, regardless of the interval since the last dose and of the type of vaccine previously received.

Previously received complete series with any one or combination of polio vaccines. Adults who are at increased risk of exposure to poliomyelitis and who have previously completed a primary series with any one or combination of polio vaccines can be given, once, a dose of OPV or IPV. The need for further doses of either vaccine has not been established.

Doses	Number of Doses	Dose Volume	Comments
Primary series	3 (IPV)	As indicated by manufacturer	Give doses 1 and 2, 4-8 weeks apart; give dose 3, 6-12 months after dose 2.
Booster	1 (IPV)		Give dose 4 to children 4-6 years of age.
Additional	1 (IPV)		Give a dose, **once**, to persons traveling to developing countries.

Figure 19.14. *Inactivated Poliovirus Vaccine (IPV)*

Side Effects and Adverse Reactions

In rare instances, administration of OPV has been associated with paralysis in healthy recipients and their contacts. Although this risk is extremely small for vaccinees and their susceptible, close contacts, they should be informed of this risk. No serious side effects of IPV have been documented. Since IPV may contain trace amounts of streptomycin and neomycin, persons with a history of an anaphylactic reaction following receipt of these antibiotics should not receive IPV. Persons with a history of reactions that are not anaphylactic are not at increased risk and can be vaccinated.

Precautions and Contraindications

Pregnancy. There is no convincing evidence of adverse effects of either OPV or IPV in pregnant women or developing fetuses; regardless, it is prudent on theoretical grounds to avoid vaccinating pregnant women. However, if immediate protection against poliomyelitis is needed, OPV, not IPV, is recommended.

Altered Immunity. Patients with a congenital immune deficiency disease, an acquired immune deficiency disease, or an altered immune state due to disease or to immunosuppressive therapy are at increased risk for paralysis associated with OPV. Therefore, if polio immunization is indicated, these persons (including asymptomatic and symptomatic HIV-infected persons) and their household members and other close contacts should receive IPV, not OPV. Although a protective immune response from receipt of IPV cannot be assured, some protection may be provided to the immunocompromised patient. Also, OPV should not be given to a member of a household in which there is a history of congenital or hereditary immunodeficiency unless the potential recipient and other household members are known to be immunocompetent. If OPV is inadvertently administered to a household or other close contact of an immunodeficient patient, close physical contact between the patient and the recipient of OPV should be avoided for approximately 1 month after vaccination. This is the period of maximum excretion of vaccine virus.

Rabies

Travelers to rabies endemic countries should be warned about the risk of acquiring rabies, although rabies vaccination is not a requirement for entry into any country. Rabies is almost always transmitted by bites which introduce the virus into wounds. Very rarely, rabies has been transmitted by non-bite exposures which introduce the virus into open cuts or mucous membranes. Although dogs are the main reservoir of the disease in many developing countries, the epidemiology of the disease in animals differs sufficiently from one region or country to another to warrant the evaluation of all animal bites. Any animal bite or scratch should receive prompt local treatment by thoroughly cleansing the wound with copious amounts of soap and water; this local treatment significantly reduces the risk of rabies. Persons who may have been exposed to rabies should always contact local health authorities immediately for advice about postexposure prophylaxis and should also contact their personal physician or State health department as soon as possible thereafter.

Preexposure vaccination with human diploid cell rabies vaccine (HDCV) (official name: Rabies Vaccine) or Rabies Vaccine Adsorbed (RVA) is recommended for persons living in or visiting (for more than 30 days) areas of the world where rabies is a constant threat, as well as for most veterinarians, animal handlers, spelunkers, and certain laboratory workers. For international travelers, the risk of rabies is highest in areas of the world where dog rabies remains highly endemic, including (but not limited to) parts of Mexico, El Salvador, Guatemala, Peru, Colombia, Ecuador, India, Nepal, Philippines, Sri Lanka, Thailand, and Viet Nam. The disease is also found in dogs in most of the other countries of Africa, Asia, Central and South America except as noted in Figure 19.15. Preexposure prophylaxis may provide protection when there is an inapparent or unrecognized exposure to rabies and when postexposure therapy is delayed. Preexposure prophylaxis is of particular importance for persons at high risk of being exposed in countries where the locally available rabies vaccines may carry a high risk of adverse reactions. Preexposure vaccination does not eliminate the need for additional therapy after a rabies exposure but simplifies postexposure treatment by eliminating the need for rabies immune globulin (RIG) and by decreasing the number of doses of vaccine required.

Figure 19.15 lists countries which have reported no cases of rabies during the most recent two-year period for which information is available (formerly referred to as "rabies free countries"). Additional information can be obtained from local health authorities of the country, or the embassy, or local consulate general's office in the United States.

Figure 19.16 provides information on preexposure and postexposure prophylaxis. Routine serologic testing is not necessary for persons who receive the recommended preexposure or postexposure regimen with human diploid cell rabies vaccine (HDCV) or rabies vaccine adsorbed (RVA). Persons previously vaccinated with other vaccines should receive the complete postexposure regimen with HDCV unless they developed a laboratory confirmed antibody response to the primary vaccination. Serologic testing is still recommended for persons whose immune response might be diminished by drug therapy or by diseases. Rabies preexposure prophylaxis is not indicated for travelers to the countries listed in Figure 19.15, and postexposure treatment is rarely necessary after exposures to terrestrial animals in these countries.

Chloroquine phosphate (and possibly other structurally related antimalarials such as mefloquine, administered for malaria chemoprophylaxis) may interfere with the antibody response to HDCV. The intramuscular (IM) dose/route of preexposure prophylaxis, however, provides a sufficient margin of safety in this setting. HDCV should not be administered by the intradermal (ID) dose/route when chloroquine, mefloquine, or other drugs which may interfere with the immune response are being used. For international travelers, the ID

473

Figure 19.15. *Countries Reporting No Cases of Rabies**

The following countries and political units stated that rabies was not present.

Region	Countries
AFRICA	Mauritius[†]; Libya[†]
AMERICAS	**North**: Bermuda; St. Pierre and Miquelon.
	Caribbean: Anguilla; Antigua and Barbuda; Bahamas; Barbados; Cayman Islands; Dominica; Guadeloupe; Jamaica; Martinique; Montserrat; Netherlands Antilles (Aruba, Bonaire, Curacao, Saba, St. Maarten, and St. Eustatius); St. Christopher (St. Kitts) and Nevis; St. Lucia; St. Martin; St. Vincent and Grenadines; Turks and Caicos Islands; Virgin Islands (U.K. and U.S.).
	South: Uruguay[†].
ASIA	Bahrain; Brunei Darussalam[†]; Japan; Republic of Korea[†]; Malaysia (Malaysia-Sabah[†]); Maldives[†]; Oman[†]; Singapore; Taiwan.
EUROPE	Bulgaria[†]; Cyprus; Denmark; Faroe Islands; Finland; Gibraltar; Greece; Iceland; Ireland; Malta; Norway (mainland); Portugal[†]; Spain; Sweden; United Kingdom (Britain and Northern Ireland).
OCEANIA[§]	American Samoa; Australia; Belau (Palau); Cook Islands; Federated States of Micronesia (Kosrae, Ponape, Truk, and Yap); Fiji; French Polynesia; Guam; Kiribati; New Caledonia; New Zealand; Niue; Northern Mariana Islands; Papua New Guinea; Samoa; Solomon Islands; Tonga; Vanuatu; Western Samoa.

Most of Pacific Oceania is "rabies-free." For information on specific islands not listed above, contact the Centers for Disease Control and Prevention, Division of Quarantine.

---

[*]Bat rabies exists in some areas that are free of terrestrial rabies.
[†]Countries whose classifications should be considered provisional.
[§]Most of Pacific Oceania is free of rabies.

This list is based on data from the following publications and information provided to the Centers for Disease Control and Prevention (CDC):

(1) World Health Organization: *World Survey of Rabies XXI* (for 1986/87); Veterinary Public Health Unit, Division of Communicable Disease, WHO, Geneva, 1989.

(2) WHO Collaborating Centre for Rabies Surveillance and Research: *Rabies Bulletin Europe*, 1991;15(1):3.

(3) Pan American Zoonoses Center. *Epidemiological surveillance of rabies for the Americas,* 1989;21(1-6)

Figure 19.16. Rabies Immunization

I. PREEXPOSURE IMMUNIZATION. Preexposure immunization consists of three doses of HDCV or RVA, 1.0 ml, IM (i.e., deltoid area), one each on days 0, 7, and 21 or 28. **ONLY HDCV may be administered by the intradermal (ID) dose/route (0.1 ml ID on days 0, 7, and 21 or 28).** If the traveler will be taking chloroquine or mefloquine for malaria chemoprophylaxis, the 3-dose series must be completed before initiation of antimalarials. If this is not possible, the IM dose/route should be used. Administration of routine booster doses of vaccine depends on exposure risk category as noted below. Preexposure immunization of immunosuppressed persons is not recommended.

Criteria for Preexposure Immunization

Risk category	Nature of risk	Typical populations	Preexposure regimen
Continuous	Virus present continuously, often in high concentrations. Aerosol, mucous membrane, bite, or nonbite exposure possible. Specific exposures may go unrecognized.	Rabies research lab workers*, Rabies biologics production workers.	Primary preexposure immunization course. Serology every 6 months. Booster immnization when antibody titer falls below acceptable level.*[†]
Frequent	Exposure usually episodic with source recognized, but exposure may also be unrecognized. Aerosol, mucous membrane, bite, or nonbite exposure.	Rabies diagnostic lab workers*, spelunkers, veterinarians, and animal control and wildlife workers in rabies epizootic areas. Certain travelers to foreign rabies epizootic areas.	Primary preexposure immunization course. Booster immunization or serology every 2 years.[†]
Infrequent (greater than population-at-large)	Exposure nearly always episodic with source recognized. Mucous membrane, bite, or nonbite exposure.	Veterinarians and animal control and wildlife workers in areas of low rabies endemicity. Veterinary students.	Primary preexposure immunization course. No routine booster immunization or serology.
Rare (population-at-large)	Exposure always episodic, mucous membrane, or bite with source recognized.	U.S. population-at-large, including individuals in rabies-epizootic areas.	No preexposure immunization.

II. POSTEXPOSURE IMMUNIZATION. All postexposure treatment should begin with immediate thorough cleansing of all wounds with soap and water.

Persons not previously immunized:
RIG, 20 I.U./kg body weight, one half infiltrated at bite site (if possible), remainder IM; 5 doses of HDCV or RVA, 1.0 ml IM (i.e., deltoid area), one each on days 0, 3, 7, 14 and 28.

Persons previously immunized:[§]
Two doses of HDCV or RVA, 1.0 ml, IM (i.e., deltoid area), one each on days 0 and 3. RIG should not be administered.

---

*Judgement of relative risk and extra monitoring of immunization status of laboratory workers is the responsibility of the laboratory supervisor (see U.S. Department of Health and Human Service's *Biosafety in Microbiological and Biomedical Laboratories, 1984*).

[†]Preexposure booster immunization consists of one dose of HDCV or RVA, 1.0 ml/dose, IM (deltoid area) or HDCV, 0.1 ml ID (deltoid). Acceptable antibody level is 1:5 titer (complete inhibition in RFFIT at 1:5 dilution). Boost if titer falls below 1:5.

[§]Preexposure immunization with HDCV or RVA; prior postexposure prophylaxis with HDCV or RVA; or persons previously immunized with any other type of rabies vaccine *and* a documented history of positive antibody response to the prior vaccination.

dose/route should be initiated early, to allow the three dose series to be completed 30 days or more before departure; otherwise the IM dose/route should be used. RVA should never be administered ID.

Precautions and Contraindications

Reactions after vaccination with HDCV or RVA. Persons may experience local reactions such as pain, erythema, and swelling or itching at the injection site, or mild systemic reactions, such as headache, nausea, abdominal pain, muscle aches, and dizziness. Approximately 6% of persons receiving booster vaccinations with HDCV experience an immune complex-like reaction characterized by urticaria, pruritis, and malaise. Once initiated, rabies postexposure prophylaxis should not be interrupted or discontinued because of local or mild systemic reactions to rabies vaccine.

Pregnancy. Pregnancy is not a contraindication to postexposure prophylaxis.

Age. In infants and children, the dose of HDCV or RVA for preexposure or postexposure prophylaxis is the same as that recommended for adults. The dose of RIG for postexposure prophylaxis is based on body weight (Figure 19.16).

Rift Valley Fever

Rift Valley Fever (RVF) is a viral disease that affects primarily livestock and humans. It is transmitted by several means including the bites of mosquitoes and other biting insects, and percutaneous inoculation or inhalation of aerosols from contaminated blood or fluids of infected animals. The risk of RVF infection to persons who travel to endemic areas generally is low. Occasionally, outbreaks occur involving large numbers of human cases, e.g., the Nile Delta, Egypt (1978 and 1993) and the lower Senegal River Basin of Mauritania (1987). Travelers can reduce their risk of exposure by avoiding contact with livestock and minimizing their exposure to arthropod bites. No commercial human vaccine is available.

Rubella

Rubella infection may be associated with significant morbidity in adults and is associated with a high rate of fetal wastage or anomalies if contracted in the early months of pregnancy. The risk of exposure to rubella outside the United States may be high. Therefore, although vaccination against rubella is not a requirement for entry into any country, all travelers, particularly women of childbearing age, should be immune to rubella. Persons should be considered to be susceptible to rubella unless they have documentation of (1) previous vaccination on or after the first birthday or (2) laboratory evidence of immunity. Because many illnesses can appear similar to rubella clinically, a history of rubella illness, even if physician-diagnosed, should not be considered sufficient evidence of immunity. A single dose of rubella virus vaccine (official name: Rubella Virus Vaccine, Live) is recommended for all susceptible children, adolescents, and adults, particularly females, unless vaccination is contraindicated. Combination with measles and mumps vaccines (MMR) is the vaccine of choice. Because there is no evidence that persons who have previously either received the vaccine or had rubella are at any risk of local or systemic reactions from receiving live rubella vaccine, testing for susceptibility before vaccination is unnecessary. (See Chapter 18 for a discussion of rubella immunization schedule modifications for infants who will be traveling.)

Side Effects and Adverse Reactions

Vaccinees can develop low-grade fever, rash, and lymphadenopathy after vaccination. Joint pain, or frank arthritis has been reported in 13-15% of adult women. Arthralgia and transient arthritis occur more frequently and tend to be more severe in susceptible women than in men or children. Transient peripheral neuritic complaints, such as paresthesias and pain in the arms and legs have occurred rarely. There is no increased risk of these reactions for persons who are already immune when vaccinated. The vaccine virus is not transmitted from vaccinees to pregnant, susceptible contacts.

There have been infrequent reports that susceptible vaccinees, primarily adult women, have developed chronic or recurrent arthralgias, sometimes with arthritis or other symptoms (paresthesias, blurred vision, carpal tunnel syndrome). While one group has reported the frequency of chronic joint symptoms in susceptible adult women to be 5 percent, other data from the United States and other countries that use the RA 27/3 strain suggest that such phenomena are rare events. In comparative studies, the frequency of chronic joint symptoms is substantially higher following natural infection than following vaccination.

Precautions and Contraindications

Pregnancy. Rubella vaccine should not be given to women known to be pregnant, nor should a vaccinated women become pregnant within 3 months of vaccination, because of theoretical risks to the developing fetus from rubella vaccine infection. Based on studies conducted in the U.S. and abroad, the Advisory Committee on Immunization Practices of the U.S. Public Health Service believes that the risk to the fetus of vaccine-associated malformations is so small as to be negligible. If, however, a pregnant woman is vaccinated, or if she becomes pregnant within 3 months of vaccination, she should be counseled on the theoretical risks. Rubella vaccination during pregnancy should not ordinarily be a reason to recommend interruption of pregnancy, although the final decision rests with the individual patient and her physician.

Febrile Illness. Although vaccination of persons with serious illness should be postponed until recovery, minor illnesses such as upper respiratory infections with or without low grade fever do not preclude vaccination.

Allergies. Hypersensitivity reactions very rarely follow the administration of live rubella vaccine. Most of these reactions are considered minor. Live rubella vaccine is produced in human diploid cell culture. Consequently, a history of an anaphylactic reaction to egg ingestion needs to be taken into consideration only if measles or mumps antigen are to be included with rubella vaccine.

Since rubella vaccine contains trace amounts of neomycin ($25\mu g$), persons who have experienced anaphylactic reactions to topically or systemically administered neomycin should not receive rubella vaccine. A history of contact dermatitis to neomycin is not a contraindication to receiving rubella vaccine. Live rubella vaccine does not contain penicillin.

Simultaneous Administration of Rubella Vaccine. Rubella vaccination may be administered simultaneously (but in a different site) with any other live or inactivated vaccine. Inactivated vaccines and oral polio vaccines may be administered at any time before or after the rubella vaccination. However, if live rubella vaccine is not given simultaneously with the yellow fever vaccine, they should be administered at least 30 days apart.

Recent Administration of Immune Globulin (IG)* or Other Antibody-Containing Blood Products (*Formerly called immune serum globulin and immunoglobulin). Vaccination should be administered at least 14 days after administration of IG or other blood products, because passively acquired antibodies might interfere with the response to the vaccine. Administration of MMR should be delayed following administration of blood product. The length of the delay varies from 3-11 months depending on the type of blood product received. Rubella vaccination using products that do not contain measles vaccine should be deferred for at least 3 months after administration of blood products.

Altered Immunity. Replication of live rubella vaccine virus may be potentiated in patients with immune deficiency diseases and by the suppressed immune responses that occur with leukemia, lymphoma, generalized malignancy, and therapy with corticosteroids, alkylating drugs, antimetabolites, and radiation. Patients with such conditions should not be given live rubella virus vaccine. However, rubella vaccination, generally given as MMR, can be considered for susceptible HIV-infected travelers, regardless of symptoms. There is no contraindication to using rubella vaccine, since limited studies of measles, mumps, and rubella (MMR) immunization in symptomatic HIV-infected patients have not documented serious or unusual adverse events.

Schistosomiasis

Schistosomiasis, an infection estimated to occur worldwide among some 200 million people, is caused by flukes whose complex life cycles utilize specific fresh water snail species as intermediate hosts. Infected snails release large numbers of minute free-swimming larvae (cercariae) which are capable of penetrating the unbroken skin of the human host. Even brief exposures to contaminated water can result in infection. Exposure to schistosomiasis is a health hazard for U.S. citizens who travel to endemic areas of the Caribbean, South America, Africa, and Asia. Outbreaks of schistosomiasis have occurred among adventure travelers participating in river trips in Africa as well as resident expatriates and Peace Corps volunteers. The countries where schistosomiasis is most prevalent include Brazil, Puerto Rico, and St. Lucia; Egypt and most of sub-Saharan Africa; and southern China, the Philippines, and Southeast Asia. Those at greatest risk are travelers who engage in wading or swimming in fresh water in rural areas where poor sanitation and appropriate snail hosts are present. Bathing with contaminated fresh water can also transmit infection. Human schistosomiasis cannot be acquired by wading or swimming in salt water (oceans or seas).

Clinical manifestations of acute infection can occur within 2-3 weeks of exposure to cercariae-infected water, but most acute infections are asymptomatic. The most common acute symptoms are: fever, lack of appetite, weight loss, abdominal pain, weakness, headaches, joint and muscle pain, diarrhea, nausea, and cough. Rarely, the central nervous system can be involved to produce seizures or transverse myelitis as a result of mass lesions of the brain or spinal cord. Chronic infections can cause disease of the lung, liver, intestines, and/or bladder. Many people who develop chronic infections can recall no symptoms of acute infection. Diagnosis of infection is usually confirmed by serologic studies or by finding schistosome eggs on microscopic examination of stool and urine. Schistosome eggs may be found 6-8 weeks after exposure but are not invariably present. Safe and effective oral drugs are available for the treatment of schistosomiasis.

Since there is no practical way for the traveler to distinguish infested from noninfested water, fresh water swimming in rural areas of endemic countries should be avoided. In such areas heating bathing water to 50°C (122°F) for 5 minutes or treating it with iodine or chlorine in a manner similar to the precautions recommended for preparing drinking water will destroy cercariae and make the water safe. Thus, swimming in chlorinated swimming pools is virtually always safe, even in endemic countries. Filtering water with paper coffee filters may also be effective in removing cercariae from bathing water. If these measures are not feasible, allowing bathing water to stand for 3 days is advisable since cercariae rarely survive longer than 48 hours. Vigorous towel drying after accidental water exposure has been suggested as a way to remove cercariae in the process of skin penetration.

Although such toweling may prevent some infections, to recommend this to travelers might give them a false sense of security; it is far safer to recommend avoiding contact with contaminated water. At this time there are no available drugs which are known to be effective as chemoprophylactic agents.

Upon return from foreign travel, if you think you may have been exposed to schistosome-infected fresh water, be sure to see a physician to undergo screening tests.

Sexually Transmitted Diseases

International travelers are at risk of contracting sexually transmitted diseases (STDs) including human immunodeficiency virus (HIV, the cause of AIDS) if they choose sexual partners who have these diseases. Travelers should be aware that the risk of STDs is high in some parts of the world. AIDS has become a global health problem and the prevalence of HIV infection in many populations continues to escalate (see Chapter 18). Also of concern are the antibiotic-resistant STD agents, particularly penicillin-, tetracycline-, and quinolone-resistant strains of *Neisseria gonorrhoeae*.

To avoid acquiring STDs, travelers should not have sexual contact with persons who may be infected. Persons most likely to be infected are those with numerous sex partners. In many places, persons who make themselves available for sex with travelers are likely to be persons, such as prostitutes, with many partners. In addition, injecting drug users are at high risk of being infected with HIV, regardless of the number of their sex partners.

Travelers choosing to have sexual contact may reduce their risk of acquiring infection by always using a latex condom during intercourse, and may reduce their risk of acquiring HIV infection by avoiding anal intercourse.

Anyone who may have been exposed to a STD who develops vaginal or urethral discharge, an unexplained rash or genital lesion, or genital or pelvic pain should cease sexual activity and promptly seek competent medical care. Because STDs are often asymptomatic, especially in women, anyone who believes that they may have been exposed to a STD should consult their physician regarding the advisability of screening for STD.

Smallpox

In May 1980, the World Health Organization (WHO) declared the global eradication of smallpox. There is no evidence of smallpox transmission anywhere in the world. The last reported case of endemic smallpox occurred in Somalia in October 1977, and the last reported case of laboratory-acquired smallpox occurred in the United Kingdom in 1978. WHO amended the International Health Regulations January 1, 1982, deleting smallpox from the diseases subject to the Regulations.

Smallpox vaccination should not be given for international travel. The risk from smallpox vaccination, although very small, now exceeds the risk of smallpox; consequently, smallpox vaccination of civilians is indicated **only for laboratory workers directly involved with smallpox or closely related orthopox viruses, e.g., monkeypox, vaccinia, and others.**

Misuse of Smallpox Vaccine

Smallpox vaccine should never be used therapeutically. There is no evidence that vaccination has therapeutic value in the treatment of recurrent herpes simplex infection, warts, or any other disease.

Tetanus (See Diphtheria, Tetanus, and Pertussis)

Tuberculosis

In many countries tuberculosis is much more common than in the United States, and it is an increasingly serious public health problem. To become infected, a person usually would have to spend a long time in a closed environment where the air was contaminated by a person with untreated tuberculosis who is coughing and has numerous *Mycobacterium tuberculosis* organisms (or tubercle bacilli) in secretions from the lungs. Tuberculosis infection is generally transmitted through the air; therefore, there is virtually no danger of its being spread by dishes, linens, and items that are touched, or by food. However, it can be transmitted through unpasteurized milk or milk products.

Travelers who anticipate possible prolonged exposure to tuberculosis should have a tuberculin skin test before leaving. If the reaction is negative, they should have a repeat test after returning to the

United States. Because persons with HIV infection are more likely to have an impaired response to the tuberculin skin test, travelers with HIV infection should inform their physician about their HIV status. Physicians can then determine whether to perform anergy testing. Except for travelers with impaired immunity (e.g., HIV infection), travelers who already have a positive tuberculin reaction are unlikely to be reinfected. All persons who are infected or who become infected with *Mycobacterium tuberculosis* can be treated to prevent tuberculosis disease. Travelers who suspect that they have been exposed to tuberculosis should inform their physician of the possible exposure and receive an appropriate medical evaluation. Tuberculosis disease can be treated successfully with multiple medications.

Typhoid Fever

Typhoid vaccination is not required for international travel, but it is recommended for travelers to areas where there is a recognized risk of exposure to *Salmonella typhi*, the organism which causes typhoid fever. *Salmonella typhi* is transmitted by contaminated food and water and is prevalent in many countries of Africa, Asia, and Central and South America. Vaccination is particularly recommended for travelers who will have prolonged exposure to potentially contaminated food and water in smaller cities and villages or rural areas off the usual tourist itineraries.

Both the oral Ty21a vaccine and several different preparations of parenteral typhoid vaccine have been shown to protect 50%-80% of recipients, depending in part on the degree of subsequent exposure. However, even travelers who have been vaccinated should use caution in selecting food and water.

Figure 19.17 provides information on dosage for both vaccines.

The oral typhoid vaccine has been licensed for use in the United States. It is a live-attenuated bacterial vaccine of the Ty21a s. *typhi* strain. The vaccine is taken as 4 separate doses over seven days. Each dose of the vaccine should be kept refrigerated until it is taken. The same dose is used for all ages. The oral vaccine is much less immunogenic in children less than 4 years of age, and its efficacy has not been demonstrated in any group of children younger than 6 years of age.

For the parenteral inactivated vaccine, when there is insufficient time for 2 doses 4 weeks apart, 3 doses of the same volumes (listed in the table) at weekly intervals may be administered, although it is recognized that this schedule may be less effective.

483

For travelers who have received one or more doses of parenteral vaccine in the past, a single parenteral booster dose is adequate, even if more than 3 years have elapsed since the last immunization. As a reasonable, although unproven alternative, an oral vaccine booster series can be given.

A purified Vi capsular polysaccharide parenteral typhoid vaccine may be licensed in the United States in the future. A single intramuscular dose of this vaccine has provided 55%-74% protection in individuals aged 5-44 years who live in highly endemic areas. It is immunogenic in children as young as one year old, but efficacy has not been demonstrated for this group.

Oral Typhoid Vaccine		
Doses	**Oral Route (≥6 years of age)**	**Comments**
Primary series	One enteric-coated capsule taken on alternate days, for four doses, with cool liquid (<37° C), one hour before a meal.	
Booster series	Sames as primary series.	Repeat series every 5 years under conditions of continued or repeated exposure.

Parenteral Inactivated Typhoid Vaccine				
	Subcutaneous Route		**Intradermal route**	
Doses	**<10 years of age**	**≥10 years of age**	**All ages**	**Comments**
Primary series: 1 & 2	0.25 ml	0.50 ml		Give 4 or more weeks apart.
Booster	0.25 ml	0.50 ml	0.1 ml*	1 dose at least every 3 years under conditions of continued or repeated exposure.

*Generally less reaction follows vaccination by the intradermal route, except when acetone-killed and dried vaccine is used. (Acetone-killed and dried vaccine should not be given intradermally).

Parenteral Vi Capsular Polysaccharide Vaccine		
Dose	**Intramuscular Route (≥2 years of age)**	**Comments**
Primary	0.5 ml	Single dose
Booster	0.5 ml	1 dose at least every 2 years under conditions of continued or repeated exposure.

Figure 19.17. *Typhoid Vaccine*

Contraindications

Information is not available on the safety of either parenteral or oral vaccine during pregnancy; therefore, it is prudent on theoretical grounds to avoid vaccinating pregnant women. Neither parenteral nor oral vaccine should be given to persons with acute febrile illness.

Live Ty21a vaccine should not be used among immunocompromised persons, including those infected with human immunodeficiency virus. Parenteral inactivated vaccine presents a theoretically safer alternative for this group. (See Chapter 18 for a discussion of typhoid immunization for infants who will be traveling.)

Theoretic concerns have been raised regarding oral Ty21a vaccine and concurrent use of oral polio vaccine (OPV) or antimalarial prophylaxis. Currently, no data are available that document interference with oral polio vaccine immunogenicity by Ty21a. However, the antimalarial prophylactic agent mefloquine has been shown to inhibit the in vitro growth of *S. typhi* strains, including Ty21a, at levels that may be achieved transiently in the gut following an oral dose of mefloquine. This has not been shown for other antimalarial agents. Therefore, it may be prudent to separate administration of prophylactic mefloquine and Ty21a by 24 hours. Simultaneous administration of Ty21a and yellow fever vaccine (YF 17D) or of Ty21a and immunoglobulin do not appear to pose a problem.

Reactions

Oral typhoid vaccination, with live-attenuated Ty21a vaccine, produces few adverse reactions. Abdominal discomfort, nausea, vomiting and rash have been reported as possible rare reactions.

Inactivated parenteral typhoid vaccination often results in discomfort at the site of injection for 1-2 days. The local reaction may be accompanied by fever, malaise, and headache. The experimental Vi capsular polysaccharide parenteral vaccine has been shown to elicit fewer local and systemic reactions than the inactivated whole cell vaccine.

Typhoid and Paratyphoid A and B Vaccines

The effectiveness of paratyphoid A vaccine has never been established, and field trials have shown that the usually small amounts of paratyphoid B antigens contained in vaccines combining typhoid and paratyphoid A and B antigens ("TAB" vaccines) are not effective. Knowing this and recognizing that combining paratyphoid A and B antigens with typhoid vaccine increases the risk of vaccine reaction, typhoid vaccine should be used alone.

Typhus Fever

Vaccination against typhus is not required by any country as a condition for entry. Several distinct rickettsiae cause a disease known as typhus in humans. Each agent has a distinct epidemiology but all cause disease with similarities of fever, headache and rash. Treatment of all forms of typhus is similar. Chloramphenicol, doxycycline or other forms of tetracycline result in rapid resolution of fever and relapses are infrequent. Murine typhus is relatively common throughout the world and is transmitted by fleas. Highest incidence of cases occurs during the summer months when rats and their fleas are most active and abundant. Epidemic typhus is rare except during periods when municipal services are disrupted as in war or natural disaster. The disease is passed from human to human by the body louse. Incidence of epidemic typhus occurs during the winter months when laundering of louse-infested clothing is absent and person-to-person spread of lice is common. Endemic foci of epidemic typhus exist in highland populations in Africa and South America, but tourists are at minimal risk of acquiring lice and disease. Scrub typhus is a common cause of fever among susceptible persons who engage in occupational or recreational behavior that bring them in contact with larval mite infested scrub brush habitats. Incidence is highest during the spring and summer when the activity of humans brings them in contact with mites seeking animal hosts. The disease is limited to Pacific islands and southeast and east Asia. Tick typhus, actually a form of spotted fever, is not uncommon in travelers who spend time trekking or on safari in Africa or the Indian subcontinent. Prompt removal of attached ticks and use of repellents to prevent tick attachment provide the best preventions against disease. Production of typhus vaccine in the United States has been discontinued and there are no plans for commercial production of a new vaccine.

Yellow Fever

Yellow fever, a viral disease transmitted by mosquitoes, occurs only in parts of Africa and South America. This illness is characterized by severe hepatitis and hemorrhagic fever. Yellow fever is a rare illness among travelers, but it is important because of its high mortality rate and because of international vaccination requirements. In addition to vaccination, travelers should take precautions against exposure to mosquitoes when traveling in areas with yellow fever transmission.

Vaccination

For purposes of international travel, yellow fever vaccine (official name: Yellow Fever Vaccine) produced by different manufacturers worldwide must be approved by WHO and administered at an approved Yellow Fever Vaccination Center. State and territorial health departments have the authority to designate nonfederal vaccination centers; these can be identified by contacting state or local health departments (CDC does not maintain a list of the designated centers). Vaccinees should receive an International Certificate of Vaccination completed, signed, and validated with the center's stamp where the vaccine is given.

A number of countries require a certificate from travelers arriving from infected areas or from countries with infected areas. Some countries in Africa require evidence of vaccination from all entering travelers. Some countries may waive the requirements for travelers coming from noninfected areas and staying less than 2 weeks. Vaccination is also recommended for travel outside the urban areas of countries which do not officially report the disease, but which lie in the yellow fever endemic zone (see maps at the end of this section). Practitioners should note that the actual areas of yellow fever virus activity far exceed the officially reported infected zones. Fatal cases of yellow fever have occurred in unvaccinated tourists visiting rural areas within the yellow fever endemic zone. Laboratory personnel who might be exposed by direct or indirect contact or by aerosols to virulent yellow fever virus also should be vaccinated.

Some countries require an individual, even if only in transit, to have a valid International Certificate of Vaccination if he or she has been in countries either known or thought to harbor yellow fever virus. Such requirements may be strictly enforced, particularly for persons traveling from Africa or South America to Asia. Travelers with a specific contraindication to the yellow fever vaccine should obtain a waiver before traveling to countries requiring vaccination.

Precautions and Contraindications

Age. Infants under 4 months of age are more susceptible to serious adverse reactions (encephalitis) than older children and should never be immunized. The risk of this complication appears to be age-related. Immunization should be delayed until age 9 months except when the risk of infection is high. (See Chapter 18 for a discussion of yellow fever immunization for infants.)

Pregnancy. A small study showed that yellow fever vaccine virus given in pregnancy can infect the developing fetus, but the potential risk of adverse events associated with congenital infection is unknown. Therefore, it is prudent on theoretical grounds to avoid vaccinating pregnant women and for non-immunized pregnant women to postpone travel to epidemic areas until after delivery. If the travel itinerary of a pregnant woman does not present a substantial risk of exposure and immunization is contemplated solely to comply with an international travel requirement, then efforts should be made to obtain a waiver letter from the traveler's physician. Pregnant women who must travel to areas where the risk of yellow fever is high should be vaccinated. It is believed that under these circumstances, the small theoretical risk for mother and fetus from vaccination is far outweighed by the risk of yellow fever infection.

Altered immune states. Infection with yellow fever vaccine virus poses a theoretical risk of encephalitis to patients with immunosuppression in association with acquired immunodeficiency syndrome (AIDS) or other manifestations of human immunodeficiency virus (HIV) infection; leukemia; lymphoma; generalized malignancy or with administration of corticosteroids, alkylating drugs, antimetabolites, or radiation. There are no data however that indicate an immunosuppressed state poses a risk to a yellow fever vaccine recipient. The decision to immunize immunocompromised patients with yellow fever vaccine should be based on a physician's evaluation of the patient's state of immunosuppression weighed against the risk of exposure to the virus. If travel to a yellow fever infected zone is necessary and immunization is contraindicated, patients should be advised of the risk, instructed in methods to avoid bites of vector mosquitoes, and a vaccination waiver letter should be supplied by the traveler's physician. Anecdotal experience suggests that low dose (10 mg prednisone or equivalent daily) or short-term (less than 2 weeks) corticosteroid therapy or intra-articular, bursal, or tendon injections with corticosteroid do not pose a risk to recipients of yellow fever vaccine. Persons with asymptomatic HIV infections who cannot avoid potential exposure to yellow fever virus should be offered the choice of immunization. Anecdotal observations indicate that HIV infected vaccinees may have a prolonged viremia with yellow fever vaccine virus. Vaccinees should be monitored for possible adverse effects. Because immunization of these individuals may be less effective than for uninfected persons, it may be desirable to measure the neutralizing antibody response following vaccination prior to travel (consult State health department or CDC, Fort Collins, Colorado (303) 221-6400).

Family members of immunosuppressed persons, who themselves have no contraindications, may receive yellow fever vaccine.

Hypersensitivity. Live yellow fever vaccine is produced in chick embryos and should not be given to persons clearly hypersensitive to eggs; generally persons who are able to eat eggs or egg products may receive the vaccine.

If vaccination of an individual with a questionable history of egg hypersensitivity is considered essential because of a high risk of exposure, an intradermal test dose may be administered under close medical supervision. Specific directions for skin testing are found in the package insert. In some instances, small test doses of vaccine administered intradermally have led to an antibody response.

If international travel regulations are the only reason to vaccinate a patient hypersensitive to eggs, efforts should be made to obtain a waiver. A physician's letter clearly stating the contraindication to vaccination has been acceptable to some governments. (Ideally, it should be written on letterhead stationery and bear the stamp used by health department and official immunization centers to validate the International Certificate of Vaccination.) Under these conditions, it is also useful for the traveler to obtain specific and authoritative advice from the embassy or consulate of the country or countries he or she plans to visit. Waivers of requirements obtained from embassies or consulates should be documented by appropriate letters and retained for presentation with the International Certificate of Vaccination.

Reactions

Reactions to yellow fever vaccine are generally mild. Two percent to 5% of vaccinees have mild headaches, myalgia, low-grade fevers, or other minor symptoms 5-10 days after vaccination. Fewer than 0.2% of vaccinees find it necessary to curtail regular activities. Immediate hypersensitivity reactions, characterized by rash, urticaria, and/or asthma, are extremely uncommon (incidence less than 1/1,000,000) and occur principally in persons with histories of egg allergy.

Simultaneous Administration of Other Vaccines and Drugs

Determination of whether to administer yellow fever vaccine and other immunobiologics simultaneously should be made on the basis of convenience to the traveler in completing the desired immunizations before travel and on information regarding possible interference. The following will help guide these decisions.

Studies have shown that the serologic response to yellow fever vaccine is not inhibited by administration of certain other vaccines concurrently or at various intervals of a few days to 1 month. Measles, and smallpox, vaccines given in combination with yellow fever vaccine did not reduce the immunogenicity of yellow fever vaccine. Bacillus Calmette Guerin (BCG) and yellow fever vaccines have been administered simultaneously without interference. Additionally, severity of reactions to vaccination was not amplified by concurrent administration of yellow fever and other live virus vaccines. If live virus vaccines are not given concurrently, 4 weeks should be allowed to elapse between sequential vaccinations.

Some data have indicated that persons given yellow fever and cholera vaccines simultaneously or 1-3 weeks apart had lower-than-normal antibody responses to both vaccines. Unless there are time constraints, cholera and yellow fever vaccines should be administered at a minimal interval of 3 weeks. If the vaccines cannot be administered at least 3 weeks apart, then the vaccines can be given simultaneously or at any time within the 3-week interval.

Hepatitis B and yellow fever vaccine and measles (Edmonton-Zagreb) and yellow fever vaccine may be given concurrently. There are no data on possible interference between yellow fever and typhoid, paratyphoid, typhus, plague, rabies, or Japanese encephalitis vaccines.

A prospective study of persons given yellow fever vaccine and 5 cc of commercially available immune globulin revealed no alteration of the immunologic response to yellow fever vaccine when compared to controls. Although chloroquine inhibits replication of yellow fever virus in vitro, it does not adversely affect antibody responses to yellow fever vaccine in humans receiving the drug as antimalarial prophylaxis.

Prevention of Mosquito Bites

Yellow fever transmission is unusual in urban areas and only occurs during an epidemic. Travelers to rural areas of Africa and South America, however, may be exposed to mosquitoes transmitting yellow fever and other mosquito-borne diseases. Mosquitoes which transmit urban yellow fever generally feed during the early morning or late afternoon hours both indoors and outdoors. Wearing long-sleeved shirts and long pants will help to prevent mosquito bites. Insect repellents containing diethyltoluamide (DEET) should be used. If the traveler will be staying in a rural area with limited facilities, use of a portable mosquito net should also be considered. (For further prevention information see section entitled "Protection Against Mosquitos and other Arthropod vectors" in Chapter 15).

YELLOW FEVER ENDEMIC ZONES

IN AFRICA

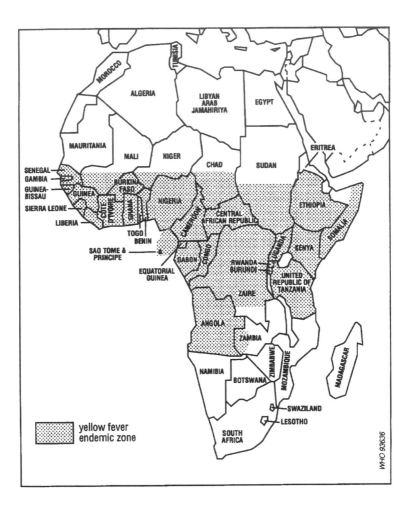

NOTE: Although the "yellow fever endemic zones" are no longer included in the International Health Regulation, a number of countries (most of them being not bound by the Regulations or bound with reservations) consider these zones as infected areas and require an International Certificate of Vaccination against Yellow Fever from travelers arriving from those areas. The above map based on information from WHO is therefore included in this publication for practical reasons.

Figure 19.18.

YELLOW FEVER ENDEMIC ZONES

IN THE AMERICAS

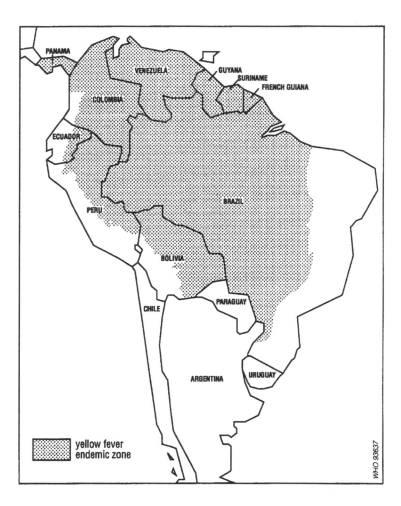

NOTE: Although the "yellow fever endemic zones" are no longer included in the International Health Regulations, a number of countries (most of them being not bound by the Regulations or bound with reservations) consider these zones as infected areas and require an International Certificate of Vaccination against Yellow Fever from travelers arriving from those areas. The above map based on information from WHO is therefore included in this publication for practical reasons.

Figure 19.19.

Chapter 20

Geographical Distribution of Potential Health Hazards to Travelers

Introduction

This [chapter] is intended to give a *broad* indication of the health risks to which travelers may be exposed in various areas of the world and which they may not encounter in their usual place of residence.

In practice, to identify areas accurately and define the degree of risk likely in each of them is extremely difficult, if not impossible. For example, viral hepatitis A is ubiquitous but the risk of infection varies not only according to area but also according to eating habits; hence, there may be more risk from communal eating in an area of low incidence than from eating in a private home in an area of high incidence. Generalizations may therefore be misleading.

Another factor is that tourism is an important source of income for many countries and to label specific areas as being of high risk for a disease may be misinterpreted. However, this does not absolve national health administrations from their responsibility to provide an accurate picture of the risks from communicable diseases that may be encountered in various parts of their countries.

Taken from HHS Pub. No. (CDC) 94-8280, *Health Information for International Travel, 1994*; reprinted from *International Travel and Health Vaccination Requirements and Health Advice—Situation as on 1 January 1994*, Published by World Health Organization.

495

Africa

Northern Africa

Northern Africa (Algeria, Egypt, Libyan Arab Jamahiriya, Morocco, and Tunisia) is characterized by a generally fertile coastal area and a desert hinterland with oases that are often foci of infections.

Arthropod-borne diseases are unlikely to be a major problem to the traveler, although dengue fever, filariasis (focally in the Nile Delta), leishmaniasis, malaria, relapsing fever, Rift Valley fever, sandfly fever, typhus, and West Nile fever do occur. Small foci of plague have been reported in the Libyan Arab Jamahiriya.

Foodborne and waterborne diseases are endemic; the dysenteries and other diarrheal diseases are particularly common. Hepatitis A occurs throughout the area. Typhoid fever is common in some areas. Schistosomiasis (bilharziasis) is very prevalent in the Nile Delta area in Egypt and in the Nile valley; it occurs focally in other countries in the area. Alimentary helminthic infections, brucellosis, and giardiasis are common. Echinococcosis (hydatid disease) may occur. Sporadic cases of cholera occur.

Other hazards include poliomyelitis, trachoma, rabies, scorpion stings, and snake bites. However, no cases of poliomyelitis have been reported from Algeria since 1990, from Libyan Arab Jamahiriya since 1991 or from Morocco since 1989.

Sub-Saharan Africa

Sub-Saharan Africa (Angola, Benin, Burkina Faso, Burundi, Cameroon, Cape Verde, Central African Republic, Chad, Comoros, Congo, Côte d'Ivoire, Djibouti, Equatorial Guinea, Ethiopia, Gabon, Gambia, Ghana, Guinea, Guinea-Bissau, Kenya, Liberia, Madagascar, Malawi, Mali, Mauritania, Mauritius, Mozambique, Niger, Nigeria, Reunion, Rwanda, Sao Tome and Principe, Senegal, Seychelles, Sierra Leone, Somalia, Sudan, Togo, Uganda. United Republic of Tanzania, Zaire, Zambia, and Zimbabwe). In this area, entirely within the tropics, the vegetation varies from the tropical rain forests of the west and center to the wooded steppes of the east, and from the desert of the north through the Sahel and Sudan savannas to the moist orchard savanna and woodlands north and south of the equator.

Many of the diseases listed below occur in localized rural foci and are confined to rural areas. They are mentioned so that the international traveler and the medical practitioner concerned may be aware of the diseases that may occur.

Arthropod-borne diseases are a major cause of morbidity. Malaria in the severe falciparum (malignant) form occurs throughout the area, except at over 3,000 meters altitude and in the islands of Cape Verde, Mauritius, Reunion, and Seychelles. Various forms of filariasis are widespread; endemic foci of onchocerciasis (river blindness) exist in all the countries listed except in the greater part of Kenya and in Djibouti, Gambia, Mauritania, Mozambique, Somalia, Zambia, Zimbabwe, and the island countries of the Atlantic and Indian Oceans. However, onchocerciasis exists in the island of Bioko, Equatorial Guinea. Both cutaneous and visceral leishmaniasis may be found, particularly in the drier areas. Visceral leishmaniasis is on the increase in Sudan. Human trypanosomiasis (sleeping-sickness), mainly in small isolated foci, is reported from all countries except Djibouti, Gambia, Mauritania, Somalia, and the island countries of the Atlantic and Indian Oceans. Relapsing fever and louse-, flea-, and tick-borne typhus occur. Natural foci of plague have been reported from Kenya, Madagascar, Mozambique, Uganda, the United Republic of Tanzania, and Zaire. Tungiasis is widespread. Many viral diseases, some presenting as severe hemorrhagic fevers, are transmitted by mosquitos, ticks, sandflies, etc., which are found throughout this region. Large outbreaks of yellow fever occur periodically in the unvaccinated population.

Foodborne and waterborne diseases are highly endemic. Schistosomiasis (bilharziasis) is present throughout the area except in Cape Verde, Comoros, Djibouti, Reunion, and the Seychelles. Alimentary helminthic infections, the dysenteries and diarrheal diseases, including cholera, giardiasis, typhoid fever, and hepatitis A and E are widespread. Dracunculiasis (Guinea-worm) infection occurs in isolated foci. Paragonimiasis (oriental long fluke) has been reported from Cameroon, Gabon, Liberia and most recently from Equatorial Guinea.

Other diseases. Hepatitis B is hyperendemic. Poliomyelitis is endemic in most countries except in Cape Verde, Comoros, Mauritius, Reunion, and the Seychelles. Trachoma is widespread. Among other diseases, certain, frequently fatal, arenavirus haemorrhagic fevers have attained notoriety. Lassa fever has a virus reservoir in a commonly found multimammate rat. Studies have shown that an appreciable reservoir exists in some rural areas of West Africa; people visiting these areas should take particular care to avoid rat-contaminated food or food containers, but the extent of the disease should not be exaggerated. The Ebola and Marburg hemorrhagic fevers are present but reported only infrequently. Echinococcosis (hydatid disease) is widespread in animal-breeding areas.

Epidemics of meningococcal meningitis may occur throughout tropical Africa, particularly in the savanna areas during the dry season.

Other hazards include rabies and snake bites.

Southern Africa

Southern Africa (Botswana, Lesotho, Namibia, St. Helena, South Africa, and Swaziland) varies physically from the Namib and Kalahari deserts to fertile plateaux and plains and to the more temperate climate of the southern coast.

Arthropod-borne diseases such as Crimean-Congo hemorrhagic fever, malaria, plague, relapsing fever, Rift Valley fever, tick-bite fever, and typhus—mainly tick-borne—have been reported from most of this area except St. Helena, but except for malaria in certain areas, they are not likely to be a major health problem for the traveler. Trypanosomiasis (sleeping sickness) may occur in Botswana and Namibia.

Foodborne and waterborne diseases are common in some areas, particularly amebiasis and typhoid fever. Hepatitis A occurs in this area. Schistosomiasis (bilharziasis) is endemic in Botswana, Namibia, Swaziland and South Africa.

Other hazards. No cases of poliomyelitis have been reported from these countries since 1988. Hepatitis B is hyperendemic. Snakes may be a hazard in some areas.

The Americas

Available data suggest that transmission of the poliomyelitis virus in the Region of the Americas may have been interrupted or is, at the very least, rapidly approaching this point. Wild virus transmission in 1991 was documented only in Colombia and Peru. However, in 1993 wild virus was detected in Canada, although, no paralytic cases have been found despite intensive surveillance.

North America

North America (Bermuda, Canada, Greenland, St. Pierre and

Miquelon, and the United States of America [with Hawaii]) extends from the Arctic to the subtropical cays of the southern USA.

The incidence of communicable diseases is such that they are unlikely to prove a hazard for international travelers greater than that found in their own country. There are, of course, health risks but in general, the precautions required are minimal. Plague, rabies in wildlife including bats, Rocky Mountain spotted fever, tularemia, and arthropod-borne encephalitis occasionally occur. Lyme disease is endemic in the northeastern United States and the upper Midwest. During recent years, the incidence of certain food-borne diseases, e.g., salmonellosis, has increased in some regions. Other hazards include poisonous snakes, poison ivy, and poison oak. In the north, a serious hazard is the very low temperature in the winter.

In the USA, proof of immunization against diphtheria, measles, poliomyelitis, and rubella is now universally required for entry into school. In addition, the school entry requirements of most states include immunization against tetanus (49 States), pertussis (44 States), and mumps (43 States).

Mainland Middle America

Mainland Middle America (Belize, Costa Rica, El Salvador, Guatemala, Honduras, Mexico, Nicaragua, and Panama) ranges from the deserts of the north to the tropical rain forests of the southeast.

Of the *arthropod-borne* diseases, malaria exists in all eight countries, but in Costa Rica and Panama it is confined to a few areas and in Mexico, mainly to the west coast. Cutaneous and mucocutaneous leishmaniasis occur in all eight countries. Visceral leishmaniasis occurs in El Salvador. Guatemala, Honduras and Mexico. Onchocerciasis (river blindness) is found in two small foci in the south of Mexico and four dispersed foci in Guatemala. American trypanosomiasis (Chagas' disease) has been reported to occur in localized foci in rural areas in all eight countries. Bancroftian filariasis is present in Costa Rica. Dengue fever and Venezuelan equine encephalitis may occur in all countries.

The *foodborne and waterborne* diseases, including amebic and bacillary dysenteries and other diarrheal diseases, and typhoid fever are very common throughout the area. All countries have reported cases of cholera in 1992, although the risk of contracting the disease in Belize, Costa Rica, Honduras and Panama is very low. Hepatitis A occurs throughout the area. Helminthic infections are common.

Paragonimiasis (oriental lung fluke) has been reported in Costa Rica, Honduras and Panama. Brucellosis occurs in the northern part of the area. Many *Salmonella typhi* infections from Mexico and *Shigella dysenteriae* type 1 infections from mainland Middle America as a whole have been caused by drug-resistant enterobacteria.

Other diseases. Rabies in animals (usually dogs and bats) is widespread throughout the area. Snakes may be a hazard in some areas.

Caribbean Middle America

Caribbean Middle America (Antigua and Barbuda, Aruba, Bahamas, Barbados, British Virgin Islands, Cayman Islands, Cuba, Dominica, Dominican Republic, Grenada, Guadeloupe, Haiti, Jamaica, Martinique, Montserrat, Netherlands Antilles, Puerto Rico, St. Christopher and Nevis, Saint Lucia, Saint Vincent and the Grenadines, Trinidad and Tobago, Turks and Caicos Islands, and the Virgin Islands (USA)). The islands, a number of them mountainous with peaks 1000-2500 m high, have an equable tropical climate with heavy rain storms and high winds at certain times of the year.

Of the *arthropod-borne* diseases, malaria occurs in endemic form only in Haiti and in parts of the Dominican Republic; elsewhere it has been eradicated. Diffuse cutaneous leishmaniasis was recently discovered in the Dominican Republic. Bancroftian filariasis occurs in Haiti and some other islands and other filariases may occasionally be found. Human fascioliasis due to Fasciola hepatica is endemic in Cuba. Outbreaks of dengue fever occur in the area, and dengue hemorrhagic fever has also occurred. Tularemia has been reported from Haiti.

Of the *foodborne and waterborne* diseases, bacillary and amebic dysenteries are common and hepatitis A is reported, particularly in the northern islands. No cases of cholera had been reported in the Caribbean at the time of printing. Schistosomiasis (bilharziasis) is endemic in the Dominican Republic, Guadeloupe, Martinique, Puerto Rico, and Saint Lucia, in each of which control operations are in progress. and it may also occur sporadically in other islands.

Other diseases. Other hazards may occur from spiny sea urchins and coelenterates (coral and jellyfish) and snakes. Animal rabies, particularly in the mongoose, is reported from several islands.

Tropical South America

Tropical South America (Bolivia, Brazil, Colombia, Ecuador,

French Guiana, Guyana, Paraguay, Peru, Suriname, and Venezuela) covers the narrow coastal strip on the Pacific Ocean, the high Andean range with numerous peaks 5000-7000 m high, and the tropical rain forests of the Amazon basin, bordered to the north and south by savanna zones and dry tropical forest or scrub.

Arthropod-borne diseases are an important cause of ill health in rural areas. Malaria (in the falciparum, malariae and vivax forms) occurs in all ten countries or areas, as do American trypanosomiasis (Chagas disease), and cutaneous and mucocutaneous leishmaniasis. There has been an increase of the latter in Brazil and Paraguay. Visceral leishmaniasis is endemic in north-east Brazil, with foci in other parts of Brazil, less frequent in Colombia, and Venezuela, rare in Bolivia and Paraguay, and unknown in Peru. Endemic onchocerciasis occurs in isolated foci in rural areas in Ecuador, Venezuela, and northern Brazil. The bites of blackflies, the vectors of onchocerciasis, may also transmit other filarial parasites or cause unpleasant and sometimes severe hemorrhagic reactions. Bancroftian filariasis is endemic in parts of Brazil, Guyana and Suriname. Plague has been reported in natural foci in Bolivia, Brazil, Ecuador, and Peru. Among the arthropod-borne viral diseases, jungle yellow fever may be found in forest areas in all countries except Paraguay and areas east of the Andes; in Brazil it is confined to the northern and western states. Epidemics of viral encephalitis and dengue fever occur in some countries of this area. Bartonellosis, or Oroya fever, a sandfly-borne disease, occurs in arid river valleys on the western slopes of the Andes up to 3,000 meters. Louse-borne typhus is often found in mountain areas of Colombia and Peru.

Foodborne and waterborne diseases are common and include amebiasis, diarrheal diseases, including cholera, helminthic infections, and hepatitis A. The intestinal form of schistosomiasis (bilharziasis) is found in Brazil, Suriname, and north-central Venezuela. Paragonimiasis (oriental lung fluke) has been reported from Ecuador, Peru and Venezuela. Brucellosis is common and echinococcosis (hydatid disease) occurs, particularly in Peru. All countries except Paraguay reported cases of cholera in 1992. Bolivia, Ecuador and Peru continue to be affected by the epidemic wave which originated in the latter country in 1991. Risk of cholera transmission is low to moderate in other countries.

Other diseases include rodent-borne arenavirus hemorrhagic fever in Bolivia. Hepatitis B and D (delta hepatitis) are highly endemic in the Amazon basin. Rabies has been reported from many of the countries in this area. Meningococcal meningitis occurs in epidemic outbreaks in Brazil.

Snakes and leeches may be a hazard in some areas.

Temperate South America

Temperate South America (Argentina, Chile, Falkland Islands (Malvinas), and Uruguay). The mainland ranges from the Mediterranean climatic area of the western coastal strip over the Andes divide on to the steppes and desert of Patagonia in the south and to the prairies of the northeast.

The *arthropod-borne* diseases are relatively unimportant except for the widespread occurrence of American trypanosomiasis (Chagas disease). Outbreaks of malaria occur in northwestern Argentina, and cutaneous leishmaniasis is also reported from the northeastern part of the country.

Of the *foodborne and waterborne* diseases, gastroenteritis (mainly salmonellosis) is relatively common in Argentina, especially in suburban areas and among children under 5 years of age. Cases of cholera have occurred in the northern provinces of Argentina and few cases have been reported from Chile. No cases of cholera have been reported from Uruguay. Typhoid fever is not very common in Argentina but hepatitis A and intestinal parasitosis are widespread, the latter especially in the coastal region. Taeniasis (tapeworm), typhoid fever, viral hepatitis, and echinococcosis (hydatid disease) are reported from the other countries.

Anthrax is an occupational hazard in the three mainland countries. Animal rabies is endemic in Argentina; it has increased in the last five years but is confined mainly to urban and suburban areas. Rodent-borne hemorrhagic fever is endemic in a limited zone of the pampas and in the center of the country.

Asia

East Asia

East Asia (China, the Democratic People's Republic of Korea, Hong Kong, Japan, Macao, Mongolia, and the Republic of Korea). The area includes the high mountain complexes, the desert and the steppes of the west, the various forest zones of the east, down to the subtropical forests of the southeast.

Among the *arthropod-borne* diseases, malaria now occurs only in China. Although reduced in distribution and prevalence, bancroftian and brugian filariasis are still reported in southern China. A resurgence of visceral leishmaniasis is occurring in China and plague may be found in China. Cutaneous leishmaniasis has been recently reported from Xinjiang, Uygur Autonomous Region. Hemorrhagic fever with renal syndrome—rodent-borne, Korean hemorrhagic fever—is endemic except in Mongolia, and epidemics of dengue fever and Japanese encephalitis may occur in this area. Mite-borne or scrub typhus may be found in scrub areas in southern China, certain river valleys in Japan, and in the Republic of Korea.

Foodborne and waterborne diseases such as diarrheal diseases and hepatitis A are common in most countries. Hepatitis E is prevalent in western China. The present endemic area of schistosomiasis (bilharziasis) is in the central Chang Jiang (Yangtze) river basin; active foci no longer occur in Japan. Clonorchiasis (oriental liver fluke) and paragonimiasis (oriental lung fluke) are reported in China, Japan, Macao and the Republic of Korea, and fasciolopsiasis (giant intestinal fluke) in China. Brucellosis occurs in China.

Other diseases. Hepatitis B is highly endemic. Poliomyelitis continues to be reported from China. Trachoma, and leptospirosis occur in China.

Eastern South Asia

Eastern South Asia (Brunei Darussalam, Cambodia, Indonesia, Lao People's Democratic Republic, Malaysia, Myanmar (formerly Burma), the Philippines, Singapore, Thailand, and Viet Nam). From the tropical rain and monsoon forests of the northwest, the area extends through the savanna and the dry tropical forests of the Indochina peninsula, returning to the tropical rain and monsoon forests of the islands bordering the South China Sea.

The *arthropod-borne* diseases are an important cause of morbidity throughout the area. Malaria and filariasis are endemic in many parts of the rural areas of all the countries or areas—except for malaria in Brunei Darussalam, and Singapore, where only imported cases occur. Foci of plague exist in Myanmar. Plague also occurs in Viet Nam. Japanese encephalitis, dengue and dengue hemorrhagic fever can occur in epidemics in both urban and rural areas. Mite-borne typhus has been reported in deforested areas in most countries.

Foodborne and waterborne diseases are common. Cholera and other watery diarrheas, amebic and bacillary dysentery, typhoid fever, and hepatitis A and E may occur in all countries in the area. Schistosomiasis (bilharziasis) is endemic in the Southern Philippines and in central Sulawesi (Indonesia) and occurs in small foci in the Mekong delta. Among helminthic infections, fasciolopsiasis (giant intestinal fluke) may be acquired in most countries in the area; clonorchiasis (oriental liver fluke) in the Indochina peninsula; opisthorchiasis (cat liver fluke) in the Indochina peninsula, the Philippines, and Thailand; and paragonimiasis in most countries. Melioidosis can occur sporadically throughout the area.

Other diseases. Hepatitis B is highly endemic. Poliomyelitis is reported throughout the area, but the incidence is low in Malaysia and it has been eliminated in Brunei Darussalam and Singapore. Trachoma exists in Indonesia, Myanmar, Thailand, and Viet Nam.

Other hazards include rabies, snake bites, and leeches.

Middle South Asia

Middle South Asia (Afghanistan, Armenia, Azerbaijan, Bangladesh, Bhutan, India, Islamic Republic of Iran, Kazakhstan, Kyrgyzstan, Maldives, Nepal, Pakistan, and Sri Lanka, Tajikistan, Turkmenistan and Uzbekistan). Bordered for the most part by high mountain ranges in the north, the area extends from steppes and desert in the west to monsoon and tropical rain forests in the east and south.

Arthropod-borne diseases are endemic in all these countries except for malaria in the Maldives. There are small foci of malaria in Azerbaijan and Tajikistan. In some of the other countries, malaria occurs in urban as well as rural areas. Filariasis is common in Bangladesh, India, and the southwestern coastal belt of Sri Lanka. Sand fly fever is on the increase. A sharp rise in the incidence of visceral leishmaniasis has been observed in Bangladesh, India and Nepal. In Pakistan, it is mainly reported from the north (Baltisan). Cutaneous leishmaniasis occurs in Afghanistan, India (Rajasthan), the Islamic Republic of Iran, and Pakistan. There are very small foci of cutaneous and visceral leishmaniasis in Azerbaijan and Tajikistan. Tick-borne relapsing fever is reported from Afghanistan, India, and the Islamic Republic of Iran, and typhus occurs in Afghanistan and India. Epidemics of dengue fever may occur in Bangladesh, India, Pakistan, and Sri Lanka and the hemorrhagic form has been reported from eastern India and Sri Lanka. Japanese encephalitis has been reported from the eastern part of the area and Crimean-Congo hemorrhagic fever from the western part. Another tick-borne hemorrhagic fever has been reported in forest areas of Karnataka State in India and in a rural area of Rawalpindi District in Pakistan.

Foodborne and waterborne diseases are common throughout the area, in particular cholera and other watery diarrheas, the dysenteries, typhoid fever, hepatitis A and E, and helminthic infections. Large epidemics of hepatitis E can occur. Giardiasis is said to be common in the Islamic Republic of Iran. A focus of urinary schistosomiasis (bilharziasis) exists in the southwest of the Islamic Republic of Iran. Foci of dracunculiasis (guinea worm) infection occur in India and in Pakistan. Brucellosis and echinococcosis (hydatid disease) are found in many countries in the area.

Other diseases. Hepatitis B is endemic. Outbreaks of meningococcal meningitis have been reported in India and Nepal. Poliomyelitis is widespread except in Bhutan and the Maldives. Trachoma is common in Afghanistan, in parts of India, the Islamic Republic of Iran, Nepal, and Pakistan. Snakes and the presence of rabies in animals are hazards in most of the countries in the area.

Western South Asia

Western South Asia (Bahrain, Cyprus, Iraq, Israel, Jordan, Kuwait, Lebanon, Oman, Qatar, Saudi Arabia, Syrian Arab Republic, Turkey, the United Arab Emirates, and Yemen). The area ranges from the mountains and steppes of the north-west to the large deserts and dry tropical scrub of the south.

The *arthropod-borne* diseases, except for malaria in certain areas, are not a major hazard for the traveler. Malaria does not exist in Kuwait and no longer occurs in Bahrain, Cyprus, Israel, Jordan, Lebanon, or Qatar. Its incidence in the Syrian Arab Republic is low, but elsewhere is endemic in certain rural areas. Cutaneous leishmaniasis is reported throughout the area; visceral leishmaniasis, although rare throughout most of the area, is common in central Iraq, in the southwest of Saudi Arabia, in the northwest of the Syrian Arab Republic, in Turkey and in the west of Yemen. Murine and tick-borne typhus can occur in most countries. Tick-borne relapsing fever may occur. Crimean-Congo hemorrhagic fever has been reported from Iraq. Limited foci of onchocerciasis are reported in Yemen.

505

The *foodborne and waterborne* diseases are a major hazard in most countries. The typhoid fevers and hepatitis A exist in all countries and cases of cholera have been reported from Iraq. Schistosomiasis (bilharziasis) occurs in Iraq, Saudi Arabia, the Syrian Arab Republic, and Yemen. Dracunculiasis (guinea worm) infection is found in some of these countries. Taeniasis (tapeworm) is reported from many of the countries. Brucellosis is widespread and there are foci of echinococcosis (hydatid disease).

Other diseases. Hepatitis B is endemic. No cases of poliomyelitis have been reported from Bahrain since 1981, from Kuwait since 1986, from Qatar since 1985 or from Israel since 1989, but is endemic in other countries. Trachoma and animal rabies are found in many countries in the area.

The greatest hazards to pilgrims to Mecca and Medina are heat and water depletion if the period of the Hajj coincides with the hot season.

Europe

Northern Europe

Northern Europe (Belarus, Belgium, Czech Republic, Denmark (with the Faroe Islands), Estonia, Finland, Germany, Iceland, Ireland, Latvia, Lithuania, Luxembourg, Netherlands, Norway, Poland, Republic of Moldova, Russian Federation, Slovakia, Sweden, Ukraine and the United Kingdom (with the Channel Islands and the Isle of Man). The area encompassed by these countries extends from the broadleaf forests and the plains of the west to the boreal and mixed forest to be found as far east as the Pacific Ocean.

The incidence of communicable diseases in most countries is such that they are unlikely to prove a hazard to international travelers greater than that found in their own country. There are, of course, health risks but in most areas very few precautions are required.

Of the *arthropod-borne* diseases, there are very small foci of malaria and cutaneous and visceral leishmaniasis in Azerbaijan and Tajikistan, and tick-borne typhus in east and central Siberia. Tick-borne encephalitis, for which a vaccine exists, Lyme disease, and Crimean-Congo hemorrhagic fever may occur throughout northern Europe. Rodent-borne hemorrhagic fever with renal syndrome is now recognized as occurring at low endemic levels in this area.

The *foodborne and waterborne* diseases reported, other than the ubiquitous diarrheal diseases [and small numbers of cases of cholera in Tajikistan—editor's note in source document.], are taeniasis (tapeworm) and trichinellosis in parts of northern Europe, diphyllobothriasis (fish tapeworm) from the freshwater fish around the Baltic Sea area. Fasciola hepatica infection can occur. Hepatitis A occurs in the Eastern European countries. The incidence of certain food-borne diseases, e.g., salmonellosis and campylobacteriosis, is increasing significantly in some of these countries.

Other diseases. Poliomyelitis continues to be reported from the Russian Federation and the Ukraine. After 14 years without any poliomyelitis the Netherlands reported an outbreak in 1992-93 among unvaccinated members of a religious group, but only one case was reported in a person outside this group. Rabies is endemic in wild animals (particularly foxes) in rural areas of northern Europe except Finland, Iceland, Ireland, Norway, Sweden, and the United Kingdom. In recent years, the Russian Federation and Ukraine have experienced extensive epidemics of diphtheria.

A climatic hazard in part of northern Europe is the extreme cold in winter.

Southern Europe

Southern Europe (Albania, Andorra, Austria, Bosnia/Herzegovina, Bulgaria, Croatia, France, Gibraltar, Greece, Hungary, Italy, Liechtenstein, Malta, Monaco, Portugal (with the Azores and Madeira), Romania, San Marino, Slovenia, Spain (with the Canary Islands), Switzerland, and the former Yugoslav Republic of Macedonia, and Yugoslavia. The area extends from the broadleaf forests in the north-west and the mountains of the Alps to the prairies and, in the south and south-east, the scrub vegetation of the Mediterranean.

Among the *arthropod-borne* diseases, sporadic cases of murine and tick-borne typhus and mosquito-borne West Nile fever occur in some countries bordering the Mediterranean littoral. Both cutaneous and visceral leishmaniasis and sandfly fever are also reported from this area. Tickborne encephalitis, for which a vaccine exists, Lyme disease, and rodent-borne hemorrhagic fever with renal syndrome may occur in the eastern and southern parts of the area.

The *foodborne and waterborne* diseases—bacillary dysentery and other diarrheas, and typhoid fever—are more common in the summer and autumn months, with a high incidence in the southeastern and southwestern parts of the area. Brucellosis can occur in the extreme southwest and southeast and echinococcosis (hydatid disease) in the southeast. Fasciola hepatica infection has been reported from different countries in the area. The incidence of certain food-borne diseases, e.g., salmonellosis and campylobacteriosis, is increasing significantly in some of these countries.

Other diseases. Poliomyelitis is reported from Croatia and Yugoslavia, hepatitis B is endemic in the southern part of eastern Europe (Albania, Bulgaria and Romania). Rabies in animals exists in most countries of southern Europe except Gibraltar, Malta, Monaco, and Portugal.

Oceania

Australia, New Zealand and the Antarctic

In Australia the mainland has tropical monsoon forests in the north and east, dry tropical forests, savanna and deserts in the center, and Mediterranean scrub and subtropical forests in the south. New Zealand has a temperate climate with the North Island characterized by subtropical forests and the South Island by steppe vegetation and hardwood forests.

International travelers to Australia and New Zealand will, in general, not be subjected to the hazards of communicable diseases to an extent greater than that found in their own country.

Arthropod-borne diseases (mosquito-borne epidemic polyarthritis and viral encephalitis) may occur in some rural areas of Australia.

Among the *foodborne and waterborne* diseases, amebic meningoencephalitis has been reported.

Other hazards. Coelenterates (corals and jellyfish) may prove a hazard to the sea-bather, and heat is a hazard in the northern and central parts of Australia.

Melanesia and Micronesia-Polynesia

Melanesia and Micronesia-Polynesia (American Samoa, Cook Islands, Easter Island, Federated States of Micronesia, Fiji, French Polynesia, Guam, Kiribati, Marshall Islands, Nauru, New Caledonia, Niue, Palau, Papua New Guinea, Pitcairn, Samoa, Solomon Islands, Tokelau, Tonga, Trust Territory of the Pacific Islands, Tuvalu, Vanuatu, Wake Island [U.S.] and the Wallis and Futuna Islands). The area covers an enormous expanse of ocean with the larger, mountainous, tropical and monsoon rainforest-covered islands of the west giving way to the smaller, originally volcanic peaks and coral islands of the east.

Arthropod-borne diseases occur in the majority of the islands. Malaria is endemic in Papua New Guinea and is found as far east and south as Vanuatu. Neither malaria nor anopheline vectors are found in Fiji or the islands to the north and as far as French Polynesia and Easter Island in the east, or in New Caledonia to the south. Filariais is widespread but its prevalence varies. Mite-borne typhus has been reported from Papua New Guinea. Dengue fever, including its hemorrhagic form, can occur in epidemics in most islands.

Foodborne and waterborne diseases such as the diarrheal diseases, typhoid fever and helminthic infections are commonly reported. Biointoxication may occur from raw or cooked fish and shellfish. Hepatitis A occurs in this area.

Other diseases. Hepatitis B is endemic. Poliomyelitis occurs in Papua New Guinea and trachoma in parts of Melanesia.

Hazards to bathers are coelenterates, poisonous fish, and sea snakes.

Indexes

General Index

0157:H7 bacteria 16, 17
7-minute frosting 133

A

A Quick Consumer Guide to Safe Food Handling 13, 77
abdominal cramps 5, 18, 61, 62, 75, 117, 348, 354, 356, 381, 436
abdominal distention 380
abscesses 24, 273, 276, 423, 468
Access Travel: Airports 332
acetaldehyde 194
acetazolamide 338
activated charcoal 353, 354
active immunization 282, 400
acupuncture 397, 440
Administration on Aging 88
adult botulism 4
Advisory Committee on Immunization Practices (ACIP) 283, 382, 395, 399, 414
Aedes aegypti 425, 426
Aedes mosquitoes 425
Aeromonas hydrophila 351
aerosolized pentamidine isethionate 71
African sleeping sickness *see* African trypanosomiasis

African trypanosomiasis 69, 422
age groups
children 14, 15, 18, 24, 29, 46, 49, 52, 53, 69, 72, 75, 76, 85, 86, 109, 113, 117, 118, 123, 140, 142-146, 152, 197, 250, 254, 274, 294, 296, 319, 324, 331, 332, 339, 349, 351, 353, 355, 356, 358, 383-387, 392, 393, 396, 400, 404, 407-410, 412-417, 426, 428, 429, 431, 432, 434, 436-438, 440, 443, 447, 450, 453, 455-457, 463, 464, 469, 470, 476, 477, 483, 484, 488, 502
diaper-aged children 76
elderly 8, 15, 18, 21, 29, 38, 44, 48, 57, 59, 85, 87, 88, 105, 113, 114, 118, 133, 223, 323, 338, 357, 358, 432
infants 4, 29, 70, 73, 113, 117, 143, 250, 339, 341, 367, 399, 400, 404, 409, 410, 412-418, 424, 428, 429, 431, 439, 443, 456, 458, 459, 464, 469, 476, 477, 485, 488
newborns 8, 21, 23, 29, 116
Agricultural Marketing Service 43, 130, 170
AIDS 8, 23, 30, 36, 44, 54, 59, 70-72, 78, 143, 260, 328, 329, 396-398, 421, 422, 481, 488
albumen 39

513

G

I

Index of Travel Destinations

531